Quick Reference to
Intravenous Drugs

J.B. Lippincott Company Philadelphia
London   Mexico City   New York   St. Louis   São Paulo   Sydney

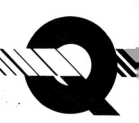

Quick Reference to

Intravenous Drugs

Diane Proctor Sager, R.N., M.S.N.
Formerly Clinical Specialist in Medical Nursing at the District of Columbia General Hospital, Washington, D.C. Presently in private practice

Suzanne Kovarovic Bomar, R.N., M.S.N.
Formerly Clinical Specialist in Medical Nursing and Critical Care at the District of Columbia General Hospital, Washington, D.C.

Special Consultant:
Joseph G. Barbaccia, Pharm.D.
Clinical Pharmacist, Washington Hospital Center, Washington, D.C.

Sponsoring Editors: Paul R. Hill, David T. Miller
Manuscript Editor: Randi Boyette
Indexer: Pamela W. Fried
Art Director: Tracy Baldwin
Production Supervisor: N. Carol Kerr
Production Assistant: J. Corey Gray
Compositor: International Computaprint Corporation
Printer/Binder: R. R. Donnelley & Sons Company

6 5

Library of Congress Cataloging in Publication Data

Sager, Diane Proctor.
    Quick reference to intravenous drugs.

    (Lippincott's quick references)
    Primarily an up-dated version of the Drug information section of the authors' Intravenous medication.
    Includes bibliographical references and index.
    1. Injections, Intravenous—Dictionaries.
I. Bomar, Suzanne Kovarovic. II. Title.
RM170.S236 1983   615.8'55   82–14811
ISBN 0–397–54411–1

The authors and publisher have exerted every effort to ensure that drug selection and dosage set forth in this text are in accord with current recommendations and practice at the time of publication. However, in view of ongoing research, changes in government regulations, and the constant flow of information relating to drug therapy and drug reactions, the reader is urged to check the package insert for each drug for any change in indications and dosage and for added warnings and precautions. This is particularly important when the recommended agent is a new or infrequently employed drug.

To our children

Preface

Recognizing the increasing number of intravenous medications being developed and the expanding role of the nurse regarding their administration, in 1980 we developed a textbook entitled *Intravenous Medications: A Guide to Preparation, Administration, and Nursing Management.* It was our hope that the book would be as complete a reference on intravenous drugs as possible. We included information on equipment, pharmacologic principles, and techniques of administration as well as information on all drugs approved for intravenous use at that time.

We remain convinced that such a comprehensive text is needed for all nurses and for medical and paramedical personnel who are involved in intravenous drug preparation or administration. Recently, however, the need for a more concise version of that text has become evident and has prompted the writing of this book. We have written *Quick Reference to Intravenous Drugs* as a quick-reference handbook primarily for use in patient-care settings where intravenous medications are prepared and administered. Much of the value of such a handbook lies in its manageable size and easy accessibility of information; thus, it has been necessary to modify our original material in several areas.

We eliminated the section on theories and techniques, focusing instead on the drugs themselves. However, pertinent material on prevention, recognition, and management of untoward drug reactions and of extravasation has been included in the Appendix, because such information is often required for on-the-spot assessment at the time of drug administration.

This book consists primarily of the Drug Information Section of the original book. While some infrequently used drugs were deleted, many newly approved medications have been added. All drugs retained from the original text have been completely updated. The same seven content areas have been maintained, although the format is changed from a columnar form to a narrative style for compactness.

Whenever a more comprehensive treatment of intravenous medications (e.g., principles, equipment, legal aspects) is needed, we suggest that our original text be consulted. However, as a readily available resource on the drugs themselves, this new work is a complete reference.

Note of Appreciation. We wish to extend our appreciation to Mr. David T. Miller, Vice President and Editor at J.B. Lippincott Company, for his assistance, support, and encouragement during the preparation of this book.

Diane Proctor Sager, R.N., M.S.N.
Suzanne Kovarovic Bomar, R.N., M.S.N.

Introduction

Ever-increasing numbers of institutions are preparing to initiate, or are now using, pharmacy-based unit-dose and intravenous admixture programs. Some members of the nursing community have voiced concerns that such programs remove the nurse from traditional involvement in drug administration. It is our belief that these programs free the nurse from those aspects of drug preparation that are more appropriately performed by other professionals, allowing her to devote more time to professional bedside nursing care.

Regardless of whether the nurse is responsible for the preparation of intravenous drugs and admixtures, she still must have a thorough understanding of all drugs she deals with, because she administers them. Because she is generally the final checkpoint through which the medication passes before being given to the patient, the nurse can help to ensure accuracy of dosage and mode of administration. And, as the professional in closest contact with the patient, the nurse is best equipped to observe for adverse reactions, to administer comfort measures when required, and to monitor for drug effectiveness.

The primary source of information in this reference is the drug manufacturer, whose guidelines are considered to be the legal standards for administration of the drug. What the maker of the drug states about a specific agent insofar as indications, dosage, mode of administration, contraindications, adverse reactions, and warnings is overseen by the Food and Drug Administration. It behooves the practitioner to use this book and updated information in drug-package inserts in conjunction with strict adherence to institutional policies and procedures, and to the policies of the pharmacy and therapeutics committee, the director of pharmacy services, a drug information center, and other pertinent sources. The nurse must also be aware of the legal implications of deviations from these standards, policies, and procedures. Chapter One of *Intravenous Medications* (Sager and Bomar, J.B. Lippincott Company, 1980) gives detailed information on the legal aspects of drug administration for nurses.

All of the drugs presented in this handbook are currently available and approved for human clinical intravenous use by the Food and Drug Administration. Agents classified for investigational use only have not been included. All drugs are listed in alphabetical order according to their generic names. The List of Drugs on page xiii has been cross-indexed to facilitate rapid location of the entry for a drug whether the generic or the trade name is known. The information on each drug is divided into seven major sections in a sequence that follows the order in which it will be needed in preparing to administer a drug. The purpose and the contents of each of the seven sections are discussed below:

Actions/Indications. The term *actions* in this book refers to the physiologic and pharmacologic effects that a drug produces within the body when it is administered intravenously. The *indications* listed for each drug are those clinical situations in which the drug's actions can produce a desired effect or response, such as the relief of pain, or the prevention, diagnosis, or treatment of a disease. In the case of the antibiotics, the indications may be listed in one of two forms: either there will be list of the organisms that the drug is active against, or there will be a list of infected organ systems and the organisms causing infections within those systems.

These indications are those currently recognized by the Food and Drug Administration. A drug may have other uses through alternate routes of administration; whenever possible these are listed, but they are not described. Besides helping to ensure the appropriateness of a drug for a particular patient, knowledge of the approved actions and indications will facilitate monitoring for drug effectiveness.

Dosage. The currently accepted adult and pediatric dosages are given. The dosages are those recommended by the manufacturer unless otherwise stated. Dosages are given for each indication. If this information is unnecessary or unavailable, one dosage is given for all indications. Pediatric dosages (and, when appropriate, adult dosages) are given by weight, age and/or body surface area (in square meters). A nomogram for adult and child body surface area and a chart for the conversion of pounds to kilograms can be found in the Appendix.

Preparation and Storage. All drugs have specific preparation requirements for reconstitution, dilution in fluids, and protection from environmental factors and perishability. Strict attention to these details is mandatory for safe and effective drug administration. Deviations can change the actions of the drug in the body.

The volume of diluent added to a drug in its powder form must be precise and according to instructions to produce an accurate concentration (mg/ml). Accuracy of the concentration of a drug solution will help to ensure the delivery of an accurate dose to the patient. Similarly, accurate preparation of a drug–fluid solution is also essential for the delivery of an accurate dose and a stable solution.

Conditions are described under which a prepared solution should not be used, *e.g.,* with the appearance of discoloration, a precipitate, opalescence, or a separation.

The stability of prepared drug solutions for stock use and infusion is also listed in this section. The preparer is encouraged to use this information in labeling vials and bottles to prevent the use of a drug after its period of known stability has passed. Special precautions to follow, such as protection of a drug or infusion solution from light, and the use of syringe and in-line filters are included.

Drug Incompatibilities. Information in this section was based, in part, on data in the second edition of Lawrence Trissel's *Handbook on Injectable Drugs,* (American Society of Hospital Pharmacists, Washington, D.C., 1977) as well as on data from the drug manufacturers. In most instances, other agents with which the drug *cannot* be combined are listed. The reader is cautioned, however, that for some drugs the list is of only the agents with which the drug *can* be mixed. The warning to avoid mixing certain drugs "in any manner" means that the two agents cannot be combined in a syringe, intravenous tubing, or fluid containers under any circumstances. Caution is advised when drugs are mixed, because incompatibility does not always produce a visible change to warn the preparer. Special flushing techniques and intravenous tubing arrangements are required when drugs that are incompatible must be given at the same time. A thorough discussion of this subject is in Chapter 8 of *Intravenous Medications* (Sager and Bomar, J.B. Lippincott Company, 1980).

Modes of IV Administration. Currently, the three accepted methods of intravenous administration of a drug are: injection, intermittent infusion, and continuous infusion. The mode or modes appropriate for each drug are indicated as "YES" at the beginning of the section. If a drug cannot be administered by one of these modes, this is indicated by a "NO."

The following are the definitions of the three modes that were used in the preparation of this material:

Injection is the administration of a relatively small volume of a concentrated solution of a drug directly into the venous system from a syringe via intravenous tubing or a cannula, or into the vein itself using a needle. Medications administered in this fashion are given over a short period of time either by rapid injection (bolus) or over several minutes.

Intermittent Infusion is the administration of a specific dose of a drug in a small, predetermined volume of fluid (50 to 200 ml) with the admixture being infused over a period of time ranging from 15 minutes to 2 hours. This technique of delivery is used to produce peaks in the blood level of the drug. Piggyback and volume-control infusion units are used.

Continuous Infusion is the administration of a medication in a large volume of fluid (250 to 1000 ml), with or without interruption, over several hours or days. Drugs may be given by this mode for titration purposes when they are administered to control a disease state. Examples of this are the administration of lidocaine or bretylium, to control a cardiac arrhythmia, and dopamine, to control systemic arterial blood pressure. This mode is also used when a drug must be highly diluted to be tolerated by the body, or when a constant blood level of the drug must be maintained, as with certain antibiotics.

Under the *Intermittent Infusion* and *Continuous Infusion* columns, the fluids that can be used as vehicles for administration are listed. Use no others. The abbreviations for these solutions are as follows:

D5W	Dextrose 5% in water
D5/NS	Dextrose 5% in normal saline (0.9% sodium chloride)
D5/0.45% Saline	Dextrose 5% in one half normal saline (0.45% sodium chloride)
NS	Normal saline (0.9% sodium chloride)
0.45% Saline	One-half normal saline (0.45% sodium chloride)
RL	Ringer's Lactate
LR	Lactated Ringer's solution

These abbreviations are used throughout the text.

Appropriate concentrations and injection or infusion times (rates) are given for each medication, and must be observed to avoid adverse reactions.

Contraindications; Warnings; Precautions; Adverse Reactions. Information in this section was based mainly on the literature from the manufacturers. Other sources were often used and are indicated as references. Where appropriate, directions for the detection and treatment of drug overdosage are included.

The practitioner should be aware that the drug manufacturer has included all known adverse reactions that have occurred with the administration of an agent, but that new, previously unreported, reactions can occur. Whenever the patient exhibits a change in condition or develops a new complication (*e.g.*, change in liver enzymes, blood count, blood pressure, blood gases, mental status), the drug(s) that the patient is receiving should be suspected as the source until proven otherwise. This is why it is vitally important for the nurse to assess the patient's condition frequently and report all findings based on her knowledge of the drugs that the patient is receiving.

Nursing Implications. A major component of the nursing intervention involved with drug administration begins after the drug has been given. The suggestions for patient care presented in this section are based on the preceding six sections of information. Primarily, the nurse must be concerned with monitoring appropriate physiologic parameters to detect desired responses and adverse reactions. Recommendations are made here on the frequency of heart rate, blood pressure, respiratory rate, arterial blood gases, urine output, etc. Naturally, modifications in such schedules must be made by the practitioner depending on the patient's condition. Expected changes in these parameters, both desirable and undesirable, are also presented. Supportive care for minor and major discomforts produced by the drug is described, as are safety precautions and the management of emergencies related to the use of the drug. The reader is referred to the Appendix on the subjects of anaphylaxis and extravasation when appropriate.

This material was written with all levels of practitioners in mind, from the student to the experienced nurse. Also, keeping in mind that available equipment and institutional policies and procedures vary, we have attempted to present the information in a manner that can be applied to all situations.

It must be remembered that the entire entry on each drug has implications for nurses, and that practitioners must not limit themselves to familiarity with only the *Nursing Implications* sections. It is our philosophy that the administration of intravenous medications requires clear, logical thinking, a knowledge of all facets of the drug being administered, and a commitment on the part of the nurse to carry out the procedure with the greatest precision.

List of Drugs by Alphabetical Order

(See also Appendix, 362, and Index, 371)

Abbokinase (See Urokinase for Injection, 346)

Acetazolamide Sodium, 1

Achromycin Intravenous (See Tetracycline Hydrochloride, 320)

ACT-D (See Dactinomycin, 94)

A.C.T.H. (See Corticotropin, 80)

Acthar (See Corticotropin, 80)

Actinomycin-D (See Dactinomycin, 94)

Actrapid (See Insulin, Regular, 180)

Adrenalin (See Epinephrine Hydrochloride, 148)

Adrenocorticotropic Hormone (See Corticotropin, 80)

Adriamycin (See Doxorubicin Hydrochloride, 135)

Adrucil (See Fluorouracil, 157)

Aerosporin (See Polymyxin B Sulfate, 283)

Aldomet Ester HCl Injection (See Methyldopate Hydrochloride, 210)

Alpen-N (See Ampicillin, Sodium, 17)

Alphaprodine Hydrochloride, 2

Amcill-S (See Ampicillin, Sodium, 17)

Amethopterin (See Methotrexate Sodium, 206)

Amicar (See Aminocaproic Acid, 7)

Amikacin Sulfate, 4

Amikin (See Amikacin Sulfate, 4)

Aminocaproic Acid, 7

Aminophyllin (See Aminophylline, 8)

Aminophylline, 8

Amobarbital Sodium, 11

Amphotericin B, 14

Ampicillin, Sodium, 17

Amytal (See Amobarbital Sodium, 11)

Ancef (See Cefazolin Sodium, 52)

Anectine (See Succinylcholine Chloride, 316)

Anileridine Phosphate, 19

Antilirium (See Physostigmine Salicylate, 280)

Apresoline Hydrochloride (See Hydralazine Hydrochloride, 172)

AquaMEPHYTON (See Phytonadione, 282)

Ara-C (See Cytarabine, 88)

Arfonad (See Trimethaphan Camsylate, 338)

Asparaginase, 21

Ativan (See Lorazepam, 189)

Atropine Sulfate, 24

Aureomycin (See Chlortetracycline Hydrochloride, 71)

Azathioprine Sodium Salt, 27

Bactocill (See Oxacillin Sodium, 256)

Bactrim Intravenous Infusion (See Trimethoprim and Sulfamethoxazole, 340)

BCNU (See Carmustine, 47)

acetazolamide sodium ■
(Diamox)

Actions/Indications
Potent carbonic anhydrase inhibitor.

In glaucoma: rapidly decreases the secretion of aqueous humor thus decreasing intraocular pressure; used preoperatively and in acute crisis to rapidly lower intraocular pressure.

In convulsive disorders: suppresses abnormal paroxysmal discharge from CNS.

As a diuretic: produces a renal loss of HCO_3—which carries with it sodium, water and potassium; used in the reduction of edema due to congestive heart failure, drug-induced edema (steroids); prior to eye surgery.

Dosage
Acute closed-angle glaucoma—250 mg every 4 hrs. May be preceded by an initial dose of 500 mg.

Convulsive disorders—children and adults: 8–30 mg/kg/24 hrs in divided doses.

Optimum dose range: 375 mg–1000 mg/24 hrs. When used concomitantly with other anticonvulsants, start with 250 mg/24 hrs; increase as indicated.

Congestive heart failure and drug-induced edema—5 mg/kg, usually 250–375 mg daily on alternate days. Overdosage will decrease diuresis.
*Not recommended for pediatric use in this situation.

Preparation and Storage
Supplied in vials containing 500 mg of drug. Reconstitute with at least 5 ml of sterile water for injection. Use within 24 hours of preparation if refrigerated.

Drug Incompatibilities
Do not mix with any other medications.

Modes of IV Administration

Injection
Yes
Preferred IV mode. No further dilution needed after reconstitution.

Should be given at a rate of 250–500 mg over 5–6 min.

Intermittent Infusion
Yes
Add to any IV fluid, 50 ml fluid for each 250 mg of drug.

Continuous Infusion
Yes
Add to any IV fluid in any volume, at least 50 ml for each 250 mg of drug.

Contraindications; Warnings; Precautions; Adverse Reactions

Contraindications
1. In hyponatremic and/or hypokalemic states
2. In cases of marked hepatic or renal dysfunction, or adrenal insufficiency
3. In hyperchloremic acidosis
4. Long-term administration in chronic noncongestive angle-closure glaucoma

Precautions
1. Should not be used in pregnancy, especially the first trimester, unless benefits outweigh potential adverse effects on the fetus.
2. May increase the diuretic effect of other diuretics.
3. Increasing dose does *not* increase diuresis but may increase drowsiness.
4. Monitor CBC throughout therapy, bone marrow depression can occur.
5. Use with caution in patients with pulmonary obstruction or emphysema when alveolar ventilation may be impaired; this drug may precipitate or aggravate acidosis.

Adverse Reactions
Rash, renal calculus, casts in the urine, fever, bone marrow depression, thrombocytopenic purpura, pancytopenia, agranulocytosis. Also mild paresthesia, tingling feelings in extremities, anorexia, drowsiness and confusion. Transient myopia (near-sightedness) may be

acetazolamide sodium
(continued)
decreased with a lower dose and is reversible with discontinuance of the drug.

☐ **Nursing Implications**
1. Monitor patient for drug effectiveness:
   a. *Acute glaucoma*—improvement in vision, decreased ocular pain, decreased ocular pressure; disappearance of nausea and vomiting.
   b. *Seizure disorders*—chart frequency, character and duration of all seizures.
   c. *In congestive heart failure* (usually used in mild failure) —weigh all patients daily and record intake and output every 8 hours to document diuresis. Monitor resting heart rate, respirations and their changes with exertion. Observe for improvement in peripheral edema (feet, legs and sacrum) and CVP.
2. Examine patient daily for rashes, fever, hematuria and melena.
3. Monitor elderly patients carefully for confusion and take precautions where indicated; e.g., side rails, light restraints, bedside light at night.
4. Instruct patient to drink water in the amount ordered by physician to prevent crystaluria.
5. Instruct patient about the possibility of myopia.
6. Monitor for signs of mild metabolic acidosis which may be induced in long-term therapy: hyperventilation (also increased depth of respiration), drowsiness, restlessness.
7. Monitor for hypokalemia: muscle weakness, postural hypotension. Administer postassium supplements as prescribed.

Suggested Readings
Newell, Frank W., and Ernest, J. Terry: *Ophthalmology, Principles and Concepts* (3rd ed.), St. Loius; C.V. Mosby Company, 1974, Chapter 20—Glaucoma.
Condl, E. D.: Ophthalmic Nursing: The Gentle Touch. *Nursing Clinics of North America,* 5:467–476, September 1970.
Seamon, F. W.: Nursing Care of Glaucoma Patients, *Nursing Clinics of North America,* 5:489–496, September 1970.

alphaprodine hydrochloride ■
(Nisentil)

Actions/Indications
Narcotic analgesic, synthetic, rapid onset of effects, short duration.

Analgesia is comparable to morphine except for duration (30–60 min when given intravenously).

Used when a short duration of analgesia is desirable such as in minor surgery, obstetrics, cystoscopic examinations, or orthopedics.

Dosage
Adults:
Range—0.4–0.6 mg/kg. Use the lower dosage initially and evaluate patient response. *Usual adult dose—* 30 mg or less.

Do not exceed 240 mg in 24 hrs.
Children:
Safety for use in children has not been established.

Preparation and Storage
Supplied in 1 ml ampuls, 40 mg/ml and 10 ml ampuls, 60 mg/ml.

This is a Schedule II drug under the Controlled Substances Act of 1970. Maintain hospital or institutional regulations guiding its use.

Drug Incompatibilities
Do not mix with any medication **other than**: atropine, scopolamine, chlorpromazine, trifluoperazine, prochlorperazine, levallorphan.

Modes of IV Administration

Injection
Yes

Administer at a rate no greater than 20 mg/min. May be given undiluted.

Intermittent Infusion
No

Continuous Infusion
No

Contraindications; Warnings; Precautions; Adverse Reactions

Contraindications
Known hypersensitivity

Warnings
1. This drug is a habit-forming narcotic.
2. Respiratory depression can occur.
3. The central nervous system depressant effects of alphaprodine are potentiated by barbiturates, general anesthetic agents, some phenothiazines and tricyclic antidepressants. Lower dosage of this agent should be used in these circumstances.
4. Use with caution in the presence of increased intracranial pressure, hepatic insufficiency, severe depression of the central nervous system, myxedema, acute alcoholism, delirium tremens, seizure disorders, and Addison's disease.
5. Use with caution if the patient is concomitantly receiving an MAO inhibitor drug because of the possibility of hypotension.
6. Do not use for the relief of chronic pain. The need for frequent administration may make addiction more likely, and frequent injections would be unpleasant for the patient.
7. The safety of the use of this drug in labor and delivery has been established. However, its use in early pregnancy has not.

Precautions
1. For use during labor and delivery, be prepared to manage respiratory depression in the newborn.

2. Respiratory depression is more likely to occur in patients with pre-existing pulmonary disease, postoperative chest surgery, chest trauma, central nervous system depression, and in the elderly and the debilitated.

Adverse Reactions
1. Respiratory depression (in obstetrics, depression may occur in the mother and infant)
2. Dizziness
3. Drowsiness
4. Diaphoresis
5. Urticaria
6. Nausea and vomiting
7. Restlessness
8. Confusion (rare)

Management of Overdosage
Toxic effects of alphaprodine include: coma, shallow and Cheyne–Stokes respirations, cyanosis, hypotension, and pinpoint pupils. If these signs develop, a narcotic antagonist agent should be administered intravenously, naloxone (Narcan). (See page 237, for further information on this drug.) Some groups routinely give naloxone prophylactically when used in obstetrics to prevent respiratory depression in the newborn. Whether or not it is used, the infant should be closely monitored for respiratory depression for the first 4–6 hours of life. In the presence of apnea, artificial ventilation and oxygen should be administered in addition to the narcotic antagonist. Body warmth and hydration should be maintained and the patient's vital signs and respiratory status monitored carefully for 24 hours (see Nursing Implications, No. 1).

☐ Nursing Implications
1. Onset of action is 1–2 min and lasts for 30–90 min. Monitor the patient continuously for respiratory depression immediately after injection (or immediately after delivery of newborn) and for the next hour. Patients with renal or hepatic failure should

alphaprodine hydrochloride
(continued)

be monitored carefully for at least 2 hours after injection because of delayed metabolism and excretion of the drug. If respiratory rate falls below 8–10/min in an adult or below normal in a child, attempt to arouse the patient and to increase the respiratory rate to 12–14/min (or normal rate in a child). Stay with the patient until the effects of the drug have diminished. A narcotic antagonist may be prescribed; keep the agent readily available. If the patient is apneic or unarousable, begin artificial ventilation using an airway and manual breathing bag. (If this equipment is not immediately available, proceed with mouth-to-mouth breathing.) Maintain respiratory support until a narcotic antagonist can be administered (see above), and spontaneous respirations of an adequate rate return. If a patient develops respiratory depression after a normal dose of this drug, any subsequent doses should be reduced in amount.

2. Patients listed above in Warnings No. 3 and No. 4 must be monitored more closely and for a longer period of time for the development of respiratory depression.
3. If the patient has received an MAO inhibitor agent within the previous 2 weeks, monitor blood pressure carefully for 1 hour after injection; hypotension may develop.
4. Keep the patient supine for at least 15 minutes after an intravenous injection, and them ambulate with caution. (Dizziness can occur.)
5. If the patient is lethargic, drowsy, or in the immediate postoperative period, take precautions to prevent aspiration in the event of nausea and vomiting.

Suggested Reading
McCaffery, Margo, and Hart, Linda L.: Undertreatment of Acute Pain with Narcotics, *American Journal of Nursing,* October 1976, pp. 1586–1591.

amikacin sulfate ■
(Amikin)

Actions/Indications
Antibiotic (semisynthetic) aminoglycoside type, derived from kanamycin.

Used to treat *serious* infections due to susceptible strains of gram-negative bacilli including: some *Proteus* species, *Pseudomonas, E. Coli, Klebsiella–Enterobacter–Serratia* species, and others (including many strains resistant to other aminoglycosides), and such gram-positive organisms as: *Staphylococcus aureus* and *epidermidis* (especially those strains resistant to other aminoglycosides).

This drug is effective in the following infections: bacteremias (including neonatal sepsis), serious infections of: respiratory tract, central nervous system, bones and joints, skin and soft tissue, and abdominal cavity; burns and postoperative infections, serious and recurrent urinary tract infections.

Use must be based on susceptibility tests, severity of the infection, and response of the patient.

Dosage
Pretreatment Weight Must be Used to Determine Dosage.
In Normal Renal Function—Adults, Children and Older Infants:
15 mg/kg/day divided into 2–3 equal doses given at evenly spaced intervals. Do not exceed 1.5 gm/day.
Newborns:
Loading dose of 10 mg/kg followed by 7.5 mg/kg every 12 hours.

The usual duration of treatment is 7–10 days; if administration continues beyond this, renal and auditory function must be monitored daily.
In The Presence of Renal Impair-

ment Determine Dosage by One of the Following Methods:

1. Normal dosage (15 mg/kg) given at prolonged intervals to allow for excretion of the drug. Multiply patient's serum creatinine × 9 to determine time interval (in hours) between doses.
2. Reduced dosage regimen at fixed time intervals: loading dose of 7.5 mg/kg, maintenance dose given every 12 hrs and determined by:

$$\frac{\text{Pt's creat clear (ml/min)}}{\text{normal creat clear (ml/min)}} \times \frac{\text{calculated}}{\text{loading dose}}$$

3. Alternative: divide normal dose (15 mg/kg) by the patient's serum creatinine, give at usual intervals.
4. After peritoneal dialysis: 3–4 mg for every 2 liters of dialysate removed.[1]
5. After hemodialysis: 7.5 mg/kg after each dialysis.[2]

Monitor serum levels (peaks and valleys); when possible, avoid concentrations over 35 mcg/ml peak.

Preparation and Storage
Available in vials with a concentration of 50 mg/ml in 2-ml, and in a concentration of 250 mg/ml in 2- and 4-ml vials.

Aqueous solutions may darken without change in potency.

Use prepared solution promptly. Store unopened vials at room temperature.

Drug Incompatibilities
Do not mix with any other medication in any manner.

Modes of IV Administration

Injection
No

Intermittent Infusion
Yes
Add dose to 200 ml (smaller volumes in children, or as tolerated by the patient) of D5W or NS (drug is compatible with most solutions). Infuse over 30–60 min in adults

and older children, and over 1–2 hours in infants.

Continuous Infusion
No

Contraindications; Warnings; Precautions; Adverse Reactions

Contraindications
Hypersensitivity to this drug or kanamycin.

Warnings

1. Both auditory (sound perception) and vestibular (equilibrium) ototoxicity can occur in patients treated with higher doses or for periods longer than recommended. This is secondary to eighth cranial nerve damage. The risk of such damage is increased in the presence of renal failure. High-frequency deafness occurs first and must be detected only by audiometric testing. Vertigo may also appear, indicating vestibular damage. The ototoxicity of this drug in infants is not known; use only when other agents cannot be used and observe closely for signs of damage.
2. This drug can cause renal damage if large doses are given at longer than recommended times. Nephrotoxicity in patients with normal renal function, receiving recommended doses and hydration, is low. Renal impairment may be indicated by decreasing creatinine clearance, proteinuria, casts and cells in the urine, oliguria, decreasing or fixed low specific gravity, rising serum creatinine and BUN. Patients with pre-existing renal impairment may develop further deterioration in renal function.
3. Evidence of drug-induced renal impairment, and auditory and/or vestibular damage requires discontinuation of the drug or reduction in dosage and close monitoring of involved systems. If renal status does not improve with reduc-

amikacin sulfate
(continued)
tion of dosage, the drug should
be discontinued.
4. Monitor serum concentrations
(peaks and valleys) when possible (see Dosage section).
5. Concurrent and/or sequential
administration of topically or
systemic neurotoxic or nephrotoxic antibiotics (kanamycin,
gentamicin, tobramycin, neomycin, streptomycin, cephaloridine,
paromomycin, viomycin, polymyxin B, colistin, or vancomycin) should be avoided.
6. Do not give concurrently with
potent diuretics (ethacrynic
acid, furosemide, meralluride
sodium, sodium mercaptomerin
or mannitol).

Precautions
1. Adequate hydration may reduce
chemical irritation to renal tubules, and therefore decrease
the likelihood of renal damage.
If urinalysis shows casts, red or
white blood cells or albumin,
hydration should be increased.
If other signs of renal damage
appear (see Warning No. 2) a
reduction in dosage should be
instituted. Further deterioration
should prompt discontinuation
of the drug.
2. The possibility of neuromuscular blockade and subsequent respiratory paralysis should be
monitored for when this drug is
given with anesthetic or neuromuscular blocking agents. If
blockade occurs, calcium gluconate may reverse the effect.
3. There may be cross-allergenicity
with other aminoglycoside
drugs (tobramycin, streptomycin, kanamycin, gentamicin, and
neomycin).
4. Overgrowth infections due to
nonsusceptible organisms may
occur.
5. It is not known whether or not
this drug may cause fetal abnormalities. Use in pregnant wom-
en must be carefully considered
and only when absolutely neces-

sary. Breast-feeding should be
discontinued during therapy
with this drug; it is not known
whether or not it is excreted in
human milk.

Adverse Reactions
1. Ototoxicity (see Warning No. 1)
2. Nephrotoxicity (see Warning
No. 2)
3. Rarely: Rash
4. Drug fever
5. Headache
6. Paresthesia
7. Muscle tremor
8. Nausea and vomiting
9. Eosinophilia
10. Arthralgia
11. Hypotension during infusion
12. Anemia

*Management of Overdosage and
Toxic Reaction*
Hemo- and peritoneal dialysis can
remove this drug from the serum.
Monitor serum concentrations to
guide dialysis frequency and duration.

☐ **Nursing Implications**
1. Weigh the patient prior to treatment to calculate dosage.
2. Obtain urine for creatinine
clearance determinations in patients with renal impairment for
dosage calculation. Be aware of
dosage modifications for patients with renal impairment.
3. Monitor for signs and symptoms
of ototoxicity, e.g., high-frequency deafness, in patients on
large doses for over 10 days.
Arrange for audiometric testing.
The patient may complain of
ringing or roaring in the ears
(this is usually a late symptom).
Instruct the patient to report
vertigo (vestibular damage), or
monitor for signs of dizziness in
patients who cannot describe
symptoms. Notify the physician.
4. Send urine for urinalysis daily.
Be aware of results. Place the
patient on intake and output
measurements. Notify the physician if the urine output falls
below 240 ml/8-hour period (30

ml/hour) in the adult. Report fall in specific gravity below 1.020 or the development of a fixed value. Be aware of the patient's serum creatinine and BUN.

5. Keep the patient hydrated via oral or intravenous routes. Monitor for signs of dehydration (concentrated urine, high specific gravity, decreased skin turgor, dry mucous membranes).

6. Patients receiving anesthetic agents or neuromuscular blocking agents while on this drug must be monitored carefully for extension of neuromuscular blockade. These patients may require respiratory support for a longer than normal period following anesthesia.

7. Monitor for signs and symptoms of overgrowth infections:
   a. Fever (take rectal temperature at least every 4–6 hours in all patients)
   b. Increasing malaise
   c. Newly appearing localized signs and symptoms—redness, soreness, pain, swelling, drainage (increased volume or change in character of pre-existing drainage)
   d. Monilial rash in perineal area (reddened areas with itching)
   e. Cough (change in pre-existing cough or sputum production)
   f. Diarrhea

References
1. Appel, Gerald B., and Neu, Harold C.: The Nephrotoxicity of Antimicrobial Agents. *New England Journal of Medicine*, 296(3):666, March 31, 1977.
2. Ibid.

aminocaproic acid ▉
(Amicar)

Actions/Indications
Inhibitor of plasminogen activator substances; also has antiplasmin activity. This inhibits fibrinolysis to help control bleeding.

Used in the treatment of excessive bleeding which results from systemic hyperfibrinolysis and urinary fibrinolysis.

Systemic hyperfibrinolysis can be associated with:
- Postsurgical complications following cardiac surgery, portacaval shunts
- Hematological disorders such as aplastic anemia
- Abruptio placentae
- Hepatic cirrhosis
- Carcinoma of the prostate, lung, stomach, and cervix
- During the administration of thrombolytic drugs i.e., streptokinase and urokinase

Urinary fibrinolysis may be associated with life-threatening complications following severe trauma, anoxia, and shock.

This drug is also used to prevent rebleeding associated with intracranial aneurysms by preventing dissolution of the hemostatic clot that occurs because of the normal fibrinolytic mechanism.

Dosage
Adults:
Loading dose—5 gm via infusion.
   Maintenance—1.0–1.25 gm/hr to obtain a plasma level of 0.13 mg/ml or until bleeding has stopped.
   Maximum 24-hr dose is 30 gm.
   In renal failure—avoid; drug is excreted primarily via the kidneys.[1]
Children:
Loading dose—100 mg/kg or 3 gm/M^2
   Maintenance—30 mg/kg or 1 gm/M^2 at hourly intervals to obtain a plasma level of .013 mg/ml.
   Maximum 24-hr dose is 18 gm/M^2.

Preparation and Storage
Available in 20-ml vials with a concentration of 250 mg/ml.

After adding desired amount to infusion fluid, discard unused portion of drug vial. Use prepared solutions promptly.

Store unopened vials at room temperature.

aminocaproic acid
(continued)
Drug Incompatibilities
Do not mix with any other medication in any manner.

Modes of IV Administration

Injection
No
Direct injection may cause hypotension, bradycardia and other life-threatening arrhythmias.

Intermittent Infusion
Yes
Add loading dose to 100 ml D5W, NS or RL and infuse over 1 hr. Maintenance doses are administered by continuous infusion.

Continuous Infusion
Yes
Add an 8-hr dose to 1000 ml D5W, NS or RL and infuse at a rate of approximately 1 gm/hr (or 1/8 of the total dose/hr) to maintain plasma drug level.

Contraindications; Warnings; Precautions; Adverse Reactions

Contraindications
Do not use if there is evidence or suspicion of an intravascular coagulation process.

Warnings
When used in women of childbearing age or in a patient who is pregnant, the potential benefits must be weighed against the possibility of harm to the fetus.

Precautions
1. Do not infuse rapidly; to do so may result in bradycardia or other arrhythmias or hypotension.
2. Do not administer without a substantiated diagnosis of hyperfibrinolysis (hyperplasminemia).
3. Administer with caution to patients with cardiac, hepatic or renal disease.

Adverse Reactions
1. Nausea
2. Abdominal cramps
3. Diarrhea
4. Dizziness
5. Tinnitus
6. Malaise
7. Nasal stuffiness
8. Headache
9. Rash
10. Thrombophlebitis at infusion site

☐ **Nursing Implications**
1. Avoid extravasation; see Appendix.
2. Change IV site at the first sign of thrombophlebitis (pain, redness, swelling along vein tract). Apply warm compresses to the area.
3. Monitor heart rate and blood pressure at hourly intervals during the infusion. Notify physician of arrhythmias or hypotension. Strict adherence to infusion rates should prevent complications.
4. Monitor urine output at 4-hour intervals or as patient's condition dictates.

Reference
1. Mullan, S., and Dawley, J.: Antifibrinolytic Therapy for Intracranial Aneurysms. *Journal of Neurosurgery*, 28:21, 1968.

Suggested Reading
Guyton, Arthur C.: *Textbook of Medical Physiology* (5th ed.), Philadelphia: W. B. Saunders Company, 1976, Chapter 9, Hemostasis and Blood Coagulation, pp. 99–111.

aminophylline ■
(Aminophyllin)

Actions/Indications
Bronchodilator, pulmonary vasodilator and smooth muscle relaxant. Works directly on spastic bronchial muscles and induces relaxation.

Can be used in any condition that produces acute bronchospasm, such as asthma (bronchial or cardiac), status asthmaticus, and pulmonary edema (when accompanied by hypertension.*), and for reversible bronchospasm associated with chronic bronchitis and emphysema.

Also used as an antispasmotic in biliary colic.

*See Contraindications.

Dosage
Adults:
Loading dose—5.6 mg/kg (250–500 mg) given over 20 min followed by 0.2–0.7 mg/kg/hr as a continuous infusion titrated with plasma theophylline levels.

(Example: 70-kg patient would receive approximately 420 mg as a loading dose followed by an infusion of 63 mg/hr)

Reduce dose by 20–25% in the presence of congestive heart failure and in the elderly. In the presence of liver impairment reduce dose by 1/2

Children over 1 year:
Loading—5–6 mg/kg or 150 mg/M^2 given over 20 min.

Maintenance—0.9 mg/kg/hr by continuous infusion. (Alternative— 20 mg/kg/24 hrs, or 600 mg/M^2/24 hrs in equally divided doses every 6 hrs.

In children and adults, collect blood samples after loading dose or any time during continuous infusion. Optimal plasma level: 10–20 mcg/ml (theophylline).

Preparation and Storage
Available in IV and IM forms; check label carefully.

Intravenous form is supplied in 10 ml and 20 ml ampuls, each containing 25 mg/ml.

Drug Incompatibilities
Do not mix in any manner with:
Amikacin
Anileridine
Ascorbic acid
Cephalothin
Cephapirin
Chlorpromazine
Cimetidine
Clindamycin
Corticotropin
Dimenhydrinate
Epinephrine
Erythromycin
Hydralazine
Hydrocortisone
Insulin (regular)
Isoproterenol
Levorphanol
Meperidine
Methylprednisolone
Morphine
Nafcillin
Nitroprusside
Norepinephrine Bitartrate (Levophed)
Oxytetracycline
Penicillin G, potassium
Pentazocine
Prochlorperazine
Promazine
Promethazine
Sulfisoxazole
Tetracycline
Vancomycin
Vitamin B complex with C

Modes of IV Administration

Injection
Yes
Only in extreme emergencies.

This drug will cause serious tachyarrhythmias, hypotension and seizures when given in concentrated form.

DO NOT INJECT AT A RATE GREATER THAN 25 mg (1 ml)/min of the undiluted preparation.

Intermittent Infusion
Yes
Dilute to at least 1 mg in 1 ml of D5W or NS. Total daily dose may be given in 4 divided doses every 6 hrs.

DO NOT EXCEED A RATE OF 25 mg/min.

Use an infusion pump.

Continuous Infusion
Yes
This is the preferred mode of administration.

Prepare a solution concentration that will simplify calculation of drip rate, e.g., 1 mg/ml in D5W or NS.

aminophylline
(continued)
SEE DOSAGE SECTION FOR
HOURLY DOSE
Use an infusion pump.

Contraindications; Warnings; Precautions; Adverse Reactions

Contraindications
1. Hypersensitivity to theophylline derivatives
2. In the presence of hypotension
3. In the presence of coronary artery disease or angina when cardiac stimulation could be harmful
4. In peptic ulcer disease

Warnings
1. Overdosage may lead to circulatory collapse.
2. Rapid injection will produce serious tachyarrhythmias, hypotension and seizures.

Precautions
1. When the patient is acutely ill and has a history of cardiac problems such as arrhythmias, use with caution and monitor ECG for PVC's, ventricular tachycardia, ventricular fibrillation, or supraventricular tachycardia.
2. Use with caution in patients with severe cardiac disease, severe hypoxemia, hypertension, hyperthroidism, acute myocardial injury, obstructive lung disease, liver disease and in the elderly and in neonates.
3. Use extreme caution when administering to an infant less than 11 kg (25 lbs).
4. This drug should not be administered concomitantly with the following: other xanthine preparations, such as theophylline, oxytriphylline, dyphylline, ephedrine or other sympathomimetics or such antibiotics as: trolandomycin (TAO), erythromycin, or clindamycin.
5. Safety for use in pregnancy has not been established. Use only if expected benefits outweigh potential hazards.

Adverse Reactions
1. Gastrointestinal: anorexia, abdominal cramps, nausea, vomiting, reactivation of a peptic ulcer, and intestinal bleeding.
2. Central nervous system: headache, nervousness, insomnia, anxiety, dizziness, confusion, seizures.
3. Cardiovascular: palpitations, tachy- and bradyarrhythmias, hypotension, chest pain.
4. Respiratory: tachypnea.
5. Renal: albuminuria, microhematuria.
6. Others: hyperglycemia, inappropriate ADH syndrome.
7. Fatalities have occurred in overdosage.

Management of Overdosage
Management of toxic symptoms:
1. Discontinue drug immediately.
2. Give supportive, symptomatic treatment (IV fluids, oxygen).
3. Avoid giving sympathomimetic drugs (for example, epinephrine).
4. For hyperthermia, use cooling blanket or sponge baths.
5. Maintain patient airway and use artificial ventilation as needed.
6. Control seizures with appropriate parenteral medications.
7. Monitor serum theophylline levels until below 20 mcg/ml.

☐ Nursing Implications
1. Be aware of hospital policy on the IV administration of aminophylline.
2. Monitor all patients electrocardiographically in an I.C.U. who:
   a. Have a history of arrhythmias
   b. Are acutely ill with pulmonary edema or status asthmaticus
   c. Are hypoxic
   d. Are acidotic
   e. Are receiving other agents that may produce arrhyth-

mias. Observe for premature ventricular contractions, premature atrial contractions, supraventricular tachycardia and ventricular tachycardia. Slow the infusion rate *immediately* if one of these arrhythmias occurs, or if the sinus rate exceeds 120/min. Notify the physician of the occurrence. Slowing or stopping an infusion will usually control these reactions. However, be prepared to actively treat arrhythmias not controlled in this manner. Keep lidocaine 100 mg at the bedside and administer in accordance with hospital regulations and physician's orders in the event of a ventricular tachyarrythmia. A defibrillator must be readily available.

3. Monitor blood pressure frequently during an infusion (all patients), especially during the first 15 minutes, or if the infusion is being given rapidly for therapeutic reasons. Hypo- and hypertension may occur. (Suggested schedule: Every 2–3 minutes the first 15 minutes of infusion, then every 10 minutes for 1 hour, then every 30 minutes, or as patient's condition dictates.)

4. Observe for drug effectiveness, e.g., decreasing respiratory effort (observable and subjective), decreased wheezing, decreased respiratory rate, decreased cyanosis or pallor. Monitor arterial blood gases for improvement of pCO_2, pO_2, pH and $pHCO_3$, when possible.

5. Monitor for all adverse reactions; all are early warnings of overdosage and toxicity. Slow or stop the infusion at the onset of any one sign. Be aware of the patient's plasma level if obtained (see Dosage section).

6. Initiate seizure precautions.

7. Be prepared to manage vomiting to prevent aspiration.

amobarbital sodium ■
(Amytal)

Actions/Indications
Barbiturate, short acting. Central nervous system depressant, hypnotic, anticonvulsant.

Used to control seizures secondary to eclampsia, chorea, meningitis, tetanus, drug reactions, and epileptiform seizures.

In psychiatry, may be used to control catatonic, negativistic and manic reactions. May also be used for narcoanalysis and narcotherapy.

Dosage
Adults and Children Over 6 Years of Age:
65–500 mg/dose (not exceeding 1 gm). Dosage should be determined by patient response and indication.
Younger Children:
3–5 mg/kg or 125 mg/M^2 per dose.

Preparation and Storage
Available in ampuls of 125, 250 and 500 mg, some accompanied by sterile water for injection, 2.5 ml. To reconstitute from powder, use sterile water for injection in the amounts listed below and on page 12.

After adding diluent, ROTATE VIAL GENTLY; DO NOT SHAKE. Dissolution may take several minutes. Do not use a solution that has not cleared within 5 minutes, or one that contains a precipitate. Use solutions within 30 minutes.

This is a Schedule II drug under the Controlled Substances Act of 1970. Maintain hospital or institutional regulations guiding its use.

Volumes of diluent needed to make specified solution concentrations for each ampul size:[1]

Percent Solution	Concentration (mg/ml)	Volume of Diluent (ml)
125-mg ampul		
1	10	12.5
2.5	25	5.0
5	50	2.5
10*	100	1.25
20	200	0.625

amobarbital sodium
(continued)

Percent Solution	Concentration (mg/ml)	Volume of Diluent (ml)
250-mg ampul		
1	10	25.0
2.5	25	10.0
5	50	5.0
10	100	2.5
20	200	1.25
500-mg ampul		
1	10	50.0
2.5	25	20.0
5	50	10.0
10	100	5.0
20	200	2.5

*Ordinarily a 10-percent solution is used.

Drug Incompatibilities

Do not mix in any manner with:
Anileridine
Cephalosporins
Chlorpromazine
Cimetidine
Clindamycin
Codeine
Dimenhydrinate
Diphenhydramine
Droperidol
Hydrocortisone
Hydroxyzine
Insulin (regular)
Isoproterenol
Levorphanol
Meperidine
Metaraminol
Methyldopate
Morphine
Norepinephrine bitartrate (Levophed)
Penicillin G
Pentazocine
Propiomazine
Succinylcholine
Tetracyclines
Thiamine
Vancomycin

Modes of IV Administration

Injection
Yes
Do not exceed a rate of 100

mg/min. for adults or 60 mg/min. for children.

Intermittent Infusion
No
Pharmacologically inappropriate.

Continuous Infusion
No
Pharmacologically inappropriate.

Contraindications; Warnings; Precautions; Adverse Reactions

Contraindications
1. Impaired liver function
2. Family or patient history of porphyria
3. Hypersensitivity to any barbiturate
4. Respiratory disease evidenced by dyspnea or obstruction
5. History of addiction to sedative/hypnotic drugs
6. In presence of acute or chronic pain; can induce paradoxical excitement or mask symptoms

Warnings
1. May be habit-forming, causing both psychic and physical dependence.
2. The central nervous system depressant effects of this drug may be potentiated by the depressant effects of other similar drugs and alcohol.
3. Safety for use in pregnancy has not been established. When given during labor, may cause depression in the infant.
4. Safety for use in children under age 6 has not been established.
5. This drug may impair the mental and physical abilities to perform potentially hazardous tasks such as ambulating (in the elderly or debilitated), climbing stairs, driving a car.
6. Rapid injection, exceeding recommended rate, or a relative overdosage may cause apnea or hypotension. Respiratory depression may occur if this drug is given concomitantly with other central nervous system depressants.

Precautions

1. The liver is the major site of metabolism of this drug. Use with caution in patients with impaired liver function. Titrate small doses with patient response.
2. Use caution in the dosage and rate of administration of this drug in patients with hypotension, respiratory disorders, cardiac disease or hypertension.
3. Pulmonary edema may accompany long periods of unconsciousness produced by this drug.
4. This drug may induce excitement or depression in elderly or debilitated patients.
5. Use with caution in patients with borderline hypoadrenal function.

Adverse Reactions

1. Respiratory depression
2. Drug idiosyncrasy: excitement "hangover" symptoms
3. Hypersensitivity: asthma, urticaria, angioneurotic edema
4. Laryngospasm (during normal induction or as the result of improper dosage)
5. Hypotension after rapid injection
6. Nausea and vomiting (uncommon)

Management of Overdosage

1. Symptoms: First, decreased body temperature; then, fever, depression of superficial and deep reflexes, respiratory depression, gradual circulatory collapse (decreased urine output, hypotension), pulmonary edema and coma.
2. Treatment: Intravenous fluids; maintenance of blood pressure, body temperature and respiratory support. Patients with respiratory depression will require intubation and mechanical ventilation until the drug has been excreted. Hemodialysis can be used to increase the rate of excretion. Antibiotics may be needed for pulmonary complications.

☐ **Nursing Implications**

1. Strictly adhere to maximum injection rate suggestions and maximum dosage limits. Patients with liver impairment should receive smaller doses and should be monitored more closely and for a longer period of time than usual.
2. Keep the patient supine during and after injection. Monitor blood pressure, heart rate and respiratory rate every 5 minutes for 1 hour following an injection. This includes fetal heart rate monitoring. Do not leave the patient unattended.
3. Patients with porphyria are sensitive to barbiturates in that they may experience an acute attack of the disease secondary to the administration of a barbiturate (see Contraindications). The onset of an acute attack is indicated by severe colicky abdominal pain radiating to the back. There is usually severe vomiting, fever and leukocytosis in addition.[2]
4. Avoid extravasion; see Appendix. Extravascular or intra-arterial injection of this drug can cause tissue necrosis and gangrene of the affected extremity, respectively. Thrombophlebitis can also occur.
5. Take anaphylaxis precautions; see Appendix
6. Monitor for symptoms of acute overdosage (listed in order of progression):
   a. Respiratory depression, i.e., decreased respiratory rate and depth
   b. Peripheral vascular collapse, i.e., fall in blood pressure, pallor diaphoresis, tachycardia
   c. Pulmonary edema (rare)
   d. Decreased or absent reflexes, pupillary constriction

amobarbital sodium
(continued)

  e. Stupor
  f. Coma
     Stop the injection immediately upon noting one of these symptoms. Notify the physician. Discontinuation of the injection is usually all that is necessary to prevent further problems. If not, see No. 7 below.
7. Management of acute overdosage:
  a. Continue to stay with the patient and monitor vital signs.
  b. Maintain an open airway and adequate ventilation.
  c. Keep the patient as alert as possible by verbal and physical stimuli. Encourage the patient to breathe at an adequate rate (12–14 breaths/minute for an adult). If necessary, initiate artificial ventilation with a manual breathing bag (Puritan, Hope, Ambu, etc.) or mouth-to-mouth breathing at a rate of 12–14 breaths/minute.
  d. Circulatory support in the form of fluids and drugs may be ordered.
8. The sedation produced by this drug may be preceded by transient changes in mental status, such as feelings of euphoria and confusion. If this occurs, attempt to calm the patient and take measures to prevent injury until the patient returns to his normal status.
9. If a patient is to be ambulatory following an injection, ambulate with assistance; there may be transient dizziness. Obtain lying, then sitting and standing blood pressures to detect postural hypotension. If this drug has been used for outpatient procedure, a responsible adult should accompany the patient home. The patient should not drive for at least the next 8 hours.

References
1. Trissel, Lawrence: *Handbook on Injectable Drugs*, American Society of Hospital Pharmacists, Washington, D.C., 1977, p. 23.
2. Beeson, Paul B., and McDermott, Walsh (editors): *Textbook of Medicine* (14th ed.), Philadelphia, W. B. Saunders Company, 1975, p. 1873.

amphotericin b ■
(Fungizone)

Actions/Indications
Antibiotic, antifungal. To be used only in patients with progressive, potentially fatal fungal infections:
• Cryptococcosis
• Blastomycosis
• Disseminated moniliasis, coccidioidomycosis and histoplasmosis
• Mucormycosis (phycomycosis)
• Sporotrichosis
• Aspergillosis
This drug may be helpful in the treatment of American mucocutaneous leishmaniasis, but is not the drug of choice.

Dosage
Adults:
An initial test dose of 1 mg may be given over 30 min in an infusion. If no adverse reactions occur, full dose may be given. Optimal dose is unknown, but amount given should be gradually increased up to 1 mg/kg/day depending on patient response. Do not exceed 1.5 mg/kg/day.
  Usual dose—0.25 mg/kg/day.
Children and Neonates:
Test dose of 0.1 mg/kg over 6 hrs. Increase the dose, if there are no adverse reactions, over the next 4 days. Do not exceed 1 mg/kg/24 hrs (30 mg/m²/24 hrs).

Preparation and Storage
Supplied in vials containing 50 mg of drug.
  To prepare from powder add 10 ml sterile water for injection to the vial.

(Do not use diluents containing bacteriostatic agents, or saline.)

Shake until solution is clear. The resultant solution is 5 mg/ml.

Store powder and reconstituted solution in the refrigerator. Discard reconstituted solution after 7 days. Protect against exposure to light. **Aseptic Technique Must Be Strictly Observed In All Handling.** No preservative or bacteriostatic agent is present in the drug.

Use only D5W for infusion vehicle; do not use if solution is not clear.

Drug Incompatibilities

This drug is incompatible with solutions with a pH less than 6. Use only D5W for infusion. Do not mix with any other medication in any manner.

(Heparin and/or hydrocortisone may be added to solution to decrease risk of infusion phlebitis.)

Do not mix in any manner with:
Amikacin
Calcium (chloride and gluconate)
Calcium disodium edetate
Carbenicillin
Chlorpromazine
Diphenhydramine
Dopamine
Gentamicin
Kanamycin
Lidocaine
Metaraminol
Methyldopate
Penicillin G (potassium and sodium)
Polymyxin B
Potassium chloride
Prochlorperazine
Tetracyclines
Vitamins

Modes of IV Administration

Injection
No
Must be highly diluted prior to administration.

Intermittent Infusion
Yes
Preferred mode of administration. Infuse total daily dose over 6 hrs. Use a concentration of .1 mg/ml; (1 mg/10 ml.); use only D5W for infusion fluid.

In-line filters can be used but the mean pore diameter should not be less than 1.0 micron in order to assure passage of the drug solution.

Protect from light during administration.

Continuous Infusion
No

Contraindications; Warnings; Precautions; Adverse Reactions

Contraindications
Hypersensitivity, unless administration of this drug is considered to be lifesaving.

Warnings
1. The possible lifesaving benefits of this drug must be weighed against its untoward and dangerous side effects.
2. Safety for use in pregnancy has not been established.

Precautions
1. Prolonged therapy is usually necessary and unpleasant reactions are common; some are dangerous. Therefore, this drug should be used only in hospitalized patients in whom potentially fatal forms of susceptible mycotic infections have been confirmed by culture.
2. Corticosteroids in large doses should not be administered concomitantly unless they are necessary to control drug reactions.
3. May cause renal damage. Serum creatinine and BUN must be monitored at weekly intervals during therapy. If BUN exceeds 40 mg/100 ml or the serum creatinine exceeds 3.0 mg/100 ml, the drug should be discontinued or reduced in dosage until renal function improves. Use with caution in the presence of pre-existing renal failure.
4. Avoid giving other nephrotoxic antibiotics and antineoplastic

amphotericin b
(continued)

agents such as nitrogen mustard except with great caution.

5. Therapy should be discontinued if liver function test results are abnormal, e.g., elevated bromsulphalein, alkaline phosphatase and bilirubin.
6. May cause hypokalemia and low serum magnesium.
7. Whenever amphotericin is discontinued for longer than 7 days, therapy should be restarted at test-dose level, and gradually increased to therapeutic levels.
8. Extravasation may cause tissue irritation.

Adverse Reactions
A. Most common:
1. Fever (shaking chills)
2. Headache
3. Anorexia, weight loss
4. Nausea, vomiting, dyspepsia
5. Malaise
6. Diarrhea
7. Muscle and joint pains
8. Pain at injection site with phlebitis and thrombophlebitis
9. Normochromic, normocytic anemia
10. Renal function abnormalities: hypokalemia, azotemia, renal tubular acidosis, nephrocalcinosis. Permanent renal impairment may occur, especially with large doses. Supplemental alkali medication may decrease renal tubular acidosis.
B. Infrequent or rare:
11. Anuria
12. Cardiac toxicity: arrhythmias, cardiac arrest, hypertension, hypotension.
13. Blood dyscrasias: thrombocytopenia, leukopenia or leukocytosis, agranulocytopenia, eosinophilia.
14. Hemorrhagic gastroenteritis
15. Rash, pruritus
16. Loss of hearing, tinnitus (transient)
17. Vertigo
18. Blurred vision or diplopia
19. Peripheral neuropathy
20. Convulsions
21. Anaphylaxis
22. Acute liver failure

□ **Nursing Implications**
1. Take anaphylaxis precautions; see Appendix
2. Monitor for symptoms of toxicity:
   a. Renal damage—measure urinary output every 4 hours; notify the physician if urine output falls below an average of 30 ml/hour; urine for analysis at least every other day to detect abnormalities.
   b. Fever—record temperature every 4 hours (mild elevations are seen in most patients.) Administer corticosteroids as ordered to decrease febrile reactions, and antipyretics as ordered if fever occurs.
   c. Nausea, vomiting, diarrhea —administer antiemetics as ordered. Maintain hydration. Measure intake and output to guide the physician in ordering fluids. Parenteral fluids may be required.
   d. Generalized and localized pain—administer analgesics as ordered.
   e. Cardiac arrhythmias—monitor heart rate and rhythm every 2 hours; notify physician of abnormalities. Continuous ECG monitoring is advisable.
   f. Neurologic changes—observe for changes in mental status, numbness of fingers, toes, or face, seizures.
   g. Blood disorders—observe for bleeding, petechiae, bruising.
   h. Hearing loss—notify the physician of any hearing loss, ringing in the ears, or dizziness.
   i. Changes in vision.
3. Avoid extravasation, see Appendix. If it occurs, discontinue in-

fusion, apply warm compresses and prevent further damage to the area.
4. Notify the physician if jaundice is observed.
5. Provide emotional support for critically ill patients receiving this drug. Their discomforts and fears will be numerous.
6. Take seizure precautions.

ampicillin, sodium ■
(Alpen-N, Amcill-S, Omnipen-N, Pen A/N, Penbritin-S, Pensyn, Principen-N, Polycillin-N, SK-Ampicillin N, Totacillin)

Actions/Indications
Antibiotic, synthetic penicillin, broad spectrum. Bactericidal against penicillin-susceptible gram-positive and gram-negative organisms.

Used to treat moderate to severe infections secondary to susceptible organisms such as *Streptococci pneumonae*, penicillin-G sensitive staphylococci, gonococci, *E. coli*, Proteus mirabilis, *H. influenzae* and others, for infections of the respiratory tract, soft tissue, skin, urinary tract, blood and central nervous system.

Dosage
This drug should not be given in doses larger than those recommended, except where indicated.
Adults:[1]
Infections of the respiratory tract, skin, and soft tissue—250–500 mg every 6 hrs.
Gastrointestinal and urinary tract infections—500 mg every 6 hrs.
(Dosage may be higher in severe infections.)
In septicemia and bacterial meningitis—8–14 gm daily or 150–200 mg/kg/day, in equally divided doses, every 3–4 hours.
Renal impairment (creatinine clearance less than 10 ml/min.)—increase the interval between doses to 8 and 12 hrs, unless a high urine concentration of the drug is needed, then give every 6 hrs.
Children:
(Children over 40 kg may receive adult dosage.)

Infections of the respiratory tract, skin and soft tissue—25–50 mg/kg/day given in equally divided doses every 6 hrs.
Gastrointestinal and urinary tract infections—50–100 mg/kg/day given in equally divided doses every 6 hrs.
Septicemia and bacterial meningitis—100–400 mg/kg/day via continuous infusion for 3 days followed by intermittent IV or IM doses.
Neonates (Term and Premature):
Less than 1 week of age in life-threatening septicemia and meningitis[2]—100 mg/kg/day in 2 equal doses 12 hrs apart. (Usually given with an aminoglycoside antibiotic).
More than 1 week of age in septicemia and meningitis[3]—200 mg/kg/day in 3 equal doses 8 hrs apart (with an aminoglycoside).

Preparation and Storage
To reconstitute 125-, 250- and 500-mg vials add 5 ml sterile water for injection.

For the 1-gm and 2-gm vials add 10 ml sterile water for injection or bacteriostatic water for injection. (If this drug is used in neonates *do not* use bacteriostatic diluent.)

Use these solutions within 1 hour of reconstitution.

For piggyback units for infusion, use sterile water for injection or NS: to the 1-gm bottle, add 49 ml of diluent, shake well. Resultant solution is 20 mg/ml. To the 2-gm bottle, add 99 ml of diluent and shake well. The resulting solution is 20 mg/ml.

Drug Incompatibilities
Do not add any other medications to ampicillin in IV fluid. Do not mix in an IV line with any other antibiotic.

Modes of IV Administration

Injection
Yes
Must be injected over at least 3–5 min for a dose of 125–500 mg. A more rapid injection can result in seizures. Inject into tubing of a running IV.

ampicillin, sodium
(continued)
Intermittent Infusion
Yes
Preferred route. Dilute each 500 mg of dose in 100 ml (5 mg/ml) of any fluid listed in the table below.

Infuse over 30 min. Do not exceed a 100 mg/min flow rate.

Continuous Infusion
Yes
Dilute dose in 500–1000 ml of any fluid listed in the table below.

Infuse within the time limit specified in that table to insure potency.

Contraindications; Warnings; Precautions; Adverse Reactions

Contraindications
Hypersensitivity to any penicillin or ampicillin

Precautions
1. There may be cross-allergenicity with cephalosporins. Administer with caution to patients with allergy to any cephalosporin; or to multiple allergens.
2. Safety for use in pregnancy has not been established. Potential risk to the fetus must be weighed against benefits to the mother.
3. There is a possibility of secondary (overgrowth) infections due to nonsusceptible mycoses or bacterial pathogens.
4. Monitor renal, hepatic and hematopoietic function before and during therapy, if prolonged therapy required.
5. A maculopapular rash and urticaria can occur in a significant percentage of all patients receiving this drug who have renal dysfunction. This is not thought to be a true penicillin allergic reaction, and is not a contraindication. However, the patient should be monitored closely for other signs of allergy or anaphylaxis.
6. With high urine concentrations, false-positive glucose reactions may occur if Clinitest is used. Clinistix or Tes-Tape should be used.

Adverse Reactions
1. Allergy: rash, urticaria, anaphylaxis.
2. Gastrointestinal: glossitis (inflammation of tongue), stomatitis (inflammation of mucous membranes of the mouth), nausea, vomiting, diarrhea. (usually occurs with oral form)
3. Liver: slight rise in SGOT, especially in infants (significance is unknown).
4. Blood cell formation: anemia, thrombocytopenia, leukopenia and agranulocytosis. (These reactions are believed to be due to allergy, and are reversible.)

☐ **Nursing Implications**
1. Take anaphylaxis precautions; see Appendix. Report all rashes to the physician. They may be prelude to anaphylaxis.

Fluid Used—Infusion Time Limit

Solution	Concentration of Infusion	Time Limit for Infusion
	(Ampicillin/ml of fluid)	
NS	up to 30 mg/ml	8 hrs
M/6 Sodium Lactate	up to 30 mg/ml	8 hrs
D5W	10–20 mg/ml	2 hrs
D5W	up to 2 mg/ml	4 hrs
D5/0.45% Sodium Chloride	up to 2 mg/ml	4 hrs
10% Invert Sugar	up to 2 mg/ml	4 hrs
Lactated Ringer's	up to 30 mg/ml	8 hrs

2. Monitor for signs and symptoms of overgrowth infections:
   a. Fever (take rectal temperature at least every 4–6 hours in all patients)
   b. Increasing malaise
   c. Newly appearing localized signs and symptoms—redness, soreness, pain, swelling, drainage (increased volume or change in character of pre-existing drainage)
   d. Monilial rash in perineal area (reddened areas with itching)
   e. Cough (change in pre-existing cough or sputum production)
   f. Diarrhea
3. Nausea, vomiting and diarrhea are fairly common side effects with ampicillin. Administer antiemetics or constipating agents as ordered. Maintain hydration. Encourage nutritional intake as allowed by the patient's condition. Record intake and output to guide the physician in ordering parenteral fluids if they are needed.
4. Be aware of the patient's blood cell count. If the white cell count falls below 2000/cu.mm., place the patient in protective (reverse) isolation. Prevent infection by maintaining bodily cleanliness (especially perineal) and avoiding invasive procedures. Monitor for signs of infection. If the platelet count falls below 100,000/cu.mm., monitor for thrombocytopenic bleeding: gum bleeding, epistaxis, hematemesis, petechiae, hematuria, melena, blood in the stools, vaginal bleeding, ecchymosis.
5. Use Clinistix or Tes-Tape for urine glucose determinations.

References
1. *American Hospital Formulary Service*, Washington, D.C.: American Society of Hospital Pharmacists. 1977, Section 8:12–16.
2. McCracken, George H., and Nelson, John D.: *Antimicrobial Therapy for Newborns*. New York: Grune and Stratton, 1977, p. 16.
3. Ibid.

anileridine phosphate ■
(Leritine)

Actions/Indications
Narcotic analgesic similar to, but more potent than, meperidine. Used for moderate to severe pain. Has sedative qualities. Can be used as an adjunct to anesthesia or as an analgesic during labor.

Onset of action is in 2–3 min, duration is 25–40 min.

Dosage
Adults and Children over 12 Years of Age:
Initially—5–10 mg by injection followed by an infusion of 0.6 mg/min titrated with patient response
Children Under 12:
Not recommended.

Preparation and Storage
Available in 25 mg/ml solutions: 1-ml and 2-ml ampuls and 30-ml multi-dose vials.

Add only to D5W for infusion.
Store at room temperature.

This is a Schedule II drug under the Controlled Substances Act of 1970. Maintain hospital or institutional regulations guiding the use of this drug.

Drug Incompatibilities
Do not mix in any manner with: aminophylline, ammonium chloride, any barbiturate, chlorothiazide, heparin, methicillin, novobiocin, phenytoin, sodium bicarbonate, sodium iodide.

Modes of IV Administration

Injection
Rapid injection of a dose greater than 10 mg may result in respiratory depression or apnea, hypotension and cardiac arrest. Use this route

anileridine phosphate
(continued)
only in emergencies. Dilute dose to
1 mg/ml with NS.
Inject Slowly Over 2–3 Min.

Intermittent Infusion
Yes
Add 50–100 mg to 500 ml D5W.
Usual rate is 0.6 mg/min titrated
with patient response.
  Use an infusion pump.

Continuous Infusion
Yes
Same as Intermittent Infusion.

Contraindications; Warnings; Precautions; Adverse Reactions

Contraindications
  1. Respiratory depression
  2. Hypersensitivity
  3. Patients under 12 years of age

Warnings
  1. Can cause respiratory
     depression; occurs more fre-
     quently in the elderly, the debil-
     itated or in the presence of
     pulmonary impairment such as
     in chronic lung disease, chest
     trauma, or chest surgery.
  2. Can cause circulatory
     depression. Administer with ex-
     treme caution to patients in
     shock; further decrease in cardi-
     ac output and blood pressure
     may occur.
  3. In the presence of deep respira-
     tory and circulatory collapse,
     naloxone will help counteract
     the effects.
  4. Use with caution in combination
     with other narcotics, sedatives,
     phenothiazines, or anesthetics.
     These drugs may potentiate re-
     spiratory and circulatory depres-
     sant effects.
  5. Rapid injection of a dose
     greater than 10 mg may result
     in severe respiratory depression
     and apnea, hypotension and
     possibly cardiac arrest. Give via
     intravenous *injection* ONLY IN
     EXTREME EMERGENCIES.
  6. Safety for use in pregnancy has

not been established in regard
to the effects on fetal development. Can be used during labor, but precautions must be
taken to prevent or to promptly
treat respiratory depression in
the newborn, using a narcotic
antagonist.

Precautions
  1. May be habit-forming
  2. Use with extreme caution in the
     presence of hepatic impairment,
     severe central nervous system
     depression, patients with head
     injuries or when intracranial
     pressure is increased, myxede-
     ma, Addison's disease, acute al-
     coholic intoxication, delirium
     tremens, seizure disorders, and
     in patients taking MAO inhibi-
     tors

Adverse Reactions
  1. Respiratory depression (see
     Warning Nos. 1, 4, and 5)
  2. Circulatory depression (see
     Warning Nos. 2, 4, and 5)
  3. Nausea, vomiting, dry mouth
  4. Slight transient hypotension and
     bradycardia
  5. Dizziness
  6. Diaphoresis
  7. Blurred vision
  8. Euphoria, restlessness, nervous-
     ness and excitement
  9. Hypersensitivity: urticaria, rash,
     anaphylaxis

Management of Overdosage
  1. Symptoms: Respiratory
     depression, i.e., decreased respi-
     ratory rate possibly leading to
     apnea, stupor, hypotension.
  2. Treatment: *Adults:* naloxone ac-
     cording to manufacturer's dos-
     age guidelines.
     Newborns: Naloxone Neonatal
     0.01 mg/kg, repeat at 2 to 3
     minute intervals until respira-
     tions are normal. Oxygen,
     assisted ventilation, intravenous
     fluids, blood pressure support
     and constant attendance are ad-
     visable until full respiratory and
     circulatory functions return and
     are stabilized.

In patients who are addicted to narcotics (including newborn of an addicted mother), the use of a narcotic antagonist agent may precipitate an acute withdrawal syndrome. See page 237 on naloxone.

☐ **Nursing Implications**
1. Adhere strictly to injection and infusion rate restrictions.
2. Monitor respiratory status during, and for 1 hour after, injection. Count respiratory rate every 2–3 minutes during the first 30 minutes and every 5–10 minutes thereafter. If the patient's respiratory rate (adult) falls below 8–10/minute, attempt to arouse the patient and stimulate a respiratory rate of at least 12–14/minute. If the patient is receiving an infusion of this drug, temporarily stop it. Call for the physician. If the patient cannot be aroused to cooperate, begin assisted ventilation either by mouth-to-mouth breathing or by using a manual breathing bag and airway. Administer oxygen as needed. See Management of Overdosage for the use of a narcotic antagonists. The patient should have complete return of spontaneous respiratory rate, gag, swallow and cough reflexes before being left unattended.
3. Monitor blood pressure before, during, and for 1 hour after injection, at 5–10 minute intervals. Report hypotension to the physician. If the patient is receiving an infusion, slow it down to a minimal rate or discontinue. Administer fluids, the narcotic antagonist, and vasopressors as needed. Discontinuation of the drug alone may allow blood pressure to return to normal.
4. Patient situations as listed in Warning No. 4 and Precaution No. 2 should be monitored continuously during and for 2 hours after injection or infusion.

These patients are more likely to develop adverse reactions.
5. Be prepared to manage vomiting to prevent aspiration.
6. Monitor patient's response to analgesia to guide infusion rate and/or additonal injections.

Suggested Reading
McCaffery, Margo, and Hart, Linda L.: Undertreatment of Acute Pain With Narcotics. *American Journal of Nursing*, October 1976, pp. 1586–1591.

asparaginase ■
(Elspar)

Actions/Indications
An antineoplastic agent that contains an enzyme L-asparagine amidohydrolase capable of inactivating the amino acid asparagine needed by some tumor cells for cell protein synthesis and replication.

The malignant cells of acute leukemia, particularly the lymphocytic type, are dependent on an outside source of asparagine for survival. This drug depletes their source of asparagine. Normal cells can synthesize it and are less affected by a depletion of it produced by the asparaginase enzyme.

This drug is used with other agents to induce remission in acute lymphocytic leukemia in children. It is not recommended for maintenance therapy.

Dosage
The following combination regimens are recommended for children and adults:
Regimen 1:
Beginning on day 1: *prednisone* 40 mg/M^2/day orally in 3 divided doses for 15 days; follow with tapering dose as follows: 20 mg/M^2/day for 2days, 10 mg/M^2/day for 2 days, 5 mg/M^2 for 2 days, 2.5 mg/M^2 for 2 days, then discontinue.

And, *vincristine sulfate* 2 mg/M^2 intravenously once a week on days 1, 8 and 15 of the treatment period.

asparaginase
(continued)
Do not exceed a maximum single dose of 2.0 mg.

And, *aparaginase* 1,000 I.U./kg/day intravenously for 10 successive days beginning on day 22 of the treatment period.

Regimen II:
Beginning on day 1: *prednisone* 40 mg/M²/day orally in 3 divided doses for 28 days. Then discontinue gradually over the next 14 days.

And, *vincristine sulfate* 1.5 mg/M² intravenously once a week for 4 doses on days 1, 8, 15, and 22 of the treatment period. Do not exceed a maximum single dose of 2.0 mg.

And, *asparaginase* 6,000 I.U./M² **intramuscularly** on days 4, 7, 10, 13, 16, 19, 22, 25, and 28 of the treatment period.

If remission is obtained, maintenance therapy should be initiated. Asparaginase is not a part of this maintenance.

Therapy should be instituted with the above regimens to prevent central nervous system leukemia.

Other regimens to induce remission have also been used. Use of this agent as a sole induction agent should be undertaken only in an unusual situation when combined therapy cannot be used because of drug toxicity or in cases that have been refractory to other therapy.

As a sole induction agent for children and adults:
200 I.U./kg/day intravenously for 28 days. The remission obtained with this is usually short in duration—1 to 3 months.

In all regimens, dosages may need to be reduced if toxicity occurs.

See Adverse Reactions for use of intradermal skin test procedure prior to drug administration.

Preparation and Storage
Supplied in 10 ml vials of 10,000 I.U. of drug powder. Keep refrigerated.

Reconstitute with 5 ml of sterile water for injection or sodium chloride injection. Resultant concentration is 2,000 I.U./ml. Solution should be clear; discard if not. Refrigerate and use within 8 hours. If administered by infusion, use NS or D5W only, and use within 8 hours.

See Adverse Reactions for preparation of skin test solution.

Drug Incompatibilities
Do not mix with any other medication in any manner.

Modes of Intravenous Administration

Injection
No

Intermittent Infusion
Yes
Using 50–100 ml of D5W or NS over 30 min. Do not use an in-line filter.

Continuous Infusion
No

Contraindications; Warnings; Precautions; Adverse Reactions

Contraindications
1. Active pancreatitis or history of pancreatitis.
2. Known hypersensitivity or history of previous episode of anaphylaxis.

Warnings
1. Hospitalization of the patient is recommended. Anaphylaxis and sudden death have occurred during administration of this drug.
2. Preparations should be made to treat anaphylaxis with each dose of asparaginase. Allergic reactions are not completely predictable from the intradermal skin test (see Adverse Reactions below).
3. Once a patient has been treated with this agent, future retreatment is associated with an increased risk of hypersensitivity. Patients who have shown to be hypersensitive through the

skin test or patients who have received a previous course of therapy should be desensitized prior to retreatment, and then only if the benefit outweighs the risk.
4. This drug may cause liver impairment and may increase preexisting liver impairment caused by previous therapy or underlying hepatic disease. This may contribute to the toxicity of other agents by interfering with their detoxification in the liver.
5. Administration of asparaginase concurrently with or immediately before vincristine or prednisone may be associated with increased toxicity.
6. Benefits of therapy should be weighed against the potential risk to the fetus when this drug is given during pregnancy. Breast-feeding should be stopped before treatment is initiated.
7. Toxicity is reported to be greater in adults than in children.

Precautions
1. There may be a fall in circulating lymphoblasts and a reduction in leukocyte count within the first few days of therapy. This can be accompanied by a marked rise in serum uric acid. This can lead to uric acid neuropathy. Preventive measures, i.e. allopurinol, increased fluid intake, and alkalinization of urine, should be carried out.
2. As a guide to therapy, the patient's peripheral blood count and bone marrow should be monitored frequently for leukemic abnormalities.
3. Frequent serum amylase levels should be obtained to detect the onset of pancreatitis. If it occurs, therapy with this drug should be stopped and not reinstituted.
4. Hyperglycemia may occur; monitor serum glucose.
5. This agent has been shown to have immunosuppressive properties in animals. It may possibly predispose humans to infection.
6. This drug may interfere with the actions of methotrexate, which requires malignant cell replication to work.

Adverse Reactions
1. Allergic reactions: rashes, urticaria, arthralgia, respiratory distress, anaphylaxis; these may occur even after a negative skin test.
2. Fatal hyperthermia.
3. Pancreatitis, during or following therapy.
4. Hyperglycemia with glycosuria and polyuria, without elevated acetone; should be treated with discontinuation of the drug and use of fluids and insulin. This complication has been fatal.
5. Hypofibrinogenemia and depression of other clotting factors, especially factors V and VIII and variable reductions in VII and IX. There may also be a reduction in platelets.
6. Central nervous system: depression, somnolence, fatigue, coma, confusion, agitation, hallucinations, a Parkinson-like syndrome, headache.
7. Elevation of serum ammonia.
8. Chills and fever (part of an allergic reaction).
9. Nausea and vomiting, anorexia, abdominal cramps, weight loss.
10. Azotemia, usually prerenal, occurs frequently; acute renal shutdown and fatal insufficiency.
11. Proteinuria.
12. Liver function abnormalities: elevation in SGOT, SGPT, alkaline phosphatase, bilirubin, depression of serum albumin, cholesterol and plasma fibrinogen. These effects are reversed with discontinuation of the drug or sometimes during therapy.
13. Malabsorption syndrome.
14. Transient bone marrow depression.

Intradermal Skin Test Procedure
This test should be performed be-

asparaginase
(continued)
fore the initiation of therapy and again if more than one week passes between doses. Prepare the following solution: reconstitute the contents of a 10,000 I.U. vial with 5 ml of sterile water for injection (resultant solution concentration will be 2,000 I.U./ml). Withdraw 0.1 ml and inject it into another vial containing 9.9 ml of sterile water for injection (solution concentration will now be 20 I.U./ml). Use 0.1 ml of this final solution. Inject intradermally. Observe the site for 1 hour. A positive reaction will be the appearance of a wheal or erythema. Note that some patients may have a full systemic reaction to the skin test. A negative test does not guarantee that an allergic reaction will not take place with drug administration.

Desensitization
This procedure should be carried out prior to the first dose of drug in patients with a positive skin test or in any patient with an increased risk of hypersensitivity. Rapid desensitization can be attempted by administering progressively increasing amounts of drug over a few hours time. Equipment and drugs necessary to treat an acute allergic reaction should be readily available.

☐ **Nursing Implications**
1. Assist with skin testing and/or desensitization procedures. Be prepared to treat anaphylaxis at these times and prior to each dose. See Appendix.
   Notify the physician at the onset of a rash or any other minor allergic manifestation.
2. Carry out preventive measures in the management of an elevated serum uric acid:
   a. increased water intake as tolerated by the patient
   b. administration of allopurinol
   c. alkalinization of the urine
3. Monitor urine glucose once daily for elevations.
4. Monitor the patient's temperature every 4 hours on the day of administration; notify the physi-

cian of elevations. Severe hyperthermia has been reported.
5. Be aware of the patient's coagulation profile. If there is a significant depression of clotting elements, take precautions to prevent trauma and observe for bleeding (petechiae, melena, hematuria, etc.)
6. In the event of central nervous system reactions, notify the physician of the onset, reassure the patient and family of the origin and take measures to prevent patient injury, e.g. side rails and close attendance. Coma is not a rare occurrence.
7. Be prepared to manage nausea and vomiting. Keep accurate intake and output records to assist in maintaining hydration. Parenteral fluids may be necessary. Nausea and vomiting is usually mild.
8. Toxicity with this drug is common and requires dosage reduction or discontinuation depending on the severity and clinical situation. Blood glucose, BUN, creatinine, clotting factors and peripheral blood count must be monitored and the nurse should be aware of the patient's status in these areas.

atropine sulfate ■

Actions/Indications
Anticholinesterase that produces the following major effects:
1. Inhibits smooth muscle contractions (gastrointestinal and genitourinary tracts)
2. Decreases salivary, bronchial, gastric and sweat-gland secretions
3. Increases heart rate and improves A-V conduction
4. Dilates pupils and can increase intraocular pressure in glaucoma
   Indications:
1. To treat pylorospasm and other spastic conditions of the gastrointestinal tract

2. As a preanesthetic medication to decrease secretions and prevent vagal stimulation with its possible slowing effect on heart rate
3. To increase heart rate in A-V block and sinus and junctional bradyarrhythmias
4. To relieve symptoms associated with organophosphorus insecticide poisoning

Dosage
Adults:
Antispasmodic, preanesthetic—0.4–1.0 mg
Bradycardia, insecticide poisoning—0.5–2.0 mg
   (Do not exceed 2.5 mg in 1 hour; rebound bradycardia may occur.)
Children:
All indications:—0.01–0.03 mg/kg repeated as necessary.

Suggested doses are:

Weight	Dosage
7–16 lbs	0.1 mg
17–24 lbs	0.15 mg
24–40 lbs	0.2 mg
40–65 lbs	0.3 mg
65–90 lbs	0.4 mg
> 90 lbs	0.4–0.6 mg

Preparation and Storage
AVAILABLE IN SEVERAL FORMS; BE CERTAIN OF STRENGTH BEING USED:
- Single-dose ampuls containing 0.5 mg/ml, 0.4 mg/ml and 0.4 mg/0.5 ml
- Single-dose vials containing 0.4 mg/ml, 1.0 mg/ml and 1.2 mg/ml
- 20 ml multi-dose vials containing 0.4 mg/ml and
- Prefilled syringes containing 0.5 mg and 1.0 mg of drug.

Drug Incompatibilities
Can be combined with most analgesics in a syringe just prior to injection.
   Do *not* mix in any manner with: sodium bicarbonate, methohexital, metaraminol, isoproterenol, norepinephrine bitartrate (Levophed), nor with any: bromides, iodides, or alkalies

Modes of IV Administration
Injection
Yes
No dilution required. Inject over 1–2 min.

Intermittent Infusion
No
Pharmacologically inappropriate.

Continuous Infusion
No
Pharmacologically inappropriate.

Contraindications; Warnings; Precautions; Adverse Reactions

Contraindications
1. Glaucoma (angle-closure and open-angle types)
2. In the presence of adhesions between the lens and iris of the eye
3. Bronchial asthma
4. Pyloric stenosis

Precautions
1. Use with caution in patients with prostatic hypertrophy; may cause urinary retention.
2. Use with caution when an excessive increase in heart rate may precipitate cardiac decompensation; e.g., congestive heart failure, acute myocardial infarction.
3. May increase intraocular pressure in patients susceptible to angle closure glaucoma or with chronic open-angle glaucoma.
4. May produce premature ventricular contractions or ventricular tachycardia, especially in patients with preexisting cardiac problems.
5. This drug may increase the size of an ischemic area of the heart in patients with acute myocardial infarction. Use only in the presence of severe and symptomatic bradycardia (heart rate less than 50/min) in such patients.

atropine sulfate
(continued)

6. Safety for use in pregnancy has not been established. Use only when clearly needed. Use with caution in nursing mothers.

Adverse Reactions
Toxic effects from even minimal overdosage are not uncommon, especially in children. These effects are dose-related as follows:

Dosage	Effect
0.5 mg	Dryness of nose and mouth
1.0 mg	Marked dryness of nose and mouth, thirst, acceleration of heart rate, dilation of pupils
2.0 mg	Extreme dryness of nose and mouth; tachycardia with palpitation; dilation of pupils; blurring of near vision; flushed, dry skin; rebound bradycardia
5.0 mg (within 1 hour)	Above symptoms, plus: difficulty speaking and swallowing; headache; hot, dry skin; restlessness
10.0 mg (within 1 hour)	Above symptoms, plus: excitement; disorientation; hallucinations; coma
65 mg (within 1–2 hours)	May be fatal due to apena.

May produce fever in children due to decreased evaporation from the body surface (even in therapeutic doses).

May produce hallucinations and disorientation in the elderly at therapeutic doses.

In atropine overdosage, administer respiratory support, physostigmine salicylate IV, ECG monitoring and symptomatic treatment until drug can be excreted.

☐ **Nursing Implications**
1. Monitor all patients for urinary retention, especially those with known prostatic hypertrophy or urethral strictures, and elderly males. Palpate bladder size every 4 hours. Monitor urinary output. Small voidings or sudden cessation of output may indicate retention.

2. Maintain continuous ECG monitoring on all patients receiving this drug for heart block or bradycardia. Observe for: increase in heart rate greater than 110 in adults or rates higher than normal in children, premature ventricular contractions, and ventricular tachycardia. Notify physician immediately if these occur. Be prepared to treat premature ventricular contractions and ventricular tachycardia by keeping lidocaine at the bedside. (Follow ICU policy for nurse's administration of this drug.) A defibrillator must be readily available.

3. If sinus tachycardia occurs, monitor for cardiac decompensation (pulmonary edema). Signs: increasing respiratory rate, orthopnea, dyspnea, elevated (engorged) external jugular veins, rales and wheezing, cyanosis, or pallor (elevated or decreased blood pressure). These signs may appear suddenly. Notify physician. Be prepared to treat: elevate the body from the waist up if possible. Administer oxygen 2–5 L/min, prepare rotating tourniquets, prepare traditional drugs (potent diuretics such as furosemide or ethacrynate, morphine, aminophylline). Provide emotional support; do not leave the patient alone.

4. Monitor for signs of an acute increase in intraocular pressure: increase in tear production, decreasing vision, severe eye pain, patient seeing rainbows around light, nausea, vomiting.[1] Notify physician at the first sign. (Doses of atropine greater than 1.0 mg may cause blurred vision in the absence of glaucoma.)

5. Be prepared to protect elderly patients from injury if hallucina-

tions and disorientation occur. Use side rails and light restraints as necessary. These changes may last for 24 hours after the last dose. Provide reassurance and close observation.
6. Maintain hydration to prevent drying of bronchial secretions that could lead to respiratory complications. Alert patients that dryness of the mouth is an expected effect. When indicated, treat dry mouth with fluids and mouth care in patients receiving this drug for indications other than preanesthesia.
7. In the comatose patient, prevent corneal damage due to dryness (decrease in tear production) by using methylcellulose eyedrops or saline and eye dressings as indicated. Corneal damage is evidenced by scleral redness and edema.
8. In patients receiving large doses, be prepared to give respiratory support. Keep the following equipment readily available: airways, suction, oxygen, endotracheal tubes and laryngoscope, manual breathing bag and mask.

Reference
1. Newell, Frank W., and Ernest, J. Terry: *Ophthalmology—Principles and Concepts* (3rd ed.), St. Louis, C. V. Mosby Company, 1974, p. 337.

Suggested Readings
Scarpa, William J.: The Sick Sinus Syndrome, *American Heart Journal,* 92(5):648–660, November 1976 (complete review article on sick sinus syndrome and the use of atropine in its early management).
Stuckey, John G.: Atropine in Bradycardia in the Coronary-Care Unit and Elsewhere. *Heart and Lung,* 2(5):666–668, September–October 1973.
DeMaria, Anthony N., et al.: Atropine: Current Concepts of its Use in Acute Myocardial Infarction. *Heart and Lung,* 3(1):135–137, January–February 1974 (references).

azathioprine sodium salt ■
(Imuran)

Actions/Indications
Immunosuppressant and antimetabolite. Used to prevent organ rejection after transplantation by depressing the antibody producing response of the lymphoid tissue occurring after the new organ has been placed in the body.

Dosage
Adults and Children:
Initial—3–5 mg/kg/day
  Maintenance—(Usually oral)—1–2 mg/kg/day in 1 or 2 doses, with periodic adjustments to prevent rejection without drug toxicity (bone marrow depression).

Preparation and Storage
Supplied in a vial containing 100 mg of drug powder.
  To prepare: Add 10-ml of sterile water for injection to azathioprine vial. Swirl gently until mixed. Use solution within 24 hours, discard unused portions. Store unopened vials at room temperature away from light (in original box).

Drug Incompatibilities
Do not mix with any other medication in any manner.

Modes of IV Administration

Injection
Yes
Inject slowly over 5 min., diluted as described in "Preparation" column.

Intermittent Infusion
Yes
Use D5W or NS in any volume, infuse over 1 to 8 hours.

Continuous Infusion
No

Contraindications; Warnings; Precautions; Adverse Reactions

Contraindications
Hypersensitivity

azathioprine sodium salt
(continued)
Warnings
1. Can produce severe irreversible bone marrow depression. CBC, including platelet counts, should be done at least daily during the initial phase of therapy and when high doses are used. Since this drug may have a delayed action, it is important to decrease or temporarily discontinue it at the *first sign* of a large fall in the leukocyte count.
2. In the presence of severe, unremitting organ rejection, it may be better to allow rejection to occur and remove the organ rather than attempt to prevent rejection with very high doses of this drug that will produce toxicity.
3. Infection is a persistent hazard. In this event, appropriate antibacterial, antifungal and antiviral therapy should be initiated and the dose of azathioprine decreased.
4. There have been reports of patients developing lymphomas while receiving immunosuppressive drugs after kidney transplantation.
5. Persistent negative nitrogen balance has been observed when the patient is concomitantly receiving corticosteroids. If this occurs, reduce the dosage of azathioprine. (Signs: weight loss, increased BUN [azotemia], loss of muscle mass.)
6. This drug should probably be withheld if signs of toxic hepatitis or biliary stasis occur (elevated bilirubin, SGOT, jaundice).
7. This drug has potential teratogenic activity (can cause fetal abnormalities), and should be avoided in pregnancy whenever feasible.

Precautions
1. In the presence of a cadaveric kidney with tubular necrosis and delayed onset of function and in other patients with impaired renal function use reduced dosage of this drug.
2. Use reduced (1/3 to 1/4) dosage in patients concomitantly on allopurinol.

Adverse Reactions
1. Hepatic: hepatitis, jaundice, bilary stasis
2. Bone marrow depression: leukopenia, anemia, thrombocytopenia, bleeding.
3. Allergy: rashes, drug fever.
4. Skin: oral lesions and hair loss.
5. Gastrointestinal: nausea, vomiting, diarrhea (especially in higher doses), pancreatitis (rare).

☐ **Nursing Implications**
1. Be aware of the patient's white cell count during administration period; a fall in leukocytes is the first sign of bone marrow depression. If count falls below 2,000 place the patient in protective (reverse) isolation, hold the next dose and notify the physician.
2. Observe for bleeding from any site; prevent trauma that may lead to bleeding.
3. Monitor temperature at least every 4 hours to detect infection or drug fever. Also observe for drainage, swelling, soreness, redness, signs of local infections. Therapy must be initiated as soon as possible after the onset of these findings.
4. Avoid any unnecessary veinpunctures, catheterizations, nasotracheal suctioning and other instrumentation that can increase the chance of infection.
5. Monitor for jaundice of skin and sclera in fair-skinned patients and sclera in dark-skinned patients. Observe for darkening of urine.
6. Examine for oral lesions. Hydrogen peroxide-saline mouthwashes may be prescribed. Order a soft, bland diet and nonirritating oral fluids.
7. Reassure the patient, if hair loss

occurs, that the hair will grow back when the drug is discontinued.

8. Be prepared to manage nausea, vomiting and diarrhea. Antiemetics may be used prior to meals.
9. Monitor for early signs of rejection (renal transplantation): decreasing urinary output, fever, increasing proteinuria, increasing blood pressure, pain and tenderness near the organ.

Suggested Readings

Ihar, Sisir K., and Smith, Earl C.: Renal Transplantation. *Heart and Lung* 4(6):897–899, November–December 1975.

Topor, Michele A.: Kidney Transplantation (Especially in Pediatrics). *Nursing Clinics of North America,* 10(3):503–516, September 1975.

Harrington, Joan DeLong, and Brener, Etta Rae: *Patient Care in Renal Failure,* Saunders Monographs in Clinical Nursing—5, Philadelphia, W. B. Saunders Company, 1973, p. 199.

betamethasone sodium phosphate ■
(Celestone Phosphate)

Actions/Indications
A synthetic adrenocorticosteroid, glucocorticoid type used in the intravenous form for the short-term treatment of the following general groups of disorders:
- Endocrine disorders
- Rheumatic disorders
- Collagen diseases
- Dermatologic diseases
- Allergic states
- Ophthalmic diseases
- Gastrointestinal diseases
- Respiratory diseases
- Hematologic disorders
- Neoplastic disease
- Nephrotic syndrome to induce diuresis
- Tuberculous meningitis
- Trichinosis with neurologic or myocardial involvement

Dosage
Adults:
Initial dose may be up to 9 mg/day depending on the clinical situation; this should be maintained until a satisfactory response is seen. Then the lowest possible dose should be used. If there is a lack of response to this drug after a reasonable time, it should be discontinued.

Preparation and Storage
Supplied in 1 ml ampuls and multiple-dose vials of a 4.0 mg/ml solution. Store at room temperature. This drug is supplied in two parenteral forms; use *only* betamethasone sodium phosphate for injection for IV use.

Incompatibilities
Do not mix with any other medication in any manner.

Modes of Intravenous Administration

Injection
Yes
Inject slowly over at least 1 minute.

Intermittent Infusion
Yes
Use D5W or NS in any desired volume.

Continuous Infusion
Yes
Use D5W or NS in any desired volume.

Contraindications; Warnings; Precautions; Adverse Reactions

Contraindications
Systemic fungal infections.

Warnings
1. Increased dosage is usually indicated in the presence of unusual stress such as surgery.
2. This agent may mask some signs of infection, and may cause reduced resistance and inability to localize infection.
3. *Prolonged* use can cause posteri-

betamethasone sodium phosphate
(continued)

or subcapsular cataracts, glaucoma, and damage to the optic nerves, and may enhance the establishment of secondary ocular infections due to fungi or viruses.

4. There may be elevation of blood pressure, salt and water retention, and increased excretion of potassium. Dietary sodium restriction and potassium supplementation may be needed.

5. Do not vaccinate against smallpox or other illnesses during therapy.

6. Use in tuberculosis should be limited to cases with fulminating or disseminated disease, and then in conjunction with antitubercular drugs. Reactivation may occur in latent TB or in reactive patients.

7. Anaphylaxis has occurred.

8. Benefits should be weighed against risks when using this drug during pregnancy. Infants born to mothers who have received substantial doses of corticosteroids during pregnancy should be carefully observed for signs of hypoadrenal activity.

Precautions

1. Gradual reduction in dosage will minimize drug-induced secondary adrenocortical insufficiency when the drug is discontinued. After discontinuation the drug may need to be reinitiated during times of stress. At the same time, salt and/or a mineralocorticoid should also be administered.

2. There is an increase in the effects of corticosteroids in the presence of hypothyroidism and in cirrhosis. Dosage may need to be reduced accordingly.

3. Use this agent with caution in patients with ocular herpes simplex; corneal perforation can occur.

4. Changes in mental status can occur during therapy such as

euphoria, insomnia, mood swings, personality changes, depression, and psychoses. Existing mental instability may be aggravated.

5. Use aspirin with caution in the presence of this drug and hypoprothrombinemia.

6. Use with caution in the presence of:
   a. Ulcerative colitis if there is the possibility of perforation abscesses or other pyrogenic infection.
   b. Diverticulitis
   c. Fresh intestinal anastomoses
   d. Active or latent peptic ulcer
   e. Renal insufficiency
   f. Hypertension
   h. Osteoporosis
   e. Myasthenia gravis
   Steroid administration in the presence of these problems can cause other complications or exacerbation of the condition.

Adverse Reactions in Short-term Intravenous Therapy

1. Fluid and electrolyte: sodium retention, fluid retention, congestive heart failure in susceptible patients (secondary to fluid and sodium retention), potassium loss, hypokalemic alkalosis, elevated blood pressure.

2. Musculosketal: muscle weakness, possible loss of some muscle mass.

3. Gastrointestinal: peptic ulcer with the possibility of perforation, pancreatitis, abdominal distention, ulcerative esophagitis.

4. Dermatologic: impaired wound healing, increased fragility of skin, petechiae, increased sweating, suppression of reactivity to skin tests.

5. Endocrine: increased insulin or oral hypoglycemic agent requirements.

6. Ophthalmic: glaucoma (increased intraocular pressure).

7. Metabolic: negative nitrogen balance due to protein catabolism.

8. Neurologic: increased intracra-

nial pressure, changes in mental status, e.g. confusion, euphoria, exacerbation of psychoses.

☐ Nursing Implications

1. The patient receiving this drug may become less resistant to infection. Monitor for obvious signs of infection:
   a. fever
   b. sore throat
   c. cough
   d. swelling of any kind
   e. erythema
   f. purulent drainage from wounds or body openings.
2. The fluid and sodium retaining properties of this drug are less than those of cortisone or hydrocortisone, but can still occur, especially in high-dose therapy. Weigh the patient daily to detect fluid retention. Monitor blood pressure for an elevation secondary to sodium and fluid retention. A sodium restricted diet may be prescribed, and intravenous fluids should be low in sodium.
3. Monitor for signs and symptoms of congestive heart failure in susceptible patients (those with a past history of CHF, cardiac valvular lesions, cardiomyopathies or coronary artery disease):
   a. weight gain
   b. peripheral (ankles, legs, sacrum) edema
   c. shortness of breath, increasing resting respiratory rate, dyspnea or exertion
   d. rales
   e. jugular venous distention
   f. onset of third and/or fourth heart sounds.
   Notify the physician of any significant findings.
4. Monitor for signs and symptoms of hypokalemia:
   a. muscle cramps
   b. weakness
   c. arrhythmias (late complication)
   d. irritability
   The potassium depleting properties of this drug are less than,

for example, those of cortisone, hydrocortisone or prednisolone, but can still be significant. Serum potassium should be monitored every other day.

5. Anaphylaxis can occur; take precautions. See Appendix
6. Maintain patient safety with the onset of changes in mental status seen in high-dose therapy. Use side rails, restraints if necessary, and close observation. Reassure the patient and family of the origin of these problems. Attempt to keep the patient oriented. In susceptible patients, monitor for rising intracranial pressure (change in mental status, change in reflexes, rising systolic blood pressure, decreased heart rate, change in pupillary reactivity).
7. Administer anti-ulcer drug as ordered to help prevent peptic ulcer. Monitor for signs and symptoms of an ulcer and gastrointestinal bleeding:
   a. hematemesis
   b. melena, postive stool guaiac
   c. abdominal pain and distention
   d. fall in hematocrit
8. The patient's skin may become frail if therapy is somewhat prolonged. Prevent skin breakdown with careful handling, good hygiene, bed appliances to relieve pressure (foam pads, water mattresses, flotation devices, sheepskin). Inspect the skin daily for signs of problems (reddened areas, blanched areas, skin openings, soreness). Wound sutures may need to be left in place for a longer than usual time period to prevent wound separation.
9. Monitor urine glucose every other day in non-diabetics to detect glycosuria.
10. Monitor for signs and symptoms of glaucoma: scleral redness, eye pain, blurred vision, rainbow vision. Notify the physician at the onset.
11. Steroids are complicated agents that affect many body systems.

betamethasone sodium phosphate
(continued)
The practitioner is urged to do additional reading to become familiar with the adrenal system and steroid therapy.

bicarbonate, sodium ■

Actions/Indications
Alkalizing sodium salt. Dissociates in solution into sodium and bicarbonate radicals ($Na+$, HCO_3^-). The bicarbonate then combines with free hydrogen ions to form H_2CO_3 a weak acid. This reduces the number of free hydrogen ions and thus increases the serum pH.

Used to treat metabolic acidosis secondary to cardiac arrest, renal failure; as an adjunct in the management of salicylate intoxication in the absence of respiratory alkalosis, and in ketoacidosis.

Dosage
Adults:
Initially—1–5 mEq/kg. Subsequent doses must be guided by arterial blood gases. Alternatively, dosage may be determined by calculation of bicarbonate deficit:

$$mEq \text{ of } HCO_3^- = \text{body wt. in kg} \times 0.3 \times (25 - \text{pts. } HCO_3^-)$$

Cardiac arrest—50 mEq is given every 5–10 min, with the frequency guided by arterial blood gases.
Infants and Children:
0.9 mEq/kg diluted 1:1 in sterile water, guided by arterial blood gases. Children over 15 kg can receive the adult dose.

Preparation and Storage
Available in the following forms:
Ampuls and prefilled syringes—50 ml of an 8.4 % solution (50 mEg, 1 mEq/ml); 50 ml of a 7.5% solution (44.6 mEq)
Bottles—500 ml of a 5% solution (297.5 mEq, 0.6 mEq/ml); 500 ml of a 1.4% solution (83 mEq, 0.16 mEq/ml).
Store at room temperature.

Drug Incompatibilities
Do not mix with the following fluids:
Alcohol 5% in
Ringer's Injection, lactated.
Ionosol B with Invert Sugar 10%
Ionosol D with Invert Sugar 10% modified
Ionosol G with Invert Sugar 10%
Ringer's Injection
Ringer's Lactate
Sodium Lactate
Other medications: Because of the alkalinity of solutions produced by sodium bicarbonate, it is advisable not to add any other medication to a solution of sodium bicarbonate for infusion.

When injecting sodium bicarbonate into intravenous tubing containing any one of the following drugs, flush the line with a compatible solution prior to injecting the sodium bicarbonate, or inject directly into the vein or intravenous catheter:
Anileridine
Ascorbic acid
Any barbiturate
Calcium preparations
Codeine phosphate
Corticotropin
Dopamine
Epinephrine
Hydromorphone
Insulin, regular
Isoproterenol
Levarterenol
Levorphanol
Magnesium sulfate
Meperidine
Methicillin
Morphine
Penicillin G potassium
Pentazocine
Procaine
Promazine
Any tetracycline
Vancomycin
Vitamin B complex

Modes of IV Administration

Injection
Yes
Using a 7.5 or 8.4% solution, undiluted (except in children, see Dosage column), injection may be rapid. This is the preferable mode for the treatment of cardiac arrest.

Intermittent Infusion
Yes
This mode is for nonemergency situations. Titrate rate with arterial blood gases.

See Incompatibility section for fluids that cannot be used for sodium bicarbonate solutions or use 500-ml bottles of prepared 5% or 1.4% sodium bicarbonate. Use an infusion pump.

Continuous Infusion
Yes
This mode is for nonemergency situations. Titrate rate with arterial blood gases.

See Incompatibility section for fluids that cannot be used for sodium bicarbonate solutions, or use 500-ml bottles of prepared 5% or 1.4% sodium bicarbonate. Use an infusion pump.

Contraindications; Warnings; Precautions; Adverse Reactions

Contraindications
Arterial blood pH greater than 7.4

Precautions
1. Patients with congestive heart failure may need a diuretic following the administration of sodium bicarbonate to enhance the excretion of the sodium contained in this agent.
2. Dosage must always be guided by arterial blood gases, when possible. Administration should stop when the pulse returns in the management of a cardiac arrest. Further injections must be guided by arterial blood gases.[1]
3. During cardiac arrest, or any severe acidotic situation, effective ventilation must accompany sodium bicarbonate to remove carbon dioxide from the blood.[2]

Adverse Reactions
Metabolic alkalosis and hyperosmolarity, secondary to excessive unguided dosage.

☐ Nursing Implications
1. This drug is indicated when the arterial blood pH is 7.3 or less.

2. Monitor for signs of excessive sodium and water retention (especially in patients with congestive heart failure or renal impairments): increased weight; dyspnea, increased respiratory rate, orthopnea, rales; increasing resting heart rate; peripheral edema.
3. Be aware of arterial blood gas values during titration of this drug. Monitor for signs of metabolic alkalosis (blood pH greater than 7.45): decreased respiratory rate, muscle spasms, hyperactive reflexes, tetany, seizures, change in mental status.

References
1. Standards for Cardiopulmonary Resuscitation (CPR) and Emergency Cardiac Care (ECC). *JAMA*, 227: Supplement, February 18, 1974, p. 857.
2. Ibid., p. 858.

bleomycin sulfate ■
(Blenoxane)

Actions/Indications
Antineoplastic, antibiotic; impairs correct DNA formation in the cell. Indicated in the treatment of:
- Hodgkin's disease (in combination with other drugs)
- Non-Hodgkin's lymphomas (in combination)
- Squamous cell carcinomas
- Testicular carcinoma (in combination)
- Malignant pleural and peritoneal effusions

Improvement of Hodgkin's disease and testicular tumors is prompt and can be noted within 2 weeks of initiation of therapy. If no improvement is seen by this time, it is unlikely that it will occur. Squamous cell cancers respond more slowly, sometimes 3–4 weeks.

Dosage
Adults:
In squamous cell carcinoma, testicular carcinoma, Hodgkin's disease, and lym-

bleomycin sulfate
(continued)
phocytic and histocytic lymphoma[1] — 0.25
–0.50 units/kg (10–20 units/M²)
weekly or twice weekly until a total
dose of 400 units has been reached.
Response is usually seen within 2
weeks or as a total dosage of 200
units is reached.

In Hodgkin's disease, after the above
dosage following a 50% regression
of tumor size, begin a dose of 1
unit/day or 5 units/week.

For regional infusion—(intra-arterial) 30–60 units/day over 1–24 hrs
into affected areas.

Dosage should be modified in the
presence of renal or hepatic failure,
usually by 25% (see Precautions for
further qualifications for dosage).

Patients with lymphoma are more
susceptible to anaphylactic reactions
to this drug and should therefore receive a 2- to 5-unit test dose for the
first 2 doses. If no acute reaction occurs, a regular dosage schedule can
be initiated.
Children:
All indications — 10–15 units/M²/week.
Do not exceed a total cumulative dose of 400 units.

Preparation and Storage
Available in ampuls containing 15
units of drug. To reconstitute from
powder, add 5 ml (or more) of D5W
or NS. 5 ml of diluent will produce
a solution of 3 units/ml. Discard unused portion.

Reconstituted solution is stable
for 24 hours at room temperature in
NS, D5W or D5W containing heparin (100 or 1000 units/ml).

Drug Incompatibilities
Do not mix with any other medication in any manner.

Modes of IV Administration

Injection
Yes
No need to further dilute
reconstituted solution. Inject over a
10-min period.

Intermittent Infusion
Yes
Add reconstituted solution to 20 ml
D5W or NS for every 15 units of
drug administered. Infuse over 10
min.

Continuous Infusion
Yes
For intra-arterial perfusion of tumor
site.
Use D5W or NS and infuse over
12–24 hrs.

**Contraindications; Warnings; Pre-
cautions; Adverse Reactions**

Contraindications
Hypersensitivity

Warnings
1. Pulmonary toxicity occurs in approximately 10% of all patients
   treated. Patients at greatest risk
   are: those over 70 years of age,
   those receiving over 400 units
   total dose and those with impaired pulmonary function.
   Toxicity can occur at lower dosages when the drug is used in
   combination with other antineoplastic agents. Initial signs and
   symptoms include cough, dyspnea, rales, abnormal chest x-
   ray (bilateral infiltrates and fibrosis occurring up to 1 month
   after discontinuing drug) and altered pulmonary function tests.
   A chest x-ray is recommended
   every 1–2 weeks. If abnormal
   findings are noted, the drug
   should be discontinued until it
   can be established whether they
   are drug-related.
2. This agent can (rarely) cause renal impairment at any time during therapy, indicated by rising
   BUN and creatinine. Use with
   extreme caution, if at all, in patients with pre-existing renal
   impairment.
3. Hepatic toxicity has also been
   reported (rarely) and is indicated by deterioration in liver
   function tests. Use with extreme
   caution in the presence of hepatic failure.

4. Idiosyncratic reactions similar to anaphylaxis have been reported in 1% of lymphoma patients treated. These reactions usually occur with the first or second dose, immediately on injection or after several hours of injection. Some groups administer a skin test, or test dose prior to full dosage.
5. Safety for use in pregnancy has not been established.

Adverse Reactions
As with all antineoplastic agents, adverse reactions are frequent and numerous.
1. Pulmonary toxicity: pneumonitis, fibrosis
2. Skin changes: vesicles, hair loss, hyperpigmentation, hyperemia, hyperkeratosis, rashes, itching, mucous membrane ulceration
3. Renal impairment (rare)
4. Liver impairment (rare)
5. Febrile reactions (seen in 25% of all patients treated)
6. Anaphylaxis and anaphylaxis-like idiosyncratic reactions (more frequent in patients with lymphomas)
7. Minimal bone marrow supression
8. Nausea, vomiting and anorexia
9. Pain at tumor site (this can be considered a favorable sign of tumor destruction)
10. Raynaud's phenomenon (rare) in patients receiving vinblastine concurrently

☐ Nursing Implications
1. The patient receiving this medication will be experiencing the emotional and physical effects of the malignancy. Knowledge of the patient's feelings about his disease and its implications will assist in helping him tolerate the chemotherapy. The incidence of uncomfortable side effects and adverse reactions is high. It is within the nurse's role to assist the patient in coping with the discomforts of the disease and its treatment, and to help him work through depression and anger toward acceptance of the disease at his own pace. Despite the unpleasantness this drug may bring, it can be a source of hope for the patient.
2. Take anaphylaxis precautions, see Appendix.
3. Monitor for febrile reaction; fever usually begins 1 hour after injection and rises slowly over the next 2–4 hours. Take temperature every hour. Acetaminophen and/or cooling baths can be given for chills and fever. Inform the patient that this is not a hazardous complication.
4. Monitor for signs and symptoms of pulmonary toxicity:
   a. First symptoms are usually dyspnea, mild chest pain, and tachypnea.
   b. First signs are x-ray changes (see under Warnings), bilateral basilar rales. Notify the physician of onset of any one of these signs or symptoms.
5. Monitor urinary output every 8 hours. Notify physician with the onset of oliguria (less than 240 ml of urine in 8 hours for an adult). Weigh the patient daily to detect onset of fluid retention. Be aware of the patient's BUN prior to each dose.
6. Management of hair loss:
   a. Use scalp tourniquet during injection, if ordered, to help prevent hair loss. This technique may be ineffective in preventing hair loss because of the prolonged presence of this drug in the blood.
   b. Counsel the patient on the possibility of hair loss to enable him to prepare for this disfigurement.
   c. Reassure him of regrowth of hair following discontinuation of the drug.
   d. Provide privacy and time for the patient to discuss his feelings.
7. Reassure the patient that pain in the tumor site may occur. This can be considered as a fa-

bleomycin sulfate
(continued)
vorable sign of drug effectiveness.

8. Management of nausea and vomiting (usually minimal):
   a. Administer antiemetics when appropriate to prevent nausea following injections and/or before meals.
   b. Small frequent meals, timed with periods when the patient feels his best, are advisable. Bland foods may be more easily tolerated. Carbohydrate and protein content should be high.
   c. If the patient is anorexic, encourage high nutrient liquids and water to maintain nutrition and hydration.
   d. Keep accurate measurements of emesis volume and total intake and output to guide the physician in ordering parenteral fluids when necessary.

References

1. Shinn, Arthur F., et al.: Dosage Modifications of Cancer Chemotherapeutic Agents in Renal Failure. *Drug Intelligence and Clinical Pharmacy,* 11:141, 1977.
2. Silver, Richard, Lauper, R. David, and Jawroski, Charles I.: *A Synopsis of Cancer Chemotherapy,* The York Medical Group, Dun-Donnelley Publishing Corporation, 1977, p. 75.

Suggested Readings

Bolin, Rose Homan, and Auld, Margaret E.: Hodgkin's Disease. *American Journal of Nursing,* 74:1982–1986, November 1974.

Bruya, Margaret Auld, and Madeira, Nancy Powell: Stomatitis After Chemotherapy, *American Journal of Nursing,* 75:1349–1352, August 1975.

Foley, Genevieve and McCarthy, Ann Marie: The Disease (Hodgkin's) and Its Treatment. *American Journal of Nursing,* 76:1109–1114, July 1976, (references).

Giadquinta, Barbara: Helping Families Face the Crisis of Cancer. *American Journal of Nursing,* 77:1583–1586, October 1977.

Gullo, Shirley: Chemotherapy—What To Do About Special Side Effects. *RN,* 40:30–32, April 1977.

Hannan, Jeanne Ferguson: Talking is Treatment, Too. *American Journal of Nursing* 74:1991–1992, November 1974.

LeBlanc, Dona Harris: People With Hodgkin Disease: The Nursing Challenge. *Nursing Clinics of North America,* 13(2):281–300, June 1978.

McMullen, Kathleen: When the Patient is on Bleomycin Therapy. *American Journal of Nursing,* 75:964–966, June 1975.

Vietti, Teresa J., and Valeriote, Frederick: Conceptual Basis for the Use of Chemotherapeutic Agents and Their Pharmacology. *Pediatric Clinics of North America,* 23:67–92, February 1976.

Showfety, Mary Patricia: The Ordeal of Hodgkin's Disease. *American Journal of Nursing,* 74:1987–1991, November 1974.

Sovik, Corinne: The Nursing Care of Lung Cancer Patients. *Nursing Clinics of North America,* 13(3):301–317, June 1978.

bretylium tosylate ■
(Bretylol)

Actions/Indications
Antiarrhythmic; causes depletion of, and inhibits norepinephrine release at the sympathetic postganglionic adrenergic neuron terminal. Ventricular fibrillation and other ventricular arrhythmias are suppressed. There is also a transient positive inotropic effect on the myocardium. Excretion is through the kidneys.

Used in the treatment of life-threatening ventricular arrhythmias that have failed to respond to lidocaine or procainamide. Onset of action is 20 minutes to 2 hours. (Sooner if given by IV injection; i.e.,

5 to 10 minutes.) Duration of action is 6 to 8 hours.

Dosage
Adults:
Life-Threatening Arrhythmias — 5 mg/kg by rapid, undiluted intravenous injection. With other standard treatment and support. If arrhythmia persists — 10 mg/kg repeated at 15 to 30 minute intervals. There has been no published experience with doses greater than 30 mg/kg.
Other Non-Life-Threatening Ventricular Arrhythmias — 5–10 mg/kg diluted in at least 50 ml NS by infusion over at least 8 minutes. Second dose in 1 to 2 hours if needed.
Maintenance — *Intermittent* infusion: 5–10 mg/kg over 8 minutes every 6 hours or, by *continuous* infusion of 1–2 mg per minute.
Reduce dosage in 3 to 5 days under ECG monitoring.
Children:
No recommendations available.

Preparation and Storage
Supplied in 10 ml ampuls of 500 mg (50mg/ml).

Drug Incompatibilities
Do not mix with any other medication in any manner.

Modes of Intravenous Administration

Injection
Yes
This mode for life-threatening arrhythmias only, inject rapidly, undiluted.

Intermittent Infusion
Yes
In at least 50 ml. D5W or NS, infuse over at least 8 minutes for maintenance therapy.

Continuous Infusion
Yes
Dilute to a concentration of 0.5–1.0 mg/ml, infuse at a rate of 1–2 mg/min. Use an infusion pump. Use this mode for maintenance therapy.

Contraindications; Warnings; Precautions; Adverse Reactions

Contraindications
None currently known.

Warnings
1. This agent usually produces postural hypotension. Some hypotension may also occur while the patient is supine. If hypotension is symptomatic, a dopamine or norepinephrine infusion may be used. The pressor effects of these drugs are enhanced by bretylium. Volume expansion or correction of dehydration must also be carried out.
2. Some patients may have transient hypertension or increased frequency of ventricular arrhythmias.
3. The initial release of norepinephrine caused by this agent may aggravate digitalis toxicity. Use only in life-threatening arrhythmias where the etiology does not appear to be digitalis toxicity, and other anti-arrhythmics have not been effective. Simultaneous initiation of therapy with digitalis and bretylium should be avoided.
4. Avoid use in patients with fixed cardiac output (severe aortic stenosis or pulmonary hypertension). Severe hypotension may occur secondary to a fall in peripheral vascular resistance without compensatory increase in cardiac output. If survival depends on this drug, administer vasoconstrictive catecholamines (dopamine, norepinephrine) if hypotension occurs.
5. Safety for use in pregnancy has not been established; however, in life-threatening situations the benefits to the mother may outweigh the potential risk to the fetus.
6. Use in children has been limited. Guidelines for dosage and use are unavailable.

bretylium tosylate
(continued)
Precautions.
1. Rapid intravenous infusion can cause nausea and vomiting; follow administration guidelines carefully.
2. Dosage should be reduced in the presence of renal impairment. Further guidelines are unavailable.

Adverse Reactions
1. Hypotension, postural and supine.
2. Nausea and vomiting (usually avoidable with correct infusion rates).
3. Bradycardia, increased frequency of PVC's, transient hypertension, precipitation of anginal attacks, sensation of substernal pressure.

☐ **Nursing Implications**
1. Continuous electrocardiographic monitoring must be maintained to observe for drug effectiveness. A transient rise in frequency of PVC's may be an initial effect of the drug.
2. Monitor peripheral blood pressure to detect hypo- or hypertension; both can occur. Be prepared to administer vasopressors for symptomatic hypotension and/or fall in cardiac output (see Warning No. 4).
3. Avoid precipitating nausea and vomiting by maintaining recommended infusion rates. Be prepared to manage these effects if they occur, to prevent aspiration.
4. Instruct the patient to report the onset of anginal pain or substernal pressure if he is able. Notify physician if these occur.

butorphanol tartrate ■
(Stadol)

Actions/Indications
Synthetic opiate, narcotic agonist/antagonist analgesic. Duration of action is 3 to 4 hours; level of analgesia equivalent to morphine in the recommended doses. Onset of action is 1 to 2 minutes after intravenous injection. Recommended for the relief of moderate to severe pain, as a supplement to anesthesia, and during labor and delivery. This agent is metabolized in the liver.

Dosage
Adults:
1 mg, every 3 to 4 hours (range: 0.5 to 2 mg).
Children:
No recommendation for children under 18 years of age.

Preparation and Storage
Supplied in 2 mg/ml, 2 ml vials; 1 mg/ml, 2 ml vials; 2 mg/ml, 1 ml vials and disposable syringes, and 2 mg/ml, 10 ml multi-dose vials.
  Store at room temperature.

Drug Incompatibilities
Do not mix with any other drug in any manner.

Modes of Intravenous Administration

Injection
Yes
Slowly, without further dilution.

Intermittent Infusion
No

Continuous Infusion
No

Contraindications; Warnings; Precautions; Adverse Reactions

Contraindications
Hypersensitivity.

Warnings
1. Because of its narcotic-antagonist properties, this drug is not recommended for known narcotic addicts; detoxification should be done prior to use.
2. Use with caution in patients vulnerable to addiction (e.g., history of drug abuse). Even though this drug has a low physical de-

pendence liability, close supervision of long-term use is advisable.
3. This drug may elevate cerebrospinal fluid pressure and obscure signs and symptoms of increased pressure. Use with caution, if at all, in patients with head injuries.
4. Use in patients with acute myocardial infarction, ventricular dysfunction, or coronary insufficiency should be limited to those patients allergic to morphine or meperidine because this agent can increase myocardial work by increasing pulmonary vascular resistance, and increasing systemic arterial pressure.

Precautions
1. This agent, in recommended doses, causes some respiratory depression that is equal to that of 10 mg of morphine. Increasing the dosage, however, does not increase respiratory depression as is seen in morphine. Administer with caution in reduced dosage in patients with respiratory depression, limited respiratory reserve, bronchial asthma, obstructive conditions, or cyanosis.
2. Liver impairment may predispose the patient to greater side effects and greater activity from usual dosage; administer with caution in reduced dosage.
3. Safety for use in patients about to undergo surgery of the biliary tract has not been established. This drug may cause spasm of the sphincter of Oddi.
4. Slight increases in systolic blood pressure may occur; use with caution in patients with a history of hypertension.
5. Safety for use in pregnancy *prior* to labor has not been established. This drug has been found to be safe for use during labor and delivery for the mother and infant. Use with caution in the delivery of *premature* in-

fants. Do not use for nursing mothers; it is not known whether or not this drug is excreted in milk.
6. Safety for use in children younger than 18 years has not been established.

Adverse Reactions
1. Sedation, lethargy
2. Nausea, diaphoresis, vomiting
3. Headache
4. Floating feeling, dizziness
5. Agitation, euphoria, confusion
6. Autonomic changes—flushing, dry mouth, sensitivity to cold
7. Cardiovascular—palpitations, increase or decrease in blood pressure
8. Slowing of respiration, shallow breathing
9. Rashes, urticaria
10. Diplopia or blurred vision

Management of Overdosage
Overdosage will produce some degree of respiratory depression, and probably fall in blood pressure and sedation. Intravenous *naloxone* will reverse the depressant effects. Supportive therapy must be maintained; e.g., oxygen, assisted breathing, vasopressors, etc., until effects have resolved. See page 237 for information on naloxone.

☐ **Nursing Implications**
1. Monitor respiratory status frequently during the first hour; e.g., rate and depth. If rate is less than 8 breaths/minute urge the patient to increase his rate. If he is unable, begin manual breathing (or mouth-to-mouth) at a rate of 12–16/minute. Administer oxygen. Do not leave the patient alone. Administer naloxone as ordered. Remain with the patient supporting respirations until naloxone has reversed depressant effects.
2. Monitor blood pressure every 15 minutes during the first hour. Report extreme deviations to the physician.
3. Monitor for rise in cerebrospinal fluid pressure in patients

butorphanol tartrate
(continued)

with head injuries. Do not depend on level of consciousness in the evaluation since this agent will alter mental status. Use pupil reaction, reflexes and grip strength.

4. Because of the sedation, visual changes, and confusion produced by this drug, provide for patient safety; e.g., use side rails, bedrest, etc. Report confusion or hallucinations to the physician; it may not be advisable to use this drug again in this patient.
5. Keep naloxone readily available.

calcium chloride ■

Actions/Indications
Electrolyte, the most potent provider of calcium ions. Calcium is necessary for the proper functioning of cell membranes, nerves, muscles, blood clotting, myocardial conductivity and excitability, maintenance of the skeletal and vascular muscle tone.

Used in the treatment of hypocalcemia when prompt increase in serum calcium is needed:
• Neonatal tetany
• Parathyroid deficiency
• Vitamin D deficiency
• Magnesium sulfate overdose
• Sensitivity reactions with urticaria and hypocalcemia
• Hypocalcemia in acute renal failure
• Electromechanical dissociation of the heart (as a positive inotropic agent)
• Maintenance therapy in parenteral nutrition
• Treatment of hyperkalemia.

Dosage
Adults:
For indications other than cardiac arrest
—6.8–13.6 mEq (5–10 ml of a 10% or 1.36 mEq/ml solution). Additional doses must be guided by serum calcium levels.
In cardiac arrest—2.7–5.4 mEq (2–

4 ml of a 1.36 mEq/ml or 10% solution). May also be administered via intracardiac injection.
Children:
Indications other than cardiac arrest—
4 mEq/kg/24 hrs. Use a 2% solution (see Preparation column).
Dosage must be guided by serum calcium levels.
In cardiac arrest—IV: 1 ml of a 10% solution/kg (maximum); Intracardiac—1 ml of a 10% solution diluted 1:1 in NS.[1]

Preparation and Storage
Store at room temperature. Discard unused portions of vials.

Supplied in ampuls of 10 ml, 1.36 mEq/ml (10% solution) and prefilled syringes.

To make a 2% solution, add 1 ml of the 10% calcium chloride solution to 4 ml of a suitable diluent (see Infusion sections).

Drug Incompatibilities
Do not mix with:
Amphotericin
Cephalosporins
Chlorpheniramine
Epinephrine
Sodium and potassium phosphate
Sodium bicarbonate
Streptomycin
Tetracyclines
Tobramycin

Modes of IV Administration

Injection
Yes
This mode is appropriate for emergency situations.

In cardiac arrest: total dose can be administered within 15–30 seconds.

All other situations: Do not exceed a rate of injection greater than 0.7–1.5 mEq/min (approximately 0.5–1.0 ml of a 10% solution).

Intermittent Infusion
Yes
Add dose to D5W, NS, D5/NS, RL in any volume.

Infusion rate should not exceed 0.7–1.5 mEq/min.

Continuous Infusion
Yes

Add dose to D5W, NS, D5/NS.
Infusion rate should not exceed
0.7–1.5 mEq/min.

Contraindications; Warnings; Precautions; Adverse Reactions

Contraindications
1. Hypercalcemia
2. Metastatic bone disease when there is a possibility of hypercalcemia
3. Ventricular fibrillation

Precautions
1. Avoid extravasation. Do not use a scalp vein when giving this drug to children.
2. Administer with caution, if at all, to patients concomitantly receiving digitalis. Myocardial tetany and/or arrhythmias may result.
3. Monitor serum calcium at frequent intervals to guide dosage.
4. Rapid administration can cause tingling sensations in the extremities and cardiac arrhythmias, hypotension, bradycardia and other arrhythmias, syncope and cardiac arrest. Follow injection and infusion rates carefully.
5. Administration of calcium to patients with high serum phosphate levels has resulted in the precipitation of dibasic calcium phosphate in vital organs, lungs, kidneys, arterial walls, thyroid gland. Death can result. Monitor serum phosphate levels during calcium therapy.
6. If bradycardia occurs during an injection or infusion, discontinue administration.
7. Administer with caution to patients with sarcoidosis.
8. Because this agent is acidifying, also administer with caution to patients with cor pulmonale, respiratory failure (acidosis) or renal disease.

Adverse Reactions
1. Venous irritation at injection site
2. Tingling sensation in face and extremities

3. Sense of oppression or waves of heat over the body
4. Chalky taste

☐ Nursing Implications
1. The normal serum calcium is 8.5–10.5 mg/100 ml (higher in children).
2. Signs and symptoms of hypocalcemia:
   a. Neuromuscular excitability, muscle twitching, convulsions
   b. Numbness and tingling of extremities
   c. Emotional lability
   d. Carpopedal spasm (muscle spasms of hands, wrists, feet and ankles). Trousseau's sign—carpopedal spasms of the hands (inability to open the hand) following inflation of blood pressure cuff to a pressure to occlude circulation for at least 3 minutes
   e. Chvostek's sign—facial muscle twitch following tap over the facial nerve just in front of the ear
   f. In infants and small children, hypotonia and abdominal distention may be seen. As the severity of hypocalcemia increases, laryngeal stridor and tetany may appear.
3. Monitor for signs of hypercalcemia secondary to overdosage of calcium chloride (these signs will appear as the serum calcium reaches 12 mg %):[3, 4]
   a. Changes in mental status secondary to central nervous system depression, e.g., lethargy, confusion, sluggish peripheral nerve reflexes, muscular weakness
   b. Decreased Q-T interval and bradycardia on ECG
   c. Anorexia, constipation, nausea, and vomiting
   d. Rise in BUN, polyuria
4. Patients who are digitalized must be observed continuously on an ECG monitor for the onset of arrhythmias such as premature atrial or ventricular

calcium chloride
(continued)

contractions, sinus bradycardia or ventricular tachycardia. Be prepared to treat such arrhythmias. Atropine and lidocaine should be readily available.

5. In the presence of hypocalcemic tetany, protect the patient from injury through the use of padded side rails. Keep the room quiet and reduce stimulation to a minimum until therapy is effective. Monitor the patient frequently for signs of laryngeal spasm and resultant airway obstruction (this rarely occurs).

6. If this preparation is being administered during cardiopulmonary resuscitation, remind the physician if the patient has been digitalized; he may decide to withhold the drug, use another agent, or use the calcium in a lower dosage.

7. Take precautions to prevent extravasation; see Appendix. Do not administer via a scalp vein in children.

8. Use an infusion pump to maintain an accurate flow rate.

9. Follow incompatibility guidelines carefully.

References

1. Standards for Cardiopulmonary Resuscitation (CPR) and Emergency Cardiac Care. *JAMA*, 227(7):859, February 18, 1974.
2. Guyton, Arthur C.: *Textbook of Medical Physiology*, (5th ed.), Philadelphia: W. B. Saunders Company, 1976, p. 1056.
3. Ibid., p. 1056.
4. Beeson, Paul, and McDermott, Walsh (editors): *Cecil-Loeb Textbook of Medicine*, (14th ed.), Philadelphia: W. B. Saunders Company, 1975, p. 1810.

calcium gluconate and calcium gluceptate ■
(Calcium Glucoheptonate)

Actions/Indications
Electrolyte, provider of calcium ions. Calcium is necessary for proper functioning of nerves, muscles, blood clotting, myocardial conductivity, maintenance of the skeletal, and vascular muscle tone. Used in the treatment of hypocalcemia when prompt increase in serum calcium is needed:

• Neonatal tetany
• Parathyroid deficiency
• Vitamin D deficiency
• Magnesium sulfate overdose
• Sensitivity reactions with urticaria and hypocalcemia
• Hypocalcemia in acute renal failure
• Electromechanical dissociation of the heart (as a positive inotropic agent); calcium *chloride* is usually the preferred preparation, but gluconate can be used.
• Treatment of hyperkalemia
• Maintenance therapy in parenteral nutrition

Dosage
Adults:
Cardiac arrest—10 ml of a 10% solution (4.8 mEq), repeated as necessary. Administer via IV injection or intracardiac injection.

For indications other than cardiac arrest—Initial dose, 10 ml of a 10% solution (4.6 mEq or 97 mg). Additional doses must be guided by serum calcium levels.

Children:
Cardiac arrest—1 ml of a 10% solution/kg, maximum dose; intracardiac: 1 ml of a 10% solution diluted in an equal volume of NS.[1]

For indications other than cardiac arrest—5–10 ml of a 10% solution (500 mg/kg/24 hrs, or 12 g/M²/24 hrs).

Dosage must be guided by serum calcium levels for all indications.

Preparation and Storage
Supplied in 5-ml and 10-ml ampuls, usually of a 10% solution, 0.9 mEq/ml.

Discard unused portions of vials. Store at room temperature.

Drug Incompatibilities
Do not mix in any manner with:
Amphotericin-B

Cephalothin
Cephazolin
Cephradine
Clindamycin
Epinephrine
Fat emulsion
Folic acid
Magnesium sulfate
Novobiocin
Oxytetracycline
Prednisolone
Prochlorperazine
Sodium bicarbonate
Sodium or potassium phosphate
Tetracycline
Tobramycin

Special mixing procedures must be followed when adding calcium to amino acid solutions where other salts will also be added. Consult hyperalimentation solution literature.

Modes of IV Administration

Injection
Yes
This mode is appropriate for emergency situations. In cardiac arrest: total dose can be administered within 15–30 seconds.

In all other situations: do *NOT* exceed a rate of injection greater than 0.5–1.0 ml/min (of a 10% solution) or 0.7–1.5 mEq/min.

Intermittent Infusion
Yes
Add dose to D5W, NS, D5/NS, RL.

Infusion should be set at a rate no greater than 0.7–1.5 mEq/min., in any convenient volume of fluid.

Continuous Infusion
Yes
Add dose to D5W, NS, D5/NS, RL or hyperalimentation fluid.

Contraindications; Warnings; Precautions; Adverse Reactions

Contraindications
1. Hypercalcemia
2. Metastatic bone disease

Precautions
1. Avoid extravasation; do not use a scalp vein when giving this drug to children.

2. Administer with extreme caution to patients concomitantly receiving digitalis. Myocardial tetany and/or arrhythmias may result.
3. Monitor serum calcium levels at frequent intervals to guide dosage.
4. Rapid administration can cause tingling sensations in the extremities and cardiac arrhythmias. Follow infusion rate suggestions.
5. Administration of calcium to patients with high serum phosphate levels has resulted in the precipitation of dibasic calcium phosphate in vital organs. This can produce soft tissue calcification, and possibly nephrotoxicity. Monitor serum phosphate levels during calcium therapy.
6. If bradycardia occurs during an injection or infusion, discontinue administration.

☐ Nursing Implications
1. The normal serum calcium is 8.5–10.5 mg/100 ml. Calcium therapy must be guided by frequent serum calcium determinations.
2. Signs and symptoms of hypocalcemia:[2]
   a. Neuromuscular excitability, muscle twitching, convulsions
   b. Numbness and tingling of extremities
   c. Emotional lability
   d. Carpopedal spasm (muscle spasms of hands, wrists, feet and ankles). Trousseau's sign—carpopedal spasms of the hands (inability to open the hand) following inflation of blood pressure cuff to a pressure sufficient to occlude circulation for at least 3 minutes
   e. Chvostek's sign—facial muscle twitch following tap over the facial nerve just in front of the ear
   f. In infants and small children, hypotonia and abdominal distention may be seen

calcium gluconate and calcium gluceptate
(continued)

As the severity of hypocalcemia increases, laryngeal stridor and tetany may appear.

3. Monitor for signs of hypercalcemia secondary to overdosage of calcium solutions (these signs will appear as the serum calcium reaches 12 mg %):[3]
   a. Changes in mental status secondary to central nervous system depression, e.g., lethargy, confusion, sluggish peripheral nerve reflexes, muscular weakness
   b. Decreased Q-T interval and bradycardia on ECG
   c. Anorexia, constipation, nausea and vomiting
   d. Rise in BUN, polyuria
4. Patients who are digitalized must be observed continuously on an ECG monitor for the onset of arrhythmias such as premature atrial or ventricular contractions, sinus bradycardia or ventricular tachycardia. Be prepared to treat such arrhythmias.
5. In the presence of tetany, protect the patient from injury through the use of padded side rails. Keep in a quiet room, reduce stimulation to a minimum until therapy with calcium infusion is effective. Monitor the patient frequently for signs of laryngospasm (stridor, increased respiratory effort, cyanosis). Keep a tracheostomy tray available for emergency use in the event of severe laryngospasm and resultant airway obstruction (this is rare).
6. During cardiac resuscitation, inform the physician if the patient has been digitalized.
7. Take precautions to prevent extravasation; see Appendix. Do not infuse via a scalp vein in children.
8. Use an infusion pump for infusion to prevent overdosage and ensure adequate dosage.
9. Make special note of incompatibilities.

References
1. Standards for Cardiopulmonary Resuscitation (CPR) and Emergency Cardiac Care. *JAMA*, 227(7):859, February 18, 1974.
2. Guyton, Arthur C.: *A Textbook of Medical Physiology* (5th ed.), Philadelphia: W. B. Saunders Company, 1976, p. 1056.
3. Ibid.

carbenicillin disodium ■
(Geopen, Pyopen)

Actions/Indications
Antibiotic, semisynthetic penicillin. Effective against several gram-positive and gram-negative organisms; particularly effective in treating urinary tract infections due to susceptible strains of *Pseudomonas*, *Proteus* species and *E. coli.*

Other indications include:
1. Severe systemic infections and septicemia due to *H. influenzae* and *S. pneumoniae.*
2. Genitourinary infections including those due to *Neisseria gonorrhoeae*, *Enterobacter* and *Strept. faecalis.*
3. Acute and chronic respiratory infections.
4. Soft-tissue infections.
5. Infections due to susceptible anaerobic bacteria including septicemia and infections of the lower respiratory tract, abdominal cavity, skin and soft tissues and female pelvis.

This drug is usually used in combination with an aminoglycoside antibiotic.

Dosage
Adults:
Range—200–500 mg/kg/day in 4–6 divided doses or continuous infusion. Maximum recommended dose is 40 gm/day.
Dosage in Renal Failure—See Table Below.

Children:
Initial—100 mg/kg followed by 50–500 mg/kg/24 hrs divided into 4–6 doses or continuous infusion.
*Neonates:**
Initial—100 mg/kg followed by 75 mg/kg every 8 hrs for 7 days for infants under 2000 gm; or 75 mg/kg every 6 hrs for 3 days for infants over 2000 gm; for all infants, subsequent doses after above regimen are 100 mg/kg every 6 hrs.

Adults with Renal Impairment[1,2]

Creatinine Clearance (ml/min)	Dosage	Intervals
80–50	Same as for normal adults	q 4 hrs
50–10	2–4 gm	q 6 hrs
10	2 gm	q 12 hrs
Combined renal and hepatic failure	2 gm	q 24 hrs
With hemo-dialysis	2 gm	After each dialysis
With peritoneal dialysis	2 gm	q 6–12 hrs [3]

*NEONATES: The mode of administration ordered may depend on the organism being treated. More detailed dosage recommendations in relation to site of injection and organism are available from manufacturers (Geopen, Roerig, Pyopen, Beecham Labs).

Preparation and Storage
Available in 1-, 2- and 5-gram vials and in 2-, 5- and 10-gram piggyback units.
Reconstitute with sterile water for injection *only*. SEE TABLES BELOW
Refrigerate reconstituted solution. Discard after 72 hours. (When stored at room temperature, discard after 24 hours.)

Piggyback Vials

Vial Size (gm)	Vol. Diluent (ml)	Vol. of 1-gm Dose
2	100	50 ml
	50	25 ml
	20	10 ml
5	100	20 ml
	50	10 ml
10	95	10 ml

Regular Vials

Vial Size (gm)	Vol. Diluent (ml)	Vol. of 1-gm Dose
1	2.0	2.5 ml
	2.5	3.0 ml
	3.6	4.0 ml
2	4.0	2.5 ml
	5.0	3.0 ml
	6.6	4.0 ml
5	9.5	2.5 ml
	12.0	3.0 ml
	17.0	4.0 ml

Drug Incompatibilities
Do not mix in IV bottle with any other antibiotic or vitamins.
Do not mix in IV tubing with:
Sodium bicarbonate
Aminophylline
Sodium iodide
Levarterenol
Isoproterenol

Modes of IV Administration

Injection
Yes
Further dilute the reconstituted solution with sterile water for injection, 20 ml/gm of drug.
Inject at a rate no greater than 200–500 mg/min.

Intermittent Infusion
Yes
Use any IV fluid. Dilute to 1 gm/20 ml (100 mg/ml for children).
Infuse over 30–60 min.

carbenicillin disodium
(continued)

Continuous Infusion
Yes
Use any IV fluid. Add 6-, 12- or 24-hour dose to 500–1000 ml depending on fluid needs of patient. This drug is stable in solution for 24 hours.

Contraindications; Warnings; Precautions; Adverse Reactions

Contraindications
Hypersensitivity to penicillin.

Warnings
1. Serious or fatal anaphylactic reactions have been reported. Inquire about previous allergy to penicillin, cephalosporins and other allergens.
2. Blood-clotting abnormalities have been reported in uremic patients on high doses of carbenicillin. Hemorrhagic manifestations disappeared on withdrawal of the drug.
3. Safety for use in pregnancy has not been established.

Precautions
1. Avoid intra-arterial injection and extravasation.
2. Monitor hepatic, renal and hematopoietic (blood cell production) systems, particularly during prolonged therapy.
3. This drug contains 5.3–6.5 mEq (122–150 mg) of sodium per gram. Monitor cardiac status when indicated.
4. Emergence of organisms resistent to this antibiotic, such as *Klebsiella* species and *Serratia* species can cause a superinfection.
5. Monitor serum potassium; hypokalemia has been reported.

Adverse Reactions
1. Allergic reactions: rash, urticaria, drug fever, anaphylaxis
2. Thrombophlebitis at injection site
3. Nausea and unpleasant taste (especially with high doses)
4. Blood dyscrasias: leukopenia, neutropenia, thrombocytopenia, hemolytic anemia
5. Elevation in SGOT and SGPT
6. Convulsions or neuromuscular excitability in patients with impaired renal function and excessively high serum levels.

☐ **Nursing Implications**
1. Take precautions to prevent extravasation; see Appendix.
2. Take anaphylaxis precautions, see Appendix.
3. Monitor for signs of bleeding, especially in patients with impaired renal function: melena or blood in stools (daily guaiacs are advisable), hematuria, nose bleeding, gum bleeding, ecchymosis with no history of trauma, vaginal bleeding (excessive menstrual flow).
4. Monitor patients with active cardiac disease, history of cardiac disease, renal dysfunction or for fluid retention by daily weights. Check for peripheral edema at least daily. Place the patient on intake and output and record at least every 8 hours, depending on the patient's general condition.
5. Monitor cardiac patients for signs of cardiac decompensation, i.e., congestive heart failure, in addition to those activities listed in No. 4 above: increasing heart rate; increasing respiratory rate, dyspnea on exertion, orthopnea, rales; engorgement of external jugular veins.
6. Take seizure precautions in patients with renal impairment.
7. Patients on high-dose infusions may have nausea and vomiting; if so, administer antiemetics as ordered, prior to meals. Instruct the patient as to the origin of the bad taste if it occurs.
8. Monitor for signs of hypokalemia: unusual weakness, increasing lethargy, irritability, abdominal distention, poor

feeding in infants, muscle cramps.
9. Monitor for signs and symptoms of overgrowth infections:
   a. Fever (take rectal temperature at least every 4–6 hours in all patients)
   b. Increasing malaise
   c. Newly appearing localized signs and symptoms — redness, soreness, pain, swelling, drainage (increased volume or change in character of pre-existing drainage)
   d. Monilial rash in perineal area (reddened areas with itching)
   e. Cough (change in pre-existing cough or sputum production)
   f. Diarrhea

References
1. Gardner, Pierce, and Provine, Harriet: *Manual of Acute Bacterial Infections*, Boston: Little, Brown and Company, 1975, p. 241.
2. Kagen, Benjamin M., *Antimicrobial Therapy*, (2nd ed.), Philadelphia: W. B. Saunders Company, 1974, p. 433.
3. Hoffman, Thomas A., et al. Pharmacodynamics of Carbenicillin in Hepatic and Renal Failure. *Annals of Internal Medicine*, 73:173, August, 1970.

Suggested Reading
Rodman, Morton J.: Antimicrobial Drugs for Septicemia, *RN*, May 1976, pp. 67–80.

carmustine ▪
(BCNU, Bis-Chlorethyl Nitrosourea, BiCNU)

Actions/Indications
Antineoplastic agent, with alkylation and protein modification actions. Used in the palliative treatment of:
- Brain tumors (glioma, astrocytoma, metastatic brain tumors and others)
- Multiple myeloma
- Hodgkin's disease
- Non-Hodgkin's lymphomas

It may be used alone or in combination therapy with other chemotherapeutic agents.

Dosage
Adults and Children:
100 mg/M^2 for 2 days or 200 mg/M^2 as a single dose every 6–8 weeks. Alternative schedule: 40 mg/M^2 daily for 5 consecutive days repeated at 6- to 8-week intervals. Subsequent doses must be adjusted according to bone marrow function.

A repeat course of this drug should not be given until circulating blood elements have returned to acceptable levels.

Subsequent doses should be adjusted according to the hematologic response to the preceding dose.

See chart below:

Manufacturer's Suggested Adjustment of Subsequent Doses

Lowest Cell Count After Prior Dose		Percentage of Prior Dose to be Given
WBC's	Platelets	
> 4000	100,000	100%
3000–3999	75,000–99,999	100%
2000–2999	25,000–74,999	70%
< 2000	< 25,000	50%

Preparation and Storage
Supplied as a powder in vials containing 100 mg.

Powder must be kept at 2–8°C until ready to use. If it is exposed to a temperature above 27°C or 80°F, it will liquify, and should be discarded.

To reconstitute add 3 ml of accompanying diluent, then 27 ml of sterile water for injection. Concentration of the solution is 3.3 mg/ml.

After reconstitution, it is stable for 2–4 hrs. Discard unused portions. Avoid contact with skin; it causes brown staining.

If this drug is added to 500 ml D5W or NS, the solution can be

carmustine
(continued)
stored in the refrigerator for 48 hours without losing stability.

Drug Incompatibilities
Do not mix with other medications in any manner.

Modes of IV Administration

Injection
No

Intermittent Infusion
Yes
Add dose to 100–500 ml D5W or NS. Infuse over 60–120 min.
   Use an infusion pump to prevent rapid infusion.

Continuous Infusion
No

Contraindications; Warnings; Precautions; Adverse Reactions

Contraindications
1. Hypersensitivity
2. Bone marrow depression producing decreased platelets, leukocytes, or erythrocytes

Warnings
Safety for use during pregnancy has not been established.

Precautions
1. Complete blood counts should be obtained frequently for at least 6 weeks following a course of therapy.
2. Do not repeat doses more frequently than every 6 weeks.
3. Bone marrow toxicity is cumulative. Dosage must be adjusted based on lowest blood count after previous dose.
4. Monitor liver function tests throughout therapy.

Adverse Reactions
1. Bone marrow depression: occurs 4–6 weeks after administration and is dose-related. The lowest level in the platelet count may occur 4–5 weeks after a single dose; the leukocyte count in 5–6 weeks. Anemia also occurs but is less severe than the thrombocytopenia (decreased platelets) or leukopenia (decreased WBC's).
2. Nausea and vomiting: occur within 2 hours of infusion and may last for 4–6 hours. This may be prevented or diminished with antiemetics.
3. Hepatotoxicity: usually reversible, manifested by elevated SGOT, alkaline phosphatase and bilirubin.
4. Burning at infusion site.
5. Rapid infusion may produce intense flushing of the skin and hyperemia of the conjunctiva within 2 hours and may last for about 4 hours.

☐ Nursing Implications
1. The patient receiving this medication will be experiencing the emotional and physical effects of the malignancy. Knowledge of the patient's feelings about his disease and its implications will assist in helping him tolerate the chemotherapy. The incidence of uncomfortable side effects and adverse reactions is high. It is within the nurse's role to assist the patient in coping with the discomforts of the disease and its treatment, and to help him work through depression and anger toward acceptance of the disease at his own pace. Despite the unpleasantness this drug may bring, it can be a source of hope for the patient.
2. Management of hematologic effects:
   a. Be aware of the patient's white blood cell and platelet counts prior to each injection.
   b. See Adverse Reaction No. 1; anticipate when blood counts will reach the lowest points.
   c. If the WBC falls to 2000/cu mm, take measures to protect the patient from infec-

tion, such as protective (reverse) isolation, avoidance of invasive procedures, maintenance of bodily (especially perineal) cleanliness, carrying out strict urinary catheter care when appropriate, etc. Monitor for infection by recording temperatures every 4 hours, examining for rashes, swelling, drainage, and pain. Explain these measures to the patient.

d. If the platelet count falls below 100,000/cu mm, monitor for thrombocytopenic bleeding: petechiae, purpura, hematuria, melena, blood in stools, gum bleeding, vaginal bleeding, epistaxis, hematemesis, etc. Avoid trauma. Transfusions may be ordered.

e. Instruct the patient and family on the importance of follow-up blood studies if this drug is being administered on an outpatient basis.

3. Management of gastrointestinal effects:

a. Administer antiemetics with each injection; the nausea and vomiting which occur usually 2–6 hours after the injection can be prevented. Repeat antiemetic in 4–6 hours to cover the duration of the nausea produced by the carmustine (4–6 hours).

b. If nausea and vomiting are not completely relieved by the antiemetics, attempt to maintain nutrient intake. Small, frequent meals, timed with periods when the patient feels his best, are advisable. Bland foods may be more easily tolerated. Carbohydrate and protein content should be high.

c. If the patient is anorexic, encourage high nutrient liquids and water to maintain hydration.

d. Keep accurate measurements of emesis volume and total intake and output to guide the physician in ordering parenteral fluids when necessary.

4. Maintain recommended infusion rate with an infusion pump. See Adverse Reaction No. 5.

5. Warn the patient that there may be local vein discomfort during the infusion.

Suggested Readings

Gullo, Shirley: Chemotherapy— What To Do About Special Side Effects, *RN*, 40:30–32, April, 1977.

Giaquinta, Barbara: Helping Families Face the Crisis of Cancer, *American Journal of Nursing*, 77:1583–1588, October, 1977.

Foley, Genevieve, and McCarthy, Ann Marie: The Disease (Hodgkin's) and Its Treatment. *American Journal of Nursing*, 76:1109–1114 (references).

Bolin, Rose Homan, and Auld, Margaret E.: Hodgkin's Disease. *American Journal of Nursing*, 74:1982–1986, November 1974.

Hannan, Jeanne Ferguson: Talking is Treatment Too. *American Journal of Nursing*, 74:1991–1992, November 1974.

Showfety, Mary Patricia: The Ordeal of Hodgkin's Disease. *American Journal of Nursing*, 74:1987–1991, November 1974.

LeBlanc, Dona Harris: People With Hodgkin Disease: The Nursing Challenge, *Nursing Clinics of North America*, 13(2):281–300, June, 1978.

Morrow, Mary: Nursing Management of the Adolescent: The Effect of Cancer Chemotherapy on Psychosocial Development, *Nursing Clinics of North America*, 13(2):319–335, June, 1978.

cefamandole nafate ∎
(Mandol)

Actions/Indications
Antibiotic, cephalosporin group, broad spectrum.

cefamandole nafate
(continued)

Active against a wide range of gram-positive and gram-negative organisms including many anaerobes.

Indicated in the treatment of the following serious infections caused by susceptible strains of the designated organisms:

- Lower respiratory: *S. pneumoniae, H. influenzae, Klebsiella* sp, *Staph. aureus*, beta-hemolytic streptococci, *P. mirabilis.*
- Urinary tract: *E. coli, Proteus* sp, *Enterobacter* sp, *Klebsiella* sp, group D streptococci and *S. epidermis.*
- Peritonitis: *E. coli, Enterobacter* sp.
- Septicemia: *E. coli, S. aureus, S. pneumoniae, S. pyogenes, H. influenzae, Klebsiella* sp.
- Skin and soft tissue: *S. aureus, S. pyogenes, H. influenzae, E. coli, Enterobacter* sp, *P. mirabilis.*
- Bone and joint: *S. aureus.*

Dosage
Adults:
500 mg–1 gm every 4 –8 hrs; (3–12 gm/day).

Septicemia—6–12 gm/day for several days then decrease according to clinical response.

Life-threatening infections or infections due to less susceptible organisms—Up to 2 gms every 4 hours.

Infants and Children:
50–100 mg/kg/24 hours; give in divided doses every 4–8 hours.

For Severe Infections—Increase to 150 mg/kg/24 hours. Do not exceed maximum adult dose.

Preparation and Storage
Supplied as powder in 10-ml-size vials containing 500 mg, 1 gm and 2 gm, and in 100-ml-size piggyback vials containing 1 gm and 2 gm.

To reconstitute, add 10 ml sterile water for injection, D5W or NS for each gm of drug. To reconstitute piggyback vials, add 100 ml of appropriate diluent. If sterile water for injection used, add 20 ml/gm to avoid a hypotonic solution.

If stored at room temperature, discard after 24 hours. If refrigerated, discard after 96 hours.

Renal Impairment (Adults)*

Renal Function	Creatinine (ml/min) Clearance	Max Dose, Life-threatening Infections	Less Severe Infections
Normal	> 80	2 gm q 4 hrs	1–2 gm q 6 hrs
Mild Impairment	80–50	1.5 gm q 4 hrs or 2 gm q 6 hrs	0.75–1.5 gm q 6 hrs
Moderate Impairment	50–25	1.5 gm q 6 hrs or 2.0 gm q 8 hrs	0.75–1.5 gm q 8 hrs
Severe Impairment	25–10	1 gm q 6 hrs or 1.25 gm q 8 hrs	0.5–1 gm q 8 hrs
Marked Impairment	10–2	0.67 gm q 8 hrs or 1 gm q 12 hrs	0.5–0.75 gm q 12 hrs
None	< 2	0.5 gm q 8 hrs or 0.75 gm q 12 hrs	0.25–0.5 gm q 12 hrs

*Courtesy of Eli Lilly and Co., Indianapolis, IN 46285

Drug Incompatibilities

Do not mix in any manner with an aminoglycoside or with: calcium gluceptate, calcium gluconate or any solutions containing magnesium ions.

Modes of Intravenous Administration

Injection
Yes
No further dilution needed. Inject over 3–5 min. directly into vein or into the tubing of a running IV when the solution is compatible with the drug (See Continuous Infusion).

Intermittent Infusion
Yes
Infuse piggyback vials as prepared over 15–30 min.

Continuous Infusion
Yes
Add dosage to any of the following fluids: NS, D5W, D10W, D5/NS, D5/0.45% saline, D5/0.2% saline, or sodium lactate 1/6 molar.

Contraindications; Warnings; Precautions; Adverse Reactions

Contraindications
Hypersensitivity to cefamandole or any cephalosporin antibiotic.

Warnings
1. Administer with caution to patients with an allergy to penicillin or any drug; there may be cross-allergenicity.
2. Safety for use in pregnancy has not been established.
3. Safety for use in prematures and infants under one month of age has not been established. Cephalosporin can accumulate, prolonging the half-life.

Precautions
1. Evaluation of renal status is recommended in seriously ill patients receiving maximum doses. This drug is excreted by the kidneys; a reduced dosage is required in renal impairment.

2. Hemodialysis removes some of the drug. Additional dosage is required after each dialysis to maintain adequate serum concentrations.[1]
3. Nephrotoxicity has been reported in patients receiving aminoglycoside antibiotics concomitantly.
4. Overgrowth of nonsusceptible organisms can occur with prolonged use.
5. False-positive urine glucose testing may occur with Clinitest tablets or Benedict's or Fehling's solution.
6. Hypoprothrombinemia, with or without bleeding, may rarely occur especially in elderly or debilitated patients. Administration of Vitamin K will promptly reverse this situation.
7. This drug contains 3.3 mEq (77 mg) of sodium per gram.

Adverse Reactions
1. Hypersensitivity: rash, urticaria, eosinophilia, drug fever.
2. Blood dyscrasias: thrombocytopenia, neutropenia, positive direct Coombs.
3. Liver: transient rise in SGOT, SGPT, alkaline phosphatase.
4. Kidney: decreased creatinine clearance; transient increase in BUN, especially in persons over age 50.
5. Local reactions: Thrombophlebitis.

☐ Nursing Implications
1. Take anaphylaxis precautions (see Appendix).
2. Monitor for signs and symptoms of overgrowth infections due to non-susceptible organisms:
   a. Fever (take rectal temperature at least every 4–6 hours in all patients).
   b. Increasing malaise.
   c. Newly appearing signs and symptoms of a localized infection: redness, soreness, pain, swelling, drainage (increasing volume or change in character of preexisting drainage).

cefamandole nafate
(continued)

d. Oral lesions (thrush) or perineal rash (monilia) due to *Candida albicans.*
e. Cough (change in preexisting cough and sputum production).
f. Diarrhea.

3. Use Tes-Tape or Keto-Diastix for urine glucose determinations.

4. Monitor renal function in patients with renal impairment, in seriously ill patients on high doses, and in those receiving aminoglycosides (gentamicin, amikacin, tobramycin) concurrently.

a. Record intake and output every 4–8 hours, depending on the patient's condition; report onset or changes in oliguria defined as: urine output less than 240 ml in 8 hours for adults.
b. Urinalysis as indicated, usually every other day.
c. Be aware of the patient's BUN and creatinine.

5. Take precautions to reduce risk of thrombophlebitis:

a. Use small cannula in large vein.
b. Rotate insertion site every 48–72 hours.
c. Examine intravenous insertion site daily for thrombophlebitis (pain, swelling, warmth, and redness along involved vein).
d. Remove the intravenous cannula if this occurs and notify physician. Apply warm compresses, elevate the extremity and avoid trauma to the area.
e. Avoid further venipunctures on that extremity until the inflammation resolves.

Reference

1. Fraser, Donald G., Drug Therapy Reviews: Antimicrobial Spectrum, Pharmacology and Therapeutic Use of Cefamandole and Cefoxitin.

American Journal of Hospital Pharmacy, 36:1503–1508, November 1979, p. 1506.

cefazolin sodium ■
(Ancef, Kefzol)

Actions/Indications
Antibiotic, cephalosporin group, broad spectrum.

Active against *Staph aureus* (penicillin-sensitive and penicillin-resistant); Group A beta-hemolytic streptococcus, *S. pneumoniae, E. coli, Proteus mirabilis, Klebsiella* species, *Enterobacter, H. influenzae* and others.

Indicated in the treatment of the following serious infections due to susceptible strains of the designated organisms:

• Respiratory tract—*S. pneumoniae, Klebsiella* sp., *H. influenzae, S. aureus* and group A beta-hemolytic streptococci.
• Genitourinary tract—*E. coli, P. mirabilis, Klebsiella* sp., and some *Enterobacter.*
• Skin and soft tissue—*S. aureus,* and group A beta-hemolytic and other streptococci.
• Biliary tract—*E. coli,* some streptococci, *P. mirabilis, Klebsiella* sp. and *S. aureus.*
• Bone and joint—*S. aureus.*
• Septicemia—*S. pneumoniae, S. aureus, P. mirabilis, E. coli,* and *Klebsiella* sp.
• Endocarditis—*S. aureus* and group A beta-hemolytic streptococci.

Also indicated for perioperative prophylaxis in patients with a high risk of postoperative infections (open-heart surgery, prosthetic arthroplasty).

Dosage
Adults:
Mild gram-positive infections—250–500 mg every 8 hrs (750–1500 mg/24 hrs).
Moderate to severe infections—500–1000 mg every 6–8 hrs (1.5–4 gm/24 hrs).
Life-threatening infections—up to 6–12 gm/24 hrs.

All doses may be given by divided doses or continuous infusions.

Perioperative prophylaxis—
a. 1 gm, 1/2 to 1 hr. before surgery
b. For procedures longer than 2 hrs, give another 0.5–1.0 gm during procedure, then
c. 0.5–1 gm every 6–8 hrs. for 24 hrs. postoperatively. (For open-heart surgery or prosthetic arthroplasty give for 3–5 days postsurgery.)

In the presence of renal impairment— see table below.

Children:
Mild to moderate infections— 25–50 mg/kg/24 hrs divided into 3–4 equal doses.

Severe infections— up to 100 mg/kg/24 hrs in 3–4 equal doses.

Manufacturer does not recommend use of this drug in infants under 1 month of age.

See manufacturer's literature for dosage in renal impairment.

Adult Dosage in the Presence of Renal Impairment[1]

Creatinine Clearance (ml/min)	Dosage Frequency
20–50	Loading dose: 500 mg followed by 250 mg every 6 hours or 500 mg every 12 hours.
10–20	Loading dose: 500 mg followed by 250 mg every 12 hours or 500 mg every 24 hours.
less than 10	Loading dose: 500 mg followed by 250 mg every 24–36 hours or 500 mg every 48–72 hours.
On Hemodialysis	500 mg after each treatment.

Preparation and Storage
Available in vials containing 250 mg, 500 mg, and 1 gm of drug.

Reconstitute from powder with sterile water for injection as follows:

Vial Size		Diluent to Be Added
250	mg	2 ml
500	mg	2 ml
1	gm	2.5 ml

Refrigerate reconstituted solution; discard after 96 hrs.

Drug Incompatibilities
Do not mix in any manner with the following drugs:
Amikacin
Barbiturates
Calcium preparations
Chlortetracycline
Erythromycin
Kanamycin
Oxytetracycline
Polymyxin B
Tetracycline

Modes of IV Administration

Injection
Yes
Further dilute 500 mg or 1 gm of reconstituted drug with minimum of 10 ml of sterile water for injection.
Inject over 3–5 min.
Injection may be into the tubing of a running IV containing any fluid listed under the Continuous Infusion section.

Intermittent Infusion
Yes
Dilute reconstituted form in 100 ml of NS or D5W for every gram of the drug. Infuse over 15–30 min.

Continuous Infusion
Yes
Add 8-, 12- or 24-hr dosage to 500–1000 ml of fluid depending on the patient's fluid needs. Solution will be stable for 24 hrs.
Use any of the following fluids:
NS
D5W
D10W
D5/RL
D5/NS
D5/0.45% or 0.2% saline

cefazolin sodium
(continued)
5% or 10% Invert Sugar
Normosol-M in D5W.
Ringer's Lactate
Ringer's Injection
Ionosol B with 5% Dextrose
Plasma-Lyte with 5% Dextrose

Contraindications; Warnings; Precautions; Adverse Reactions

Contraindications
Hypersensitivity to any cephalosporin.

Warnings
1. Administer with caution to patients with an allergy to penicillin; there may be cross-allergenicity.
2. Safety for use in pregnancy has not been established.
3. Safety for use in infants under 1 month of age or in premature infants has not been established, and use is not recommended by the manufacturer.

Precautions
1. Overgrowth of nonsusceptible organisms can occur with prolonged use.
2. False-positive urine glucose testing may result with the use of Benedict's or Fehling's solution, or with Clinitest tablets.
3. This drug contains 2 mEq (46 mg.) of sodium per gram.
4. Patients with impaired renal function require a lower dosage.

Adverse Reactions
1. Allergic reactions: rash, urticaria, drug fever, anaphylaxis, vulvar pruritus
2. Blood dyscrasias: neutropenia, leukopenia, thrombocytopenia, positive direct and indirect Coombs' tests
3. Renal and hepatic changes: transient rise in SGOT, SGPT, BUN, and alkaline phosphatase levels have been seen without evidence of organ damage

4. Gastrointestinal: anorexia, nausea, vomiting, diarrhea, oral candidiasis (oral thrush infection)
5. Thrombophlebitis at injection site
6. Vaginitis, anogenital pruritus, genital monilial infections

☐ Nursing Implications
1. Take anaphylaxis precautions; see Appendix.
2. Monitor for signs and symptoms of overgrowth infections due to nonsusceptible organisms:
   a. Fever (take rectal temperature at least every 4–6 hours in all patients)
   b. Increasing malaise
   c. Newly appearing signs and symptoms of a localized infection: redness, soreness, pain, swelling, drainage (increased volume, or change in character of pre-existing drainage)
   d. Oral lesions (thrush) or perineal rash (monilia) of *Candida albicans*
   e. Cough (change in character or volume of pre-existing sputum)
   f. Diarrhea
3. Use Tes-Tape or Keto-Diastix for urine glucose determinations.
4. Monitor for signs and symptoms of cardiac decompensation in patients with congestive heart failure because of the sodium content of this drug:
   a. Weight gain—weigh these patients daily; report a gain over pretreatment values to the physician
   b. Increase in resting heart rate —take pulse every 4 hours
   c. Increasing respiratory rate, dyspnea, orthopnea, rales
   d. Peripheral edema

References
1. Leroy, Annie, et al.: Pharmacokinetics of Cefazolin, a New Cephalosporin Antibiotic, in Normal and Uremic Patients.

Current Therapeutic Research, 16(9):887, September 1974.

cefotaxime sodium ▪
(Claforan)

Actions/Indications
Antibiotic, cephalosporin, broad spectrum. Effective against a wide range of gram-positive and gram-negative organisms including some anaerobic species.

Indicated in the treatment of the following serious infections caused by susceptible strains of the designated organisms:
- Lower respiratory tract: *Strept. pneumoniae, S. pyogenes* and other streptococci, *Staph. aureus, E. coli, Klebsiella* species, *H. influenzae* and *Enterobacter* species.
- Urinary tract: *E. coli, Klebsiella* species, *Enterobacter* species, *P. mirabilis,* and other Proteus and *Staph. epidermis.*
- Gynecological: *E. coli,* streptococci, *Peptostreptococcus* species.
- Bacteremia/Septicemia: *E. coli, Klebsiella* species.
- Skin and soft tissue: *Staph. aureus, Strept. pyogenes* and other streptococci, *E. coli, P. mirabilis* and indole-positive Proteus.

Dosage
Adults:
Uncomplicated Infections—2 gms/24 hours (1 gm every 12 hrs).
Moderate to Severe Infections—3–6 gms/24 hours (1–2 gms every 6–8 hours).
Septicemia—6–8 gm/24 hours (2 gm every 6–8 hrs).
Life-threatening Infections—Up to 12 gm/24 hours (2 gm every 4 hours). Do not exceed 12 gm/24 hours.
Renal Impairment—It is recommended that 1/2 usual dosage be given to patients with creatinine clearance of less than 20 ml/min.
Children:
Not recommended.

Preparation and Storage
Supplied as a powder in vials containing 500 mg, 1 gm and 2 gm of drug and in infusion bottles containing 1 gm and 2 gm of drug.

To reconstitute all strengths in vials, add at least 10 ml sterile water for injection. For infusion bottles, add 50 or 100 ml sterile water for injection, NS or D5W.

Shake to dissolve. Check for particulate matter and discoloration before use. Solutions range from light yellow to amber. After reconstitution, if stored at room temperature, discard after 24 hours; if refrigerated, discard after 10 days.

If further diluted for continuous infusion, discard after 24 hours at room temperature, or 5 days under refrigeration.

Drug Incompatibilities
Do not mix in any manner with sodium bicarbonate or any diluent having a pH above 7.5 or with any aminoglycoside antibiotic.

Modes of Intravenous Administration

Injection
Yes
No further dilution needed. Inject slowly over 3–5 minutes.

Intermittent Infusion
Yes
Dilute reconstituted solution in 50–100 ml compatible fluid. (See Continuous Infusion.) Infusion bottles may be administered as prepared. Infuse over 15–30 minutes.

Continuous Infusion
Yes
Add dose to 500–1000 ml of the following fluids:
NS
D5W, D10W
D5/NS
D5/0.45% saline
D5/0.2% saline
RL
Sodium Lactate, 1/6 molar
10% Invert sugar
Freamine II Injection

cefotaxime sodium
(continued)

Contraindications; Warnings; Precautions; Adverse Reactions

Contraindications
Hypersensitivity to cefotaxime sodium or any cephalosporin.

Warnings
1. Administer with caution to patients with known allergy to penicillin or any drug; there may be cross-allergenicity.
2. Studies have not shown harm to animal fetuses but data regarding safety in human pregnancy is incomplete. Use in pregnancy only if clearly needed.
3. This drug is excreted in breast milk; use with caution in nursing mothers.
4. Safety and efficacy in infants and children have not been established.

Precautions
1. This drug has not been shown to be nephrotoxic but high serum concentrations can occur in patients with renal insufficiency. A reduced dosage is required in these patients.
2. Overgrowth of nonsusceptible organisms can occur with prolonged use.
3. Increased nephrotoxicity has been reported in patients receiving cephalosporins and aminoglycosides concurrently.
4. This drug contains 2.2 mEq (50.5 mg) sodium per gram.

Adverse Reactions
1. Local: inflammation at injection site.
2. Hypersensitivity: rash, pruritus, fever.
3. Gastrointestinal: colitis, diarrhea, nausea and vomiting.
4. Blood: granulocytopenia, eosinophilia, neutropenia, positive direct Coombs' test.
5. Genitourinary: moniliasis, vaginitis.
6. CNS: headache.
7. Hepatic/Renal: transient elevations in SGOT, SGPT, LDH, alkaline phosphatase and BUN.

☐ Nursing Implications
1. Take anaphylaxis precautions. (See Appendix.)
2. Monitor for signs and symptoms of overgrowth infections due to nonsusceptible organisms:
   a. Fever (take rectal temperature at least every 4–6 hours in all patients).
   b. Increasing malaise.
   c. Newly appearing signs and symptoms of localized infections, redness, soreness, pain, swelling, drainage (increased volume or change in character of preexisting drainage).
   d. Oral lesions (thrush) or perineal rash (monilia) due to *Candida albicans.*
   e. Cough (change in preexisting cough and sputum production).
   f. Diarrhea.
3. Monitor renal function in patients with renal impairment and in those receiving aminoglycoside antibiotics (gentamicin, amikacin, tobramycin) concomitantly.
   a. Record intake and output every 4–8 hours, depending on the patient's condition. Report onset or changes in oliguria defined as: Adults—urinary output less than 240 ml in 8 hours.
   b. Urinalysis as indicated, usually every other day.
   c. Be aware of the patient's BUN and creatinine.
4. Take precautions to reduce risk of irritation at injection site:
   a. Use scalp vein needle, or small cannula in large vein.
   b. Rotate insertion site every 48–72 hours.
   c. If inflammation noted, remove intravenous cannula and notify physician.

cefoxitin sodium ■
(Mefoxin)

Actions/Indications
Antibiotic, cephamycin type, broad spectrum. Active against a wide range of gram-positive and gram-negative organisms including many anaerobes.

Indicated in the treatment of the following serious infections caused by susceptible strains of the designated organisms:
- Lower respiratory tract: *S. pneumoniae*, other streptococci, *Staph. aureus, E. coli, Klebsiella* species, *H. influenzae*, and *Bacteroides* species.
- Genitourinary tract: *E. coli, Klebsiella* species, *P. mirabilis*, other Proteus, *Providentia* species, and *N. gonorrhoeae*.
- Intra-abdominal: *E. coli, Klebsiella* species, *Bacteroides fragilis* and *Clostridium* species.
- Gynecological: *E. coli, N. gonorrhoeae, Bacteroides* species, *Clostridium* species, Group B streptococci and others.
- Septicemia: *S. pneumoniae, Staph. aureus, E. coli, Klebsiella* species, and *Bacteroides* species.
- Bone and Joint: *Staph. aureus.*
- Skin and soft tissue: *Staph. aureus, Staph. epidermidis*, some streptococci, *E. coli, P. mirabilis, Klebsiella* species, *Bacteroides* species, *Clostridium* species and others.

Culture and sensitivity studies should be done to determine the susceptibility of the causative organism to cefoxitin.

Also indicated for prophylaxis in patients undergoing surgical procedures which are contaminated or potentially contaminated (e.g., gastrointestinal surgery, vaginal hysterectomy, cesarean section, prosthetic arthroplasty).

Dosage
Adults:
Infection—3–12 gm/24 hours (1 gm–3 gm every 6–8 hours). Specific dosage determined by severity of infection and susceptibility of causative organisms.

Prophylaxis—2 gms 1-1/2 hours before surgery, then 2 gms every 6 hours for 24 hours (72 hours for prosthetic arthroplasty).

Cesarean Section—2 gms as soon as umbilical cord is clamped; repeated 4 hours and 8 hours after first dose; then every 6 hours for no more than 24 hours.

Children (over 3 Months)
Infection—80–160 mg/kg/24 hours given in 4–6 equal doses. Do not exceed 12 gms/day total dosage.

Prophylaxis—30–40 mg/kg 1-1/2 hours before surgery, then 30–40 mg/kg every 6 hours for 24 hours.

See manufacturer's literature for dosage in renal impairment.

Preparation and Storage
Supplied as a powder in vials containing 1 gm and 2 gm of drug and in infusion bottles containing 1 gm and 2 gm of drug.

To reconstitute add 10 ml sterile water for injection to the 1 gm vial (yields 95 mg/ml) or 10 ml or 20 ml to the 2 gm vial (yields 180 mg or 95 mg/ml respectively).

To reconstitute infusion bottles add 50 to 100 ml of any compatible fluid (see Continuous Infusion section) to either the 1 gm bottle (yield 20–10 mg/ml) or the 2 gm bottle (yields 40–20 mg/ml).

After reconstitution, if stored at room temperature, discard after 24 hours; if refrigerated, discard after 7 days.

If further diluted for continuous infusion, refrigerate and discard after 48 hours.

Drug Incompatibilities
Do not mix in any manner with the following:
- Amikacin
- Gentamicin
- Tobramycin
- Other aminoglycosides

Modes of Intravenous Administration

Injection
Yes

cefoxitin sodium
(continued)
No further dilution needed. Inject over 3–5 min.

Intermittent Infusion
Yes
Dilute reconstituted form in 50–100 ml of compatible fluid (see Continuous Infusion). Infusion bottles may be infused as prepared. Infuse over 15–30 min.

Continuous Infusion
Yes
Add to 500–1000 ml of any of the following fluids:
D5W, NS
D5/NS
D5W w/ 0.02% sodium bicarbonate
D10W
D5/.0.2% saline
D5/.45% saline
Ringers Injection
RL
D5/RL
5% or 10% Invert Sugar
5% Sodium Bicarbonate
Neut
Sodium lactate, 1/6 molar
Aminosol
Normosol-M
Ionosol-B
Polyonic M
Mannitol–5%; 2.5%; & 10%
Isolyte E
Type and volume of fluid used depends on patient's needs. A scalp-vein needle is preferred for this mode of administration.

Contraindications; Warnings; Precautions; Adverse Reactions

Contraindications
Hypersensitivity to cefoxitin or to the cephalosporins.

Warnings
1. Administer with caution to patients with known allergy to penicillin or any drugs; there may be cross-allergenicity.
2. Data regarding safe use in pregnancy is incomplete. Use in pregnancy only when expected benefits outweigh potential harm.
3. This drug is excreted in breast milk.
4. Safety and efficacy for use in infants under 3 months of age has not been established. Use in older children has been associated with eosinophilia and elevated SGOT.

Precautions
1. Patients with renal insufficiency require reduced dosage since high serum concentrations can occur in these patients.
2. Overgrowth of nonsusceptible organisms can occur with prolonged use.
3. Increased nephrotoxicity has been reported in patients receiving aminoglycoside antibiotics concomitantly with cephalosporins.
4. False increases of serum creatinine can occur if done within 2 hours of drug administration.
5. False-positive reaction for urine glucose can occur with Clinitest tablets.
6. This drug contains 2.3 mEq (53.8 mg) of sodium per gram.

Adverse Reactions
1. Thrombophlebitis.
2. Hypersensitivity: rash, pruritus, fever, eosinophilia.
3. Gastrointestinal: nausea, vomiting, diarrhea (rare).
4. Blood: transient eosinophilia, leukopenia, neutropenia, hemolytic anemia. Positive direct Coombs.
5. Hepatic: transient increase in SGOT, SGPT, LDH, alkaline phosphatase.
6. Renal: elevated serum creatinine, BUN.

☐ **Nursing Implications**
1. Take anaphylaxis precautions (see Appendix).
2. Monitor for signs and symptoms of overgrowth infections due to nonsusceptible organisms:
   a. Fever (take rectal tempera-

tures at least every 4–6 hrs
in all patients.
b. Increasing malaise.
c. Newly appearing signs and
symptoms of a localized infection: redness, soreness,
pain, swelling, drainage (increasing volume or change
in character of preexisting
drainage.
d. Oral lesions (thrush) or perineal rash (monilia) due to
Candida albicans.
e. Cough (change in
preexisting cough and sputum production).
f. Diarrhea.
3. Use Tes-Tape or Keto-Diastix
for urine glucose determinations.
4. Monitor renal function in patients with renal impairment,
seriously ill patients on high
doses and those receiving an
aminoglycoside antibiotic (gentamicin, amikacin, tobramycin)
concomitantly.
a. Record intake and output
every 4–8 hrs depending on
the patient's condition; report onset or changes in oliguria, defined as: urine
output less than 240 ml in 8
hours for adults.
b. Urinalysis as indicated; usually every other day.
c. Be aware of the patient's
BUN and creatinine.
5. Take precautions to reduce the
risk of thrombophlebitis:
a. Use scalp-vein needle or
small cannula in large vein.
b. Rotate insertion site every
48–72 hours.
c. Examine insertion site daily
for signs of thrombophlebitis (pain, swelling, warmth
and redness along involved
vein).
d. Remove intravenous cannula
if any signs are present and
notify physician. Apply warm
compresses, elevate the extremity and avoid trauma to
the area.
e. Avoid further venipunctures

in that extremity until the inflammation resolves.

cephalothin sodium ■
(Keflin, Keflin Neutral)

Actions/Indications
Antibiotic, cephalosporin group,
broad spectrum. Active against
Staph. aureus (coagulase positive and
negative), group A beta-hemolytic
streptococcus, *Strep. pneumoniae,*
Clostridia, *H. influenzae, E. coli;* Proteus, *Klebsiella, Salmonella* sp. and *Shigella* sp.
Indicated in the treatment of the
following serious infections due to
susceptible strains of the designated
organisms:
• Respiratory tract—*S. pneumoniae,*
Staphylococci, group A beta-hemolytic Streptococci, *Klebsiella* and
H. influenzae.
• Skin and soft tissue —staphylococci, group A beta-hemolytic
streptococci, *E. coli, P. mirabilis,*
and *Klebsiella.*
• Genitourinary tract–*E. coli, P. mirabilis,* and *Klebsiella.*
• Septicemia, including endocarditis
—*S. pneumoniae,* staphylococci,
group A beta-hemolytic strepto-
cocci, *S. viridans, E. coli, P. mirabilis,*
and *Klebsiella.*
• Gastrointestinal—*Salmonella* and
Shigella sp.
• Meningitis—*S. pneumoniae,* group
A beta-hemolytic streptococci and
staphylococci (when more reliably
effective antibiotics cannot be
used).
• Bone and joint—staphylococci.
Also indicated for perioperative
prophylaxis in patients with a high
risk of postoperative infections (vaginal hysterectomy, open-heart surgery, prosthetic arthroplasty).

Dosage
Adults:
Usual range—500–1000 mg every 4–
6 hrs. Up to 12 gm/24 hours for serious infections.
In the presence of renal impairment
(adults)—see table below.

cephalothin sodium
(continued)
   Perioperative prophylaxis—
1. 1 to 2 gm 1/2 to 1 hr before start of surgery.
2. 1 to 2 gm during surgery (depending on duration of procedure).
3. 1 to 2 gm every 6 hrs, for 24 hrs after surgery.
Children:
Most susceptible infections —40–150 mg/kg/24 hrs; give in divided doses every 4–6 hrs.
   Serious infections or in lowered resistance—80–225 mg/kg/24 hrs given in divided doses every 4–6 hrs.
Neonates:
0–7 days of age—40 mg/kg/24 hrs (20 mg/kg every 12 hrs). Over 7 days of age—60 mg/kg/24 hrs (20 mg/kg every 8 hrs).[1]

Dosage in Renal Impairment (Adults)*

Degree of Impairment	Creatinine Clearance	Dosage and Frequency
Mild	80–50 ml/min	2 gm q 6 hrs
Moderate	50–25 ml/min	1.5 gm q 6 hrs
Severe	25–10 ml/min	1 gm q 6 hrs
Marked	10–2 ml/min	0.5 gm q 6 hrs
No function	<2 ml/min	0.5 gm q 8 hrs

*Courtesy of the Eli Lilly Co., Indianapolis, IN

Preparation and Storage
Available in vials containing 1 gm, 2 gm, 4 gm and 20 gm of drug.
   To reconstitute from powder add 4 ml of sterile water for injection for each gram of drug. If drug does not dissolve completely add an additional small amount of diluent and warm the vial in the hands.
   After reconstituting, store in refrigerator. Discard after 96 hours. If solution precipitates, can be redissolved by constantly agitating vial until warmed to room temperature.

Drug Incompatibilities
Many incompatibilities; do not mix with other drugs in any manner, except hydrocortisone.

Modes of IV Administration

Injection
Yes
Further dilute reconstituted form with sterile water for injection, 10 ml/gm of drug. Inject over 3–5 min.

Intermittent Infusion
Yes
Dilute reconstituted form in 50 ml D5W or NS. Infuse over 15–20 min.
   For smaller volumes dilute to 1 gm/10 ml.
   Discontinue other solutions while infusing this drug.

Continuous Infusion
Yes
Add 8-, 12- or 24-hour dose to 500–1000 ml of any of the following fluids, depending on patient fluid needs:
NS
D5W
D5RL
RL
Normosol M in D5W
Acetated Ringers
Ionosol B in D5W
Isolyte M with 5% Dextrose
Plasma-Lyte Injection
Plasma-Lyte M in 5% Dextrose
Ringer's Injection
   Solution is stable for 24 hours.

Contraindications; Warnings; Precautions; Adverse Reactions

Contraindications
Hypersensitivity to any cephalosporin.

Warnings
1. Before administering, inquire about previous allergic reactions to cephalosporins or to penicillin; there may be cross-allergenicity.

2. Safety for use during pregnancy has not been established.

Precautions
1. Monitor renal status during therapy, especially in the seriously ill who are receiving maximal doses. Use suggested dosage modifications in the presence of renal impairment.
2. Thrombophlebitis at injection site can be minimized by adding 10–25 mg of hydrocortisone to continuous infusion preparations. Also, use a small cannula in a larger vein and rotate the insertion site at least every 72 hours.
3. Overgrowth of nonsusceptible organisms can occur with prolonged use.
4. False-positive urine glucose testing may result with the use of Benedict's or Fehling's solution, or with Clinitest tablets.
5. Administer with caution to patients receiving aminoglycoside antibiotics concurrently; an increased incidence of nephrotoxicity in such patients has been reported.

Adverse Reactions
1. Allergic reactions: rash, urticaria, drug fever, anaphylaxis
2. Blood dyscrasias: neutropenia, thrombocytopenia, and hemolytic anemia; positive direct Coombs' test (usually seen in the presence of azotemia)
3. Hepatic: transient rise in SGOT and alkaline phosphatase without organ damage
4. Renal:
   a. Rise in BUN and decrease in creatinine clearance, especially in the presence of pre-existing renal impairment.
   b. Rise in BUN without a decrease in creatinine clearance, renal damage is not likely, and BUN will return to normal after discontinuation of therapy. Permanent renal damage rarely occurs.
5. Thrombophlebitis at injection site with continuous infusions of large doses.
6. Gastrointestinal: nausea, anorexia, diarrhea, vomiting, oral Candida infection
7. Perineal: monilial infections

☐ **Nursing Implications**
1. Take anaphylaxis precautions; see Appendix.
2. Monitor for signs and symptoms of overgrowth infections due to nonsusceptible organisms
   a. Fever (take rectal temperature at least every 4–6 hours in all patients)
   b. Increasing malaise
   c. Newly appearing signs and symptoms of a localized infection: redness, soreness, pain, swelling, drainage (increasing volume, or change in character of pre-existing drainage)
   d. Oral lesions (thrush) or perineal rash (monilia) due to *Candida albicans*
   e. Cough (change in pre-existing cough and sputum production)
   f. Diarrhea
3. Use Tes-Tape or Keto-Diastix for urine glucose determinations.
4. Monitor renal function in patients with renal impairment:
   a. Intake and output recordings every 4–8 hours, depending on the patient's condition; report onset or changes in oliguria, defined as urine output less than 240 ml in 8 hours in adults
   b. Urinalysis as indicated, usually every other day
   c. Be aware of the patient's BUN and creatinine

Reference
1. McCracken, George H. and Nelson, John D.: Antimicrobial Therapy for Newborns: Practical Application of Pharmacology to Clinical Usage, New York: Grune and Stratton, 1977, p. 28.

cephapirin sodium ■
(Cefadyl)

Actions/Indications
Antibiotic cephalosporin group, broad spectrum.

Active against beta-hemolytic streptococci, *Staph. aureus, Staph. epidermis, S. pneumoniae, H. influenzae, Klebsiella* species, *P. mirabilis, E. coli* and others.

Indicated in the treatment of the following serious infections due to susceptible strains of the designated organisms:

* Respiratory tract—*S. pneumoniae, Staph. aureus, Klebsiella* sp., *H. influenzae*, and group A beta-hemolytic streptococci.
* Skin and soft tissue—*Staph. aureus, Staph. epidermis, E. coli, P. mirabilis, Klebsiella* sp. and group A beta-hemolytic streptococci.
* Urinary tract—*Staph. aureus, E. coli, P. mirabilis* and *Klebsiella* sp.
* Septicemia—*Staph. aureus, S. viridans, E. coli, Klebsiella* sp. and group A beta-hemolytic streptococci.
* Endocarditis—*S. viridans*, and *S. aureus*.
* Osteomyelitis—*S. aureus, Klebsiella* sp., *P. mirabilis* and group A beta-hemolytic streptococci.

Dosage
Adults:
500–1000 mg. every 4–6 hrs depending on the severity of the infection. Life-threatening infections may require doses up to 12 gm daily.

In the presence of renal impairment, severe oliguria or steady-state serum creatinine greater than 5 mg/100 ml, a dose of 7.5–15.0 mg/kg every 12 hrs (when appropriate, just prior to dialysis, and every 12 hrs. thereafter).
Children (Over 3 Months of Age):
40–80 mg/kg/24 hrs in 4 divided doses.
Severe infections—100 mg/kg/24 hrs in 4 divided doses.

Therapy for beta hemolytic streptococcal infections should continue for at least 10 days.

Neonates:
Not recommended for infants under 3 months of age or in premature infants.

Preparation and Storage
Available in vials containing 500 mg, 1 gm, 2 gm and 4 gm and in piggyback vials containing 1 gm, 2 gm and 4 gm of drug.

To reconstitute from powder add 10 ml of sterile water for injection or Bacteriostatic Water for injection to the 1-gm or 2-gm vials.

Dilute piggyback packages with at least 10 ml of the above diluents.

Solutions may be light yellow.

Store in refrigerator, discard after 10 days. If stored at room temperature, discard after 12 hrs.

Drug Incompatibilities
Do not mix with:
Mannitol
Aminoglycoside antibiotics
Aminophylline
Tetracyclines
Phenytoin
Barbiturates

Modes of IV Administration

Injection
Yes
Inject reconstituted drug over 3–5 min.

Intermittent Infusion
Yes
Further dilute prepared 1- and 2-gm vials with 50 ml NS or D5W. For smaller volumes, dilute to 1 gm/10 ml.

Piggyback vials may be infused, as prepared, over 15–20 min.

Discontinue other solutions while infusing this drug.

Continuous Infusion
Yes
Add 8-, 12- or 24-hour dosage to 500–1000 ml of any IV fluid, except sodium bicarbonate, depending on patient fluid needs.

Solution is stable for 24 hours.

Contraindications; Warnings; Precautions; Adverse Reactions

Contraindications
Hypersensitivity to any cephalosporin.

Warnings
1. Administer with caution to patients with an allergy to penicillin; there may be partial cross-allergenicity.
2. Safety for use in pregnancy has not been established.
3. Safety for use in infants under 3 months of age or in premature infants has not been established and use is not recommended.

Precautions
1. Renal status should be evaluated before and during therapy. Renal impairment is rarely produced by this drug.[1] However, renal impairment is an indication for reduced dosage (see Dosage section). Increased renal toxicity has been reported in patients receiving aminoglycoside antibiotics concomitantly.
2. Prolonged use of this drug may result in the overgrowth of nonsusceptible organisms; major and minor superinfections may be produced.
3. With high urine concentrations of cephapirin, false-positive glucose reactions may occur with the use of Clinitest, Benedict's solution, or Fehling's solution. Clinistix or Tes-Tape should be used.
4. Each 500 mg of this drug contains 1.18 mEq (28 mg.) of sodium.

Adverse Reactions
1. Hypersensitivity: maculopapular rash, urticaria, drug fever, serum sickness-like reaction, anaphylaxis
2. Blood dyscrasias: neutropenia, leukopenia, anemia (secondary to depression of blood cell formation) are rare. Occasionally, patients with azotemia (increased BUN) have developed a positive direct Coombs' test
3. Liver: transient elevation of SGOT and SGPT, alkaline phosphatase, and bilirubin have been reported
4. Kidney: transient elevation of BUN, especially in patients over 50 years of age

☐ Nursing Implications
1. Take anaphylaxis precautions; see Appendix.
2. Use Clinistix or Tes-Tape for urine glucose determinations.
3. Monitor for signs and symptoms of nonsusceptible organism overgrowth infection.
   a. Fever (take rectal temperature at least every 4–6 hours)
   b. Increasing malaise
   c. Localized signs and symptoms of newly developing infection: redness, soreness, pain, swelling, drainage (change in volume or character of pre-existing drainage)
   d. Cough (change in character or amount of sputum production)
   e. Diarrhea
   f. Oral lesions (thrush) or perineal rash (monilia) due to *Candida albicans*
4. Monitor for the onset of renal damage:
   a. Measure urine output at least every 8 hours. A urine output less than 30 ml/hour for 2–3 consecutive hours in an adult should be reported to the physician.
   b. Send urine for analysis daily or on alternate days.
   c. Be aware of the patient's pretreatment BUN and any changes during therapy.
5. The incidence of venous irritation is low.

Reference
1. Appel, Gerald B., and Neu, Harold C.: The Nephrotoxicity of Antimicrobial Agents. *New England Journal of Medicine,* 296(13):722, March 31, 1977.

cephradine ■
(Velosef for Infusion—Sodium-Free,
Velosef for Injection)

Actions/Indications
Antibiotic, of the cephalosporin
type. Indicated in the treatment of
the following infections when caused
by susceptible strains of the designated organisms:
Respiratory tract—Group A beta-
hemolytic streptococci, *Strep. pneumoniae,* *Klebsiella* Sp., *H. influenzae,*
Staph. aureus.
Skin and soft tissue—*Staph. aureus*
and group A beta-hemolytic streptococci.
Urinary tract—*E. coli, Proteus mirabilis, Klebsiella* species.
Bone infections—*Staph. aureus*
(penicillin-susceptible and resistant).
Septicemia—*Strep. pneumoniae,
Staph. aureus, P. mirabilis,* and *E. coli.*
Sensitivity testing should be carried out prior to therapy.

Dosage
Adults:
500–1000 mg every 6 hrs; do not
exceed 8 gm/day.
Adults with Impaired Renal Function:
Each patient must be considered in-
dividually.
*Loading dose—*750 mg.
*Maintenance dose—*500 mg at the
following intervals:

Creatinine Clearance (ml/min.)	Time Interval
> 20	6–12 hrs
15–19	12–24 hrs
10–14	24–40 hrs
5–9	40–50 hrs
< 5	50–70 hrs

Children and Infants: Over 1 Year:
50–100 mg/kg/day in equally divided doses every 6 hrs, regulated by
age of the patient and severity of the
infection. Maximum dose should not
exceed 8 gm/day.

Preparation and Storage
Cephradine is available in two forms:
1. Sterile cephradine, sodium-free,
   supplied in 200 ml. size infusion
   bottles containing 2 gm of drug
   and

2. Cephradine for Injection [con-
   taining 6 mEq (136 mg) sodium
   per gram], supplied in vials containing 250 mg, 500 mg or 1
   gm of drug and 100 ml. infusion bottles containing 2 gm or
   4 gm of drug.
To reconstitute sterile cephradine,
sodium free—add 150 *or* 200 ml. of
compatible fluid (see Continuous In-
fusion-below) DO NOT USE STER-
ILE WATER FOR INJECTION.
Shake well until dissolved. This provides concentrations of 13.3 mg/ml.
or 10 mg/ml. The solution may be
colorless or light yellow. Protect
from concentrated light or direct
sunlight. Discard after 48 hours at
room temperature or 1 week if refrigerated.
To reconstitute Cephradine for
Injection add the following amounts
of sterile water for injection, D5W
or NS. DO NOT USE LACTATED
RINGERS. Final concentration will
be 100 mg/ml:

Vial Size	Volume
250 mg	5 ml
500 mg	5 ml
1 gm	10 ml
2 gm	20 ml
2 gm piggyback	40 ml
4 gm piggyback	80 ml

Use within 2 hours or if stored in
refrigerator discard after 48 hours.
Protect solutions from concentrated
light or direct sunlight.

Drug Incompatibilities
Do not mix with any other antibiot-
ics in IV bottle, do not mix in any
manner with:
Epinephrine
Lidocaine
Aminoglycoside antibiotics
Calcium preparations

Modes of IV Administration

Injection
Yes
Cephradine for Injection Only!
Directly into the vein or into the

tubing of a running IV when the intravenous solution is compatible with the drug.
Inject over 3–5 min.

Intermittent Infusion
Yes
Add reconstituted solution to enough D5W or NS to make a 30 mg/ml concentration.
Infuse over 30–60 min. If infused at the same time as other infusions, these other fluids must be compatible with cephradine, or be stopped during administration of this drug; see under Continuous Infusion below.

Piggyback preparations may be infused as prepared under Preparation and Storage above.

Continuous Infusion
Yes
Add reconstituted solution to any of the following IV solutions in an amount determined by fluid and electrolyte needs of the patient:
D5W
D10W
NS
Sodium Lactate 1/6 molar
D5/NS
D5/.45% sodium chloride
10% invert sugar
Normosol-R
Ionosol-B
RL-sterile cephradine, sodium-free
only
Use *no* other IV solutions.
Prepare fresh solution every 10 hrs.

Contraindications; Warnings; Precautions; Adverse Reactions

Contraindications
Hypersensitivity to any cephalosporin.

Warnings
1. Administer with caution to patients with an allergy to penicillin; there may be partial cross-allergenicity.
2. Safety for use in pregnancy has not been established.
3. This drug is secreted in breast milk during lactation.

4. Safety for use in premature infants or infants under one month of age has not been established. Use with caution in infants one month to one year of age.

Precautions
1. Prolonged use may promote the overgrowth of nonsusceptible organisms.
2. Monitor renal function and adjust dosage accordingly. Renal failure is rarely caused by this drug.
3. Patients with marked renal impairment require lower dosage since this drug in the usual dose will accumulate in the serum and tissues
4. Increased nephrotoxicity has been reported in patients receiving aminoglycoside antibiotics concomitantly.
5. False-positive urine glucose reactions may occur if Clinitest tablets, Benedict's solution or Fehling's solution is used.
6. Positive direct Coombs test has been reported to occur during therapy with this drug.
7. To reduce the risk of phlebitis, rotate cannula insertion site frequently during therapy (every 48 to 72 hours).

Adverse Reactions
1. Gastrointestinal: glossitis (inflammation of the tongue), nausea, vomiting, diarrhea, abdominal pain, tenesmus (spasmotic contraction of anal or bladder sphincter, accompanied by pain and desire to empty bowel or bladder)
2. Hypersensitivity: maculopapular rash, urticaria, erythema, joint pains, drug fever, anaphylaxis
3. Blood dyscrasias: mild transient eosinophilia, leukopenia, and neutropenia
4. Liver: transient elevations in SGOT or SGPT, total bilirubin, alkaline phosphatase and LDH. These values return to normal after discontinuation of therapy.
5. Renal: mild elevations in BUN,

cephradine
(continued)
more frequently in patients over 50 years or under 3 years of age.
6. Other: headache, dizziness, dyspnea, paresthesia, candidal overgrowth and vaginitis, hepatomegaly (rare) and thrombophlebitis at injection site.

☐ **Nursing Implications**
1. Take anaphylaxis precautions; see Appendix.
2. Check label carefully to be certain which form of drug is being used.
3. Use Clinistix or Tes-Tape for urine glucose determinations.
4. Monitor for signs and symptoms of nonsusceptible organism overgrowth infection
   a. Fever (take rectal temperature at least every 4–6 hours)
   b. Increasing malaise
   c. Localized signs and symptoms of newly developing infection: redness, soreness, pain, swelling, drainage (change in volume or character of pre-existing drainage)
   d. Cough (change in character or amount of sputum production)
   e. Diarrhea
   f. Oral lesions (thrush) or perineal rash (monilia) due to *Candida albicans.*
5. Monitor renal function in patients with renal impairment:
   a. Record intake and output every 4–8 hours, depending on the patient's condition; report onset or changes in oliguria, defined as: adults — urine output less than 240 ml in 8 hours.
   b. Urinalysis as indicated, usually every other day.
   c. Be aware of the patient's BUN and creatinine.
6. Monitor for the onset of inflammation of the tongue (glossitis). The patient will complain of soreness, and the tongue will be reddened and inflamed. Report this to the physician. Provide a soft diet, analgesics and mouthwashes as ordered. Maintain hydration.
7. Administer antiemetics and/or constipating agents as ordered if gastrointestinal disturbances occur. Maintain hydration and nutritional intake. Record urine output and emesis to assist the physician in ordering fluids if necessary.
8. Examine for thrombophlebitis at the infusion site. Discontinue the IV if this occurs. Apply warm compresses, elevate the extremity, and avoid trauma to the area. Venipunctures should not be performed on that extremity until the inflammation resolves.

chloramphenicol sodium succinate ■
(Chloromycetin)

Actions/Indications
Antibiotic, intended for use in serious infections **only** when less toxic drugs are ineffective or are contraindicated.
Examples:
• Acute infections caused by *Salmonella typhi* (not carrier state)
• Serious infections caused by susceptible strains of:
   a. *Salmonella* species
   b. *H. influenzae* (meningeal)
   c. Rickettsia
   d. Lymphogranuloma-psittacosis group
   e. Gram-negative organisms causing bacteremia and meningitis
   f. Other susceptible organisms which have been demonstrated to be resistant to all other appropriate drugs
• Cystic fibrosis regimens
This drug can be used to initiate antibiotic therapy if one of the above conditions is suspected. It should be discontinued if a less toxic agent will be effective as indicated by sensitivity tests.

Dosage

Adults:
50 mg/kg/24 hrs in divided doses at 6-hr intervals. Some resistant infections may require up to 100 mg/kg/24 hrs.

Dosage should be reduced in patients with impaired hepatic or renal function.

Children:
50 mg/kg/24 hrs in divided doses at 6-hr intervals. When adequate cerebrospinal fluid concentrations are needed: 100 mg/kg/24 hrs. Dosage should be reduced as soon as possible.

Dosage should be reduced in the presence of impaired hepatic or renal function.

Neonates and Premature Infants (Less than 2 Weeks of Age):
10–25 mg/kg/24 hrs in 3–4 equally divided doses or 6 mg/kg/dose every 6 hrs. Dosage should be reduced in the presence of impaired hepatic or renal function.

Full-Term Infants Older than 2 Weeks:
50 mg/kg/24 hrs in 3–4 equally divided doses or 12 mg/kg/dose every 6 hrs.

Preparation and Storage

Available in vials containing 1 gm of drug.

To reconstitute from powder, add 10 ml of sterile water for injection or D5W. The resulting solution will be 100 mg/ml (10%). Do not use cloudy solutions.

Store at room temperature; discard after 30 days.

Drug Incompatibilities

Do not mix in IV bottle with:
Methicillin
Gentamicin
Nitrofurantoin
Do not mix in any manner with:
Chlorpromazine
Hydroxyzine
Novobiocin
Oxytetracycline
Polymyxin-B
Prochlorperazine
Promethazine
Sulfadiazine
Tetracycline
Vancomycin
Carbenicillin
Erythromycin

Modes of IV Administration

Injection
Yes
Use a 10% solution (100 mg/ml). See Preparation section.

Inject over at least 1 min. May be injected into the tubing of a running IV.

Intermittent Infusion
Yes
Add dose to 50–100 ml of D5W. Infuse over 15–30 min.

Continuous Infusion
Yes
Add 6-, 12-, or 24-hr dose to 1000 ml of any IV fluid except protein hydrolysate, depending on the patient's fluid needs.

Solution is stable for 24 hrs.

Contraindications; Warnings; Precautions; Adverse Reactions

Contraindications
1. History of hypersensitivity or toxic reaction to chloramphenicol
2. Use as a prophylactic agent to prevent bacterial infections or to treat trivial infections such as colds, influenza, sore throats, etc.

Warnings
1. SERIOUS AND POTENTIALLY FATAL BLOOD DYSCRASIAS, SUCH AS APLASTIC ANEMIA, HYPOPLASTIC ANEMIA, THROMBOCYTOPENIA AND GRANULOCYTOPENIA, HAVE OCCURRED FOLLOWING ADMINISTRATION OF THIS DRUG. Aplastic anemia attributed to this drug has terminated in leukemia. These blood dyscrasias have occurred following short- and long-term therapy.
2. Dose-related bone marrow

chloramphenicol sodium succinate
(continued)

depression, which is reversible, has also been reported. This type of blood dyscrasia is characterized by vacuolization (development of clear air of fluid-filled spaces in a cell) of the erythroid cells, by reduction of reticulocytes, and leukopenia (decreased white blood cells). These changes disappear with discontinuation of the drug.

Precautions
1. Blood cell production must be monitored at least every 2 days throughout therapy.
2. Such studies cannot be relied upon to detect irreversible bone marrow depression that occurs prior to development of aplastic anemia.
3. Discontinue this drug with the appearance of reticulocytopenia, leukopenia, thrombocytopenia, or anemia.
4. Avoid repeated courses of this drug. Treatment should not be continued longer than required to produce a cure and to prevent relapse.
5. Avoid concurrent use of other bone marrow depressing agents.
6. Excessive blood levels of this drug will develop in patients with impaired liver or kidney function, including the immature function of these organs in premature or young infants.
7. Safety for use in pregnancy has not been established. This drug crosses the placental barrier and can produce the gray-baby syndrome in the infant (see Adverse Reaction No. 5).
8. Use with extreme caution in premature and full-term infants; high serum drug levels can produce toxic effects. See Adverse Reaction No. 5 on the gray-baby syndrome.
9. Overgrowth of nonsusceptible organisms may occur.
10. Each gram of this drug contains approximately 2.25 mEq (52 mg.) of sodium.

Adverse Reactions
1. Blood dyscrasias:
   a. Idiosyncratic irreversible and potentially fatal bone marrow depression producing aplastic anemia, hypoplastic anemia, thrombocytopenia, and granulocytopenia
   b. Reversible, dose-related bone marrow depression
   c. Paroxysmal, nocturnal hemoglobinuria
2. Gastrointestinal:
   a. Nausea, vomiting, diarrhea
   b. Glossitis (inflammation of the tongue) and stomatitis (inflammation of oral mucous membranes)
   c. Enterocolitis (rare)
3. Neurotoxic:
   a. Headache
   b. Mild depression, mental confusion
   c. Optic and peripheral neuritis (usually in long-term therapy; if this occurs, the drug should be discontinued)
4. Hypersensitivity: fever, rash, angioedema, urticaria, anaphylaxis, Herxheimer reaction in typhoid patients
5. Gray-baby syndrome: Seen in premature and full-term newborns receiving this drug or when the mother has received it during labor. This syndrome occurs most frequently when the drug has been used during the first 48 hours after delivery. Symptoms appear after 3–4 days of continued therapy with high doses in the following order:
   a. Abdominal distention with or without vomiting
   b. Progressive, pallid cyanosis
   c. Poor feeding, refusal to suck
   d. Circulatory collapse
   e. Irregular respirations
   f. Flaccidity.
Infants become gravely ill within 24 hours. Death can occur within the next 12 hours unless the drug is discontinued. The process can frequently be reversed with discontinuation of therapy.

6. Overgrowth infection secondary to organisms not susceptible to chloramphenicol.

☐ **Nursing Implications**
1. Take anaphylaxis precautions; see Appendix.
2. Assist the physician in monitoring for the onset of blood dyscrasias:
   a. Complete blood counts should be done every 2 days during therapy (see Precautions No. 1–3).
   b. Be aware of blood count results prior to each dose of the drug.
   c. Monitor for bleeding if the platelet count falls below 100,000/cu mm.
   d. If the white blood cell count falls below 2000, place the patient in protective (reverse) isolation and monitor for signs and symptoms of infection. Avoid invasive procedures and maintain bodily (especially perineal) cleanliness.
   e. Monitor for nocturnal hematuria.
3. Care of the infant on chloramphenicol:
   a. Monitor for signs of the gray-baby syndrome (see adverse reaction No. 5). Notify the physician immediately on suspicion of the onset of this syndrome. Hold the next dose of the drug until a medical decision is made.
   b. Administer supportive care as needed, e.g., prevention of aspiration, provision of respiratory support.
4. Examine the patient daily for the onset of oral lesions (glossitis or stomatitis). Report the occurrence to the physician. Order a soft, bland diet and nonirritating fluids. Administer mouthwashes as ordered (usually half saline, half hydrogen peroxide).
5. Monitor for depression and/or mental confusion. Reassure the patient as to the origin of these problems. Take precautions to prevent patient injury when indicated (e.g., side rails, soft restraints).
6. Observe for signs and symptoms of optic neuritis:
   a. loss of visual acuity
   b. central scotoma (loss of an area of the center of the visual field)
   c. pain on eye movement
   d. tenderness around the eye[1]
   Notify the physician at the onset of these findings; the drug should be discontinued.
7. Observe for signs and symptoms of peripheral neuritis:
   a. Localized neurologic pain
   b. Pain on motion of hands, fingers, feet, toes
   c. Tingling, numbness
   d. Weakness of extremities
   Notify the physician at the onset of these findings; the drug should be discontinued. Reassure the patient as to the origin of the symptoms and their transient nature.
8. If gastrointestinal disturbances occur, notify the physician. If such symptoms are pronounced, the drug will probably be discontinued. Antiemetics, antacids, and a constipating agent can be ordered. Monitor intake and output to assist the physician in planning for parenteral fluid replacement. Maintain hydration orally when possible.
9. Monitor for signs and symptoms of overgrowth infections:
   a. Fever (take rectal temperature at least every 4–6 hours in all patients)
   b. Increasing malaise
   c. Newly appearing localized signs and symptoms: redness, soreness, pain, swelling, drainage (increased volume or change in character of pre-existing drainage)
   d. Monilial rash in perineal area (reddened areas with itching)
   e. Cough (change in pre-existing cough or sputum production)
   f. Diarrhea

chloramphenicol sodium succinate
(continued)
Reference
1. Newell, Frank W., and Ernest, J. Terry: *Ophthalmology—Principles and Concepts*, (3rd ed.), St. Louis, C. V. Mosby Company, 1974, p. 307.

chlordiazepoxide hydrochloride ■
(Librium)

Actions/Indications
Central nervous system depressant; acts on the limbic system involved in emotional reactions. Also depresses the brain stem reticular formation, the cerebral cortex, and the reflex arcs of the spinal cord.

Used to control agitation, tremor, impending or active delirium tremens resulting from alcohol withdrawal, and for the general relief of anxiety.

Dosage
Adults:
Alcohol withdrawal—50–100 mg initially repeated in 2–4 hrs as necessary.

Acute anxiety—50–100 mg initially, followed by 25–50 mg, 3–4 times daily. Do not exceed 300 mg in 24 hrs.

Reduce dosage for elderly or debilitated patients, usually 25–50 mg.
Children Over Age 12:
25–50 mg. Lowest dose should be used initially, increasing as necessary. *Use of this drug in children less than 12 years of age is not recommended.*

Preparation and Storage
Supplied in 5-ml ampuls containing 100 mg of drug in crystalline form.

Prepare by adding 5 ml NS or sterile water for injection. *DO NOT USE DILUENT PROVIDED FOR IM SOLUTION PREPARATION.* Inject diluent slowly into the vial. Agitate gently until powder is completely dissolved. Do not use the solution if it is hazy or opalescent. Mix again using sterile water for injection. Use solution *immediately*; discard unused portion. Store dry form in refrigerator.

Drug Incompatibilities
Do not mix with any other medication.

Modes of IV Administration

Injection
Yes
Slowly, over 1 min. Do not mix with fluids.

Intermittent Infusion
No
This drug is unstable in solution and ineffective.

Continuous Infusion
No
This drug is unstable in solution and ineffective.

Contraindications; Warnings; Precautions; Adverse Reactions

Contraindications
Known hypersensitivity

Warnings
1. Withdrawal symptoms have been reported following sudden discontinuation of this drug, usually after extended therapy with high doses. Symptoms may include convulsions.
2. Use of this drug in the first trimester of pregnancy may carry an increased risk of congenital malformations. Its use during this period should almost always be avoided.
3. The signs and symptoms of overdosage include somnolence, confusion, coma, decreased reflexes.

Precautions
1. Any patient receiving intravenous chlordiazepoxide should be kept under close observation and at bedrest during administration and for 3 hours after the dose.
2. Use of other psychotropic agents during therapy with this drug is not recommended.

3. Caution should be exercised when administering to patients with hepatic or renal insufficiency; toxic or adverse effects may be more pronounced.
4. Reduced dosage is recommended for the elderly, debilitated and children over age 12.
5. Paradoxical reactions such as increased agitation, excitement, and acute rage have occurred in psychiatric patients and hyperactive children.
6. Variable effects on blood coagulation have been reported in patients concomitantly receiving oral anticoagulants.
7. Should not be given to patients in shock or comatose states.
8. Use with caution in patients with porphyria.

Adverse Reactions
1. Mental confusion, syncope, hypotension, tachycardia, skin eruptions, nausea, extrapyramidal symptoms, and blurred vision have been observed. These situations are usually controlled by a reduction in dosage.
2. Blood dyscrasias, including agranulocytosis, and hepatic dysfunction have been reported.

☐ Nursing Implications
1. Keep the patient at rest during the administration of this drug and for 2 hours after the last dose, and then ambulate with assistance. While the patient is on bedrest take precautions to prevent injury, e.g. side rails and restraints as indicated.
2. Be prepared to manage agitation, excitement, or acute rage in psychiatric patients, hyperactive children, or in the elderly.
3. Monitor for signs of overdose: extreme lethargy, stupor, confusion, decreasing reflexes, eventually, coma. If any one of these signs appears, notify the physician and initiate frequent monitoring of vital signs. Be prepared to manage vomiting to prevent aspiration; keep suction at the bedside. Maintain an open airway and adequate ventilation.

chlortetracycline hydrochloride ■
(Aureomycin)

Actions/Indications
Antibiotic, indicated in infections caused by the following microorganisms:
• Rickettsiae
• *Mycoplasma pneumoniae*
• Agents of psittacosis and ornithosis
• Agents of lymphogranuloma venereum
• Spirochetal agent of relapsing fever
• Gram-negative organisms: *Haemophilus ducreyi, Pasteurella pestis, Pasteurella tularensis*
• *Bartonella bacilliformis*
• Bacteriodes
• *Vibrio comma*
• *Vibrio fetus*
• *Brucella* species
This drug is also effective against certain gram-positive and other gram-negative organisms. Sensitivity tests are required.

Dosage
Adults:
500 mg at 12-hr intervals. Maximum of 500 mg every 6 hrs.
Children:
Older infants and children under 40 Kg: 10–15 mg/kg/24 hrs in 2 equally divided doses.
Children over 40 Kg: 10–20 mg/kg/24 hrs in 2 equally divided doses.
Generally not recommended in pediatrics except when another drug is not suitable. See Warning No. 5.
Not recommended for neonates or premature infants.

Preparation and Storage
Supplied in vials of 500 mg of drug.
To reconstitute from powder, add 50 ml sterile water for injection, NS, D5W, or D5/NS; do not use any diluent containing a preservative. Shake vigorously.
Solution contains 10 mg/ml. Use

chlortetracycline hydrochloride
(continued)
immediately; discard unused portions.

Drug Incompatibilities
Do not mix with:
solutions containing
calcium (except
Ringer's Injection)
Cephalothin
Cephaloridine
Cefazolin
Ammonium chloride
Dextran
Fructose
Polymyxin B
Promazine
Colistimethate
Penicillin G potassium

Modes of IV Administration

Injection
Yes
Dilute each 100 mg in at least 10 ml
sterile water for injection, NS, or
D5W. Inject over at least 5 min for
each 100 mg.

Intermittent Infusion
Yes
Add to NS or D5W, 10 ml/100 mg
of drug. Complete the infusion within 1 hr, but no more rapidly than
100 mg/5 min.

Continuous Infusion
Yes
Add to NS, D5/NS or D5W only, 10
ml/100 mg of drug. Infuse no more
rapidly than 20 mg/min.

Contraindications; Warnings; Precautions; Adverse Reactions

Contraindications
Hypersensitivity to any tetracycline.

Warnings
1. In the presence of renal failure,
   particularly during pregnancy,
   intravenous doses exceeding 1
   gm/day have been associated
   with deaths due to hepatic failure.
2. This drug should be avoided in
   patients with renal insufficiency.

Accumulation of the drug in the
presence of decreased excretion
can cause further renal damage,
a catabolic state with acidosis,
increasing azotemia and death.
If the patient requires a tetracycline, doxycycline may be used
with safety.[1]
3. When therapeutic needs outweigh the dangers (during pregnancy, renal or hepatic dysfunction), hepatic and renal function
   tests should be carried out before, during and after therapy.
   Monitor serum phosphate,
   BUN, and chlortetracycline levels.
4. A photoallergic reaction may
   occur if the patient is exposed
   to natural or artificial sunlight.
   If this occurs, the drug should
   be discontinued.
5. This drug crosses the placental
   barrier and has been related to
   retardation of skeletal development. Tetracyclines are also secreted in breast milk and may
   cause permanent discoloration
   of the infant's teeth. Use of the
   drug during the last trimester of
   pregnancy, neonatal period and
   early childhood can cause such
   discoloration.
6. The use of this drug may cause
   increased intracranial pressure.

Precautions
1. There may be overgrowth of
   nonsusceptible organisms leading to a superinfection.
2. Tetracyclines depress plasma
   prothrombin activity, thus decreasing dosage requirements in
   concomitant anticoagulation
   therapy.
3. In long-term therapy, hematopoietic, renal and hepatic studies should be performed.
4. The use of tetracyclines can
   decrease the activity of penicillin and should be avoided when
   penicillin is strongly indicated.

Adverse Reactions
1. Gastrointestinal: nausea,
   vomiting, diarrhea, enterocolitis,
   glossitis

2. Inflammatory lesions, with monilial growth in the perineal area
3. Skin: rashes, both maculopapular and erythematous
4. Renal toxicity is usually dose-related; see Warnings No. 1, 2, and 3
5. Hypersensitivity reactions include urticaria, angioneurotic edema, anaphylaxis, pericarditis, and exacerbation of lupus erythematosus
6. Bulging fontanels have been reported in infants receiving doses in the therapeutic range. This disappears after the drug is discontinued.
7. Hematologic changes: thrombocytopenia, hemolytic anemia, neutropenia, and eosinophilia

☐ **Nursing Implications**
1. Take anaphylaxis precautions; see Appendix.
2. If gastrointestinal disturbances occur, notify the physician. If disturbances such as nausea, vomiting and diarrhea are pronounced, the drug will probably be discontinued. Antiemetics, antacids, and constipating agents can be ordered to control symptoms. Monitor intake and output to assist the physician in planning for parenteral fluid replacement. Maintain hydration orally when possible.
3. If the patient will be taking the oral form of this drug as an outpatient, instruct him/her on the possibility of photosensitivity and the advisability of avoiding exposure to the sun (sun-block lotions may be of help if exposure cannot be avoided).
4. Women of childbearing age and potential, and mothers of children who may receive this drug, should be informed of Warnings No. 1 and 5 by the physician. Assist in the interpretation of these warnings to the patient.
5. Even though blood dyscrasias are infrequently caused by this agent, be aware of the patient's complete blood cell count dur-

ing therapy. If the platelet count begins to fall, the drug will probably be discontinued. Bleeding secondary to a low platelet count usually begins only after the count falls below 100,000/cu mm.
6. Monitor for signs and symptoms of overgrowth infections:
   a. Fever (take rectal temperature at least every 4–6 hours in all patients)
   b. Increasing malaise
   c. Newly appearing localized signs and symptoms: redness, soreness, pain, swelling, drainage (increased volume or change in character of pre-existing drainage)
   d. Monilial rash in perineal area (reddened areas with itching)
   e. Cough (change in pre-existing cough or sputum production)
   f. Diarrhea
7. Report the onset of any rash to the physician. If a rash occurs, keep the patient's environment comfortably cool and the skin clean. Diphenhydramine (Benadryl) may be ordered to relieve itching.
8. Report the onset of jaundice to the physician.
9. Report the onset of bulging fontanels, and other signs of increasing intracranial pressure, to the physician.
10. Be aware of this drug's relationship with renal function. Tetracyclines are usually not given to patients with renal impairment because:
   a. The drug accumulates in the body because of decreased excretion
   b. The presence of the drug may cause further deterioration in renal function
   c. It may cause a catabolic state with metabolic acidosis, increasing BUN, and possibly death due to uremia.
   Know what the patient's pretreatment BUN and creatinine levels are. Monitor for changes

chlortetracycline hydrochloride
(continued)
in these values with initiation of treatment. Monitor urine output in renal patients receiving this drug. Report increasing oliguria to the physician. Send urine for analysis at least every other day.

References
1. Barza, Michael, and Schiefe, Richard T.: Antimicrobial Spectrum, Pharmacology and Therapeutic Use of Antibiotics. Part I: Tetracyclines, *American Journal of Hospital Pharmacy*, 34:51, January 1977.
2. Ibid.

cimetidine hydrochloride ■
(Tagamet)

Actions/Indications
Histamine H_2 receptor antagonist, suppresses gastric acid secretion, promotes healing and thus reduces pain of peptic ulcers.
Used for:
• Short-term (less than 8 weeks) treatment of active duodenal ulcer.
• Hypersecretory conditions; systemic mastocytosis, multiple endocrine adenomas, and Zollinger-Ellison syndrome (tumor of the nonbeta cells of the pancreas which stimulates hypersecretion of gastric acid).

Dosage
Adults:
300 mg every 6 hrs. If patient requires an increased dosage, increase the frequency of the 300-mg dose. Do not exceed 2400 mg/day.
In the presence of renal failure—300 mg every 8–12 hrs. Administer at the end of dialysis.
Children:
Use for children under 16 years of age is not recommended (see Precaution no. 3).

Preparation and Storage
Supplied in 2-ml single-dose vials and 8-ml multiple dose vials, each containing 150 mg/ml.

Discard unused portions.
When mixed with fluid, the drug is stable for 48 hours at room temperature.

Drug Incompatibilities
Do not mix in any manner with aminophylline or barbiturates.

Modes of IV Administration

Injection
Yes
Dilute in 20 ml of NS or other compatible fluid and inject over 2 min.

Intermittent Infusion
Yes
Dilute dose in 100 ml of NS, D5W, RL or 5% Sodium Bicarbonate and infuse over 15–20 min.

Continuous Infusion
Yes
Use an appropriate volume of D5W, NS, or RL and add an 8-, 12-, or 24-hour dose or infuse at a rate of 1–4 mg/kg/hr.

Contraindications; Warnings; Precautions; Adverse Reactions

Contraindications
None currently known.

Precautions
1. This drug crosses the placental barrier and should not be used in pregnant women unless in the judgment of the physician, benefits outweigh risks.
2. This drug is excreted in human milk. Nursing should be discontinued while the patient is on therapy.
3. This drug is not recommended for children under 16 years of age unless potential benefits outweigh potential risks. In limited experience, doses of 20–40 mg/kg/day have been used.
4. Confusional states have been observed in elderly or debilitated patients; these have generally cleared within 48 hours after discontinuing drug.
5. Antacids should be given concomitantly for relief of pain.

6. This drug can interact with warfarin-type anticoagulants to further prolong prothrombin time.
7. Blood levels of some benzodiazepine derivatives (theophylline and propranolol) have been reported to increase in patients taking them concomitantly.
8. The effects of the following drugs are potentiated by cimetidine: beta-blocking agents, chlordiazepoxide (Librium), diazepam (Valium), lidocaine, phenytoin (Dilantin), theophylline, and warfarin.

Adverse Reactions
1. Mild, transient diarrhea, muscular pain, dizziness, somnolence and rash.
2. Mild to severe headache, clearing when drug is discontinued.
3. Mild gynecomastia (not associated with alterations in endocrine function).
4. Decreased white blood count, agranulocytosis, thrombocytopenia and aplastic anemia have been reported (rare).
5. Slight increase in plasma creatinine and SGOT (disappears when drug is discontinued).
6. Fever, interstitial nephritis, hepatitis and pancreatitis (clear when drug discontinued).

☐ **Nursing Implications**
1. Reassure the patient as to the transient nature of diarrhea, muscular pain, dizziness, and gynecomastia, if they occur.
2. Take precautions to prevent patient injury if dizziness or confusion are present.
3. For patients who are receiving warfarin-type anticoagulants concomitantly; be aware of prothrombin times and monitor for signs of bleeding from all sites.
4. Emotional tension, particularly repressed anger, frustration, and aggression, has been cited as predisposing to peptic ulcers. Increased emotional stress is known to aggravate pre-existing peptic ulcer.[1] When possible, assist the patient in identifying factors which produce emotional tension in his/her life. Recognition of the existence of tension or stress may lead the patient to constructive management of the problem, which will subsequently assist in healing and preventing recurrence of a peptic ulcer. Assist in referrals to appropriate supportive agencies as needed.

Reference
1. Smith, Dorothy W., and Germain, Carol P. Hanley: *Care of the Adult Patient* (4th ed.), Philadelphia, J. B. Lippincott Company, 1977, p. 737.

cisplatin ■
(Platinol)

Actions/Indications
An antineoplastic agent with properties similar to alkylating agents. Used in palliative therapy of germinal cell malignancies in the following ways:
1. Metastatic testicular malignancies: in established combination therapy with other agents in patients who have already received surgery and/or radiation.
2. Metastatic ovarian malignancies: in established combination therapy with other agents in patients who have already received surgery and/or radiation. Also this drug may be used as secondary therapy in patients who have been refractory to other chemotherapy and have not already received cisplatin.
3. Some groups have also used this drug in the treatment of lymphoma and squamous cell carcinomas of the head and neck.

Excretion is through the kidneys and liver (gastrointestinal tract).

Dosage
The patient should be hydrated with 1–2 liters of fluid as tolerated by in-

cisplatin
(continued)
travenous infusion 8 to 12 hours before the drug is administered.
Adequate hydration and urinary output should also be maintained during the 24 hours after administration of the drug.

As a single agent (Adults & Children)
—100 mg/M² once every 4 weeks.

In testicular tumors—The following *combination regimen* has been effective in producing remissions:
Cisplatin—20 mg/M² once daily intravenously for 5 days (days 1–5) every 3 weeks for 3 courses.
Bleomycin—30 units intravenously weekly (day 2 of each week) for 12 consecutive doses.
Vinblastine—0.15 to 0.20 mg/kg intravenously twice a week (days 1 and 2) every 3 weeks for 4 courses, a total of 8 doses.

Maintenance therapy—For patients who respond to the above:
Vinblastine—0.3 mg/kg intravenously every 4 weeks for a total of 2 years.

In ovarian tumors—The following *combination regimen* has been effective:
Cisplatin—50 mg/M² once every 3 weeks (on day 1).
Doxorubicin—50 mg/M² once every 3 weeks (on day 1).
See information on bleomycin on page 33, doxorubicin on page 135, and vinblastine on page 355.

Repeat courses of this drug should not be attempted until the serum creatinine is below 1.5 mg/100 ml, and/or the BUN is below 25 mg/100 ml, circulating blood elements are at an acceptable level (e.g., platelets > 100,000/mm³, WBC > 4,000/mm³), and until an audiometric analysis shows that the patient's auditory acuity is within normal limits. See Adverse Reactions nos. 1, 2, and 3.

Preparation and Storage
Supplied in 10- and 50-mg vials of drug powder. Store in the refrigerator.
Use gloves when handling this drug; discard syringes and needles carefully to avoid human contact.

When reconstituting or transferring this drug to intravenous fluids, do *not* use needles with aluminum parts. Contact with aluminum will cause a black precipitate formation and loss of drug potency. Stainless steel or brass does not react in this manner.
Reconstitute the 10- and 50-mg vials with 10 ml and 50 ml of sterile water for injection respectively. Each ml of drug will then contain 1 mg. Use only clear, colorless solutions. Use within 20 hours; store at *room* temperature.
To prepare for infusion, add 37.5 gm of mannitol to each of 2 1000-ml bottles of 5% dextrose in 0.45% or 0.33% normal saline. Then to each of these 2 bottles add one half of the total dose of cisplatin. Infuse the 2000 mls over 6 to 8 hours. The mannitol is added to assist in clearing the drug through the kidneys and thus decrease the chances of renal tubular damage. The volume of the infusion may need to be reduced in the presence of cardiac disease to prevent cardiac decompensation. This reduction may then increase the chances of renal damage, however. Some groups concurrently give furosemide in addition to the mannitol to prevent fluid retention and to maintain tubular clearance of the drug. New protocols are published frequently; be familiar with insitutional protocol as it compares to the manufacturer's above.

Drug Incompatibilities
Do not mix with any other medication in any manner.

Modes of IV Administration

Injection
No
Not currently recommended by the manufacturer.

Intermittent Infusion
Yes
Infuse over 6–8 hours. Note specific fluid dilution requirements described under Preparation and Storage. This mode is thought to help reduce nephrotoxicity.

Continuous Infusion
No
Not currently recommended by the manufacturer.

Contraindications; Warnings; Precautions; Adverse Reactions

Contraindications
1. Preexisting renal impairment.
2. In patients with bone marrow suppression.
3. In patients with hearing impairment.

Warnings
1. This drug produces cumulative nephrotoxicity. Obtain serum creatinine, BUN and creatinine clearance before therapy is initiated, and prior to each subsequent course. Do not administer more frequently than every 3 to 4 weeks. Patients who are also receiving gentamicin or cephalothin may be at greater risk of developing renal failure. Damage is usually reversible but can be permanent.
2. Anaphylaxis has occurred, rapid onset type, within a few minutes of administration.
3. Ototoxicity is cumulative. Perform audiometric testing before therapy and prior to each subsequent dose. It is thought that adequate hydration helps to reduce the chances of this reaction.
4. Safety for use in pregnancy has not been established; birth defects and chromosomal changes have been produced in animals.

Precautions
1. Monitor peripheral blood counts weekly.
2. Monitor liver function periodically during therapy.
3. Monitor for neurologic changes (see Adverse Reactions).

Adverse Reactions
1. Nephrotoxicity (renal tubular damage): this is the major dose-limiting toxicity; usually seen in the second week after a dose; becomes more severe and prolonged with repeated courses of therapy. See Warning No. 1. Damage is usually reversible.
2. Ototoxicity: manifested by tinnitus and/or hearing loss (high frequency range); may be more severe in children; can be unilateral or bilateral; becomes more severe with repeated doses; it is unclear whether or not this is reversible.
3. Hematologic: bone marrow suppression in the form of reduced leukocytes and platelets peaks between days 18 to 23, recovery is usually seen by day 39; problem is more pronounced in high doses (> 50 mg/M^2); anemia is also seen in the same frequency and timing as leukopenia and thrombocytopenia.
4. Gastrointestinal: nausea and vomiting; may be severe enough to require discontinuation of the drug; usually begins within 1–4 hours of initiation of the infusion and lasts up to 24 hours; nausea and anorexia may last for up to 1 week.
5. Hyperuricemia: more pronounced with doses greater than 50 mg/M^2; peak levels are seen between 3 to 5 days after administration; allopurinol will control this.
6. Neurotoxicity: peripheral neuropathies, loss of the sense of taste, seizures; therapy should be discontinued at the first appearance of symptoms.
7. Anaphylaxis.
8. Elevated SGOT.

☐ Nursing Implications
1. Be familiar with the other antineoplastic agents that are administered with this drug. See page number references under Dosage.
2. Maintain the hydration regimen prior to each dose as described, and for 24 hours following each dose. This is designed to help prevent renal tubular damage. Encourage a high water intake. Parenteral fluids may be neces-

cisplatin
(continued)

sary if nausea and vomiting are severe. See Adverse Reaction No. 4.

3. Administer antiemetics with the drug to prevent nausea and vomiting; they may be of little value however. Record intake and output to assist in maintaining hydration.

4. Monitor urine output; report oliguria (less than 240 ml in 8 hours for adults). Be familiar with the patient's BUN and creatinine values.

5. Take anaphylaxis precautions. Stay with the patient during the first 15–30 minutes after initiation of the drug infusion. See Appendix.

6. Be aware of audiometric test results prior to each dose. Instruct the patient to report the onset of a hearing problem or ringing in the ears.

7. If the platelet count falls below 500,000/mm^3, observe for all types of bleeding and help the patient to avoid trauma.

8. If the WBC falls below 2,000/mm^3 initiate protective isolation to prevent infection. Monitor temperature every 4 hours and watch for signs of infection.

9. Instruct the patient to report the onset of numbness, tingling, sensory loss, a burning sensation in the extremities, or a loss of the sense of taste. Notify the physician.

10. Seizures can occur in patients with prior history, take precautions.

clindamycin phosphate ■
(Cleocin)

Actions/Indications
Antibiotic, semisynthetic.

Active against susceptible strains of anaerobic bacteria and susceptible strains of gram-positive cocci (streptococci, pneumococci and staphylococci). Used for penicillin-allergic patients and those in whom a penicillin is inappropriate.

Indicated for serious infections in the following sites:
• Respiratory tract (empyema, anaerobic pneumonitis)
• Skin and soft tissue
• Septicemia
• Intra-abdominal cavity (peritonitis or abscess)
• Female pelvis and genital tract (endometritis, nongoncoccal tuboovarian abscess, pelvic cellulitis, vaginal cuff infection)
• Bone and joints (acute hematogenous osteomyelitis)

Dosage
Adults:
Serious infections—600–1200 mg/day in 2, 3, or 4 divided doses.
More severe infections—1200–2700 mg/day in 2, 3, or 4 divided doses.
Life-threatening infections—4.8 gm/day in 2, 3, or 4 divided doses.
The first dose may be given as a single rapid infusion.
Children over One Month of Age:
Serious infections—15–25 mg/kg/day in 3–4 equal doses.
More severe infections—25–40 mg/kg/day in 3–4 doses. (Also square meters of body surface may be used: 350 mg/M^2/day for serious infections, 450 mg/M^2/day for more severe.)

In severe infections, it is advised that the child be given no less than 300 mg/day regardless of body weight.

Not usually recommended for use in newborn infants.

Preparation and Storage
Available in 2-ml ampuls containing 300 mg of drug and 4-ml ampuls containing 600 mg.

Add to any IV fluid.

Store unopened vials at room temperature. Discard unused portions.

Drug Incompatibilities
May be mixed in-line with most other medications and vitamins *except*:
Ampicillin
Phenytoin sodium

Barbiturates
Aminophylline
Calcium gluconate
Magnesium sulfate

Modes of IV Administration

Injection
No
Must be diluted; cardiac arrest has been reported associated with this mode.

Intermittent Infusion
Yes
Dilute with any IV fluid. Minimum volumes and infusion times are as follows:

Dose		Diluent		Time	
300	mg	50	ml	10	min
600	mg	100	ml	20	min
900	mg	150	ml	30	min
1200	mg	200	ml	45	min

Do not give more than 1200 mg (1–2 gm) in a single 1 hour infusion.

Continuous Infusion
No

Contraindications; Warnings; Precautions; Adverse Reactions

Contraindications
Hypersensitivity to clindamycin or lincomycin.

Warnings
1. MAY CAUSE A POSSIBLY FATAL COLITIS. RESERVE THIS DRUG FOR CASES WHERE LESS TOXIC AGENTS ARE INAPPROPRIATE. Discontinue use if diarrhea occurs. Onset varies during therapy to several weeks after. Anti-peristaltic agents such as opiates or diphenoxylate (Lomotil) may prolong or worsen the condition. Simple cases may respond to discontinuation of the drug. Severe cases may respond to corticosteroids (systemic and/or enemas).
2. Do not use for nonbacterial infections.
3. Safe use in pregnancy has not been established.
4. Administer with caution to newborns and infants less than 1 month of age. Monitor renal and hepatic function. Observe for the onset of colitis; discontinue if this occurs.
5. This drug is secreted in breast milk. Nursing should be discontinued while patient is on therapy.
6. Clindamycin does not diffuse adequately enough into the cerebrospinal fluid to be used in the treatment of meningitis.
7. Do not administer concurrently with erythromycin.

Precautions
1. Monitor carefully for onset of diarrhea, especially the elderly or seriously ill.
2. Use with caution in patients with active or past history of gastrointestinal disease.
3. Use with caution in patients with numerous allergies, asthma, hayfever, other drug allergies etc.
4. Use with caution in patients with severe renal or hepatic disease. Monitor serum drug levels during high-dose therapy. Hemo- and peritoneal dialysis do not remove the drug from the blood.
5. During prolonged therapy, monitor renal and hepatic function and blood counts periodically.
6. Monitor for overgrowth infections due to nonsusceptible organisms, especially yeasts.
7. This drug has neuromuscular blocking properties that may potentiate neuromuscular blocking agents such as decamethonium, succinylcholine, d-tubocurarine.

Adverse Reactions
1. Gastrointestinal: nausea, vomiting, diarrhea, abdominal pain, colitis (see Warning No. 1)
2. Hypersensitivity: maculopapular rash and urticaria have been re-

clindamycin phosphate
(continued)
ported; anaphylaxis; rarely, erythema multiforme
3. Hepatic: jaundice and alteration of liver function tests
4. Hematopoietic: leukopenia, eosinophilia, agranulocytosis and thrombocytopenia have been reported.
5. Thrombophlebitis can occur after prolonged infusion
6. Musculoskeletal: polyarthritis (rare)

☐ **Nursing Implications**
1. Monitor for the onset of colitis, from the beginning of therapy through 1 month after termination, i.e., abdominal pain, nausea, vomiting and diarrhea, particularly with passage of mucus or blood. **Constipating drugs are not to be given.** Notify physician at the first suspicion of this complication. Administer corticosteroids as ordered. Maintain hydration orally when possible. Monitor intake and output to assist the physician in planning parenteral fluid replacement. Observe for symptoms of hypokalemia (secondary to diarrhea), e.g., weakness and muscle cramps. Potassium replacement may be necessary (parenterally).
2. Take anaphylaxis precautions; see Appendix.
3. Patients receiving this drug and a neuromuscular blocking agent (see Precaution No. 5) may require respiratory support longer than usual following administration of the neuromuscular blocking agent (see Nursing Implications under individual drugs).
4. Monitor for signs and symptoms of nonsusceptible organism overgrowth infection:
   a. Fever (take rectal temperatures at least every 4–6 hours)
   b. Increasing malaise
   c. Localized signs and symptoms of a newly developing infection: redness, soreness, pain, swelling, drainage (increased volume or change in character of pre-existing drainage)
   d. Cough (change in sputum production)
   e. Diarrhea
   f. Oral lesions (thrush) or perineal rash (monilia) due to *Candida albicans.*
5. Notify the physician at the onset of jaundice.
6. Complete blood counts should be performed during therapy. If the platelet count begins to fall, the drug will probably be discontinued. Bleeding secondary to a low platelet count usually begins if the count falls below 100,000/cu mm. If this occurs, monitor for bleeding and avoid invasive procedures.
   If the white blood cell count decreases, the drug may be discontinued. Infections secondary to a low white count usually occur only if the count reaches 2000/cu mm or less. If this occurs (it rarely does), place the patient in protective (reverse) isolation, monitor for infection, avoid invasive procedures and maintain bodily (especially perineal) cleanliness.
7. To reduce risk of thrombophlebitis, rotate the cannula insertion site every 48–72 hours. Monitor for signs and symptoms of thrombophlebitis at the infusion site, e.g., redness, swelling and pain along the vein tract. If these appear, discontinue the infusion and use another vein. Apply warm compresses and elevate the extremity until symptoms subside. Do not use this extremity for venipunctures until the phlebitis resolves.

corticotropin ■
(Adrenocorticotropic Hormone, A.C.T.H., Acthar)

Actions/Indications
Anterior pituitary hormone; stimulates the functioning adrenal cortex

to produce and secrete the adrenalcortical hormone: cortisol (the major glucocorticoid) and aldosterone (the mineralocorticoid).

Intravenous mode is used in the diagnostic testing of adrenocortical function.

Dosage
Adults:
Diagnostic—10–25 units infused over 8 hrs.

See Nursing Implications section for interpretation of test results.

Preparation and Storage
Available as a powder in vials containing 25 or 40 units of the drug. Reconstitute by adding sterile water for injection or NS in the following amounts:
25-unit vial: 1 ml.
40-unit vial: 2 ml.

Refrigerate reconstituted solution and use within 24 hours.
Be Certain That Brand And Preparation Being Used Are For Intravenous Use Only; Do NOT Use Repository Gel.

Drug Incompatibilities
Do not mix in any manner with:
Aminophylline,
Novobiocin,
Sodium bicarbonate.

Modes of IV Administration

Injection
No
Maximum diagnostic effects are only obtained via continuous infusion.

Intermittent Infusion
Yes
Add dose to 500–1000 ml D5W; infuse over 8 hrs. (May also use NS for infusion.)

Continuous Infusion
No

Contraindications; Warnings; Precautions; Adverse Reactions

Contraindications
1. Scleroderma
2. Osteoporosis
3. Systemic fungal infections
4. Ocular herpes simplex
5. Recent surgery
6. History or presence of peptic ulcer
7. Congestive heart failure
8. Hypertension
9. Sensitivity to pork, beef or equine products (check the origin of the preparation used)

Warnings
1. Safety for use in pregnancy has not been established; may cause fetal abnormalities.
2. Can cause: retention of sodium and water, an increased excretion of potassium and calcium, and elevation of blood pressure.
3. The usual difficulties encountered with prolonged steroid therapy do not apply when this drug is used for diagnostic purposes, except for those effects listed above.

Precautions
1. Perform a skin test with this drug prior to administration to patients with suspected hypersensitivity to pork, beef or equine products, depending on preparation used.
2. Observe all patients carefully for allergic reactions.
3. There is an enhanced effect of this drug in patients with hypothyroidism and in those with cirrhosis.

Adverse Reactions in Short-Term Intravenous Use
1. Hypersensitivity: dizziness, nausea, vomiting, shock, skin reactions
2. Fluid and electrolyte disturbances, e.g., sodium retention, water retention, potassium loss, calcium loss
3. Cardiac: precipitation of congestive heart failure due to sodium and fluid retention
4. Endocrine: rise in blood glucose, increased requirement for insulin or oral hypoglycemic agents

corticotropin
(continued)
5. Neurologic:
   a. Increased intracranial pressure
   b. Seizures (increasing frequency in patients with pre-existing seizure disorder)
6. Eye: Increased intraocular pressure

□ **Nursing Implications**
When This Drug Is Used as a Diagnostic Agent:
1. Perform skin testing on all individuals suspected of pork, beef or equine allergy.
2. Monitor for signs of allergic reaction; take anaphylaxis precautions (see Appendix).
3. When used as a diagnostic agent, adrenal responsiveness to this drug will produce a rise in urinary and plasma corticosteroid levels. Obtain a 24-hour urine for 17-ketosteroids and 17-hydroxyketosteroids before and after testing period. Normal response is 3–5 times an increase on the first day of the test infusion, and further increases on successive days if testing is continued.

cosyntropin ■
(Cortrosyn)

Actions/Indications
A diagnostic agent, synthetic subunit of ACTH. Acts as a corticosteroid stimulating agent in the same manner as ACTH.
   Used to diagnose patients with primary adrenocortical insufficiency. Can be used to perform a 30-min test where cosyntropin is injected and plasma cortisol levels are determined as response. To be used solely for diagnosis.

Dosage
Usual test dose for adults and children over 2 years: 0.25–0.75 mg.
Children Under 2 Years: 0.125 mg
   The most convenient test method is as follows:

1. Control blood sample taken for basal cortisol level
2. The above dose of the drug is injected intravenously.
3. In exactly 30 min a second blood sample is taken and both are refrigerated. (Some sources advocate that the second blood sample be taken after 60 min.)
4. In an alternative test technique the dosage of drug is infused at a rate of 40 mcg/hour, after an initial blood sample is taken. A second blood sample is taken at the end of the infusion.

The normal cortisol response is:
1. Control cortisol level is greater than 5 mcg/100 ml.
2. 30-min level should then be at least 7 mcg/100 ml greater than control, and exceed 18 mcg/100 ml. A response in cortisol levels less than this can indicate adrenocortical insufficiency. This test can be performed any time of day as long as the 30-min technique is used.
3. If the dose has been given by the infusion technique, the above response criteria do not apply.

Preparation and Storage
Read package insert to confirm that preparation being used can be given INTRAVENOUSLY.
   Reconstitute using diluent provided by the manufacturer. Concentration of resulting solution is 0.25 mg/ml.
   Store unopened vials at room temperature. Refrigerate reconstituted solutions and use within 48 hours. Use infusion solutions within 12 hours. Cosyntropin 0.25 mg is equivalent to 25 U.S.P. units of corticotropin.

Drug Incompatibilities
Do not add to blood or plasma.

Modes of IV Administration

Injection
Yes
Inject over 2-min period.

Intermittent Infusion
Yes
Use D5W or NS. Infuse dose at a rate of 40 mcg/hour. Use any desired volume. Plasma cortisol levels are taken before and immediately after infusion.

Continuous Infusion
No

Contraindications; Warnings; Precautions; Adverse Reactions

Contraindications
History of previous adverse reaction to this drug

Precautions
1. Patients receiving cortisone, hydrocortisone or spironolactone should omit their pretest doses on the day of testing.
2. In patients with raised bilirubin or with free hemoglobin in the plasma, falsely high fluorescence measurements will result.
3. Hypersensitivity reactions can occur in susceptible patients.

Adverse Reactions
Adverse reactions have rarely been reported; those known have been hypersensitivity reactions in patients with known pre-existing allergic disease and/or a previous reaction to natural ACTH.

☐ Nursing Implications
1. Assist in obtaining an accurate allergy history.
2. Determine if the patient and/or parents fully understand the purpose and technique of the test; supplement information as necessary.
3. Monitor patients closely during the injection or infusion and for at least 1 hour following. Make note of any sign of allergic reaction from erythema around the injection site to overt manifestations of hypersensitivity, e.g., urticaria, itching, cough, tightness in the chest, wheezing, hypotension.
4. Be prepared with drugs and respiratory support equipment to treat an allergic reaction.
5. Assist in interpretation of the test results and their significance to the patient and/or parents.

cyclophosphamide ■
(Cytoxan, Endoxan)

Actions/Indications
Antineoplastic agent, interferes with growth of neoplastic cells; the mechanism of action is unknown.
Indicated in:
• Malignant lymphomas, primary drug in induction and maintenance therapy. (Stages III and IV Hodgkin's lymphosarcomas, histiocytic lymphoma, etc.)
• Multiple myeloma
• Chronic and acute leukemias (to induce and maintain remissions)
• Mycosis fungoides
• Some solid tumors (disseminated neuroblastoma, adenocarcinoma of the ovary,retinoblastoma, oat cell lung carcinoma)

Dosage
Adults and Children:
Induction of Remission—40–50 mg/kg usually given in divided doses over 2–5 days.
Patients with bone marrow depression due to drugs, x-ray therapy, or tumor infiltration should have a dose reduced by 1/3 to 1/2.
Maintenance—A variety of schedules have been suggested: 10–15 mg/kg every 7–10 days or 3–5 mg/kg twice weekly or 50 mg/kg every 3–4 weeks.
The largest dose tolerated by the patient is usually given. Children may tolerate larger doses than adults. The total leukocyte count can be used to guide dosage. A suppression of the WBC to 3000–4000 cells/cu mm can be tolerated by most patients. (See Adverse Reactions, No. 1.)

Preparation and Storage
Available in vials containing 100 mg, 200 mg and 500 mg of drug.

cyclophosphamide
(continued)

To reconstitute powder, use sterile water for injection or bacteriostatic water for injection (paraben preserved only), in the following amounts:
100-mg vial: 5 ml.
200-mg vial: 10 ml.
500-mg vial: 25 ml.

Resulting solution contains 20 mg/ml. Shake vial to dissolve; do not heat. Discard reconstituted solution after 24 hours if unrefrigerated, or 6 days if stored in the refrigerator. If the solution does not contain a bacteriostatic agent, care must be taken during preparation to maintain sterility.

Drug Incompatibilities
Do not mix with any other medication in any manner.

Modes of IV Administration

Injection
Yes
A solution of 20 mg/ml can be given without further dilution.

Intermittent Infusion
Yes
Add dose to 100–500 ml D5W, NS or D5/NS and infuse over 1 hr.

Continuous Infusion
No

Contraindications; Warnings; Precautions; Adverse Reactions

Contraindications
None currently known. See Warning No. 7.

Warnings
1. In patients who are postadrenalectomy, adjustment of the doses of both replacement steroids and cyclophosphamide may be necessary to prevent toxicity due to the cyclophosphamide.
2. The rate of metabolism and the leukopenic activity of this drug are increased by chronic administration of phenobarbital. Combined drug actions may occur with other agents.
3. This drug may interfere with normal wound healing.
4. This drug can cause fetal abnormalities. Do not use in pregnancy, especially the first trimester, unless potential benefits outweigh risks to the fetus.
5. Cyclophosphamide is excreted in human milk. Breast-feeding must be discontinued prior to instituting therapy.
6. Both male and female patients capable of conception must be warned of the possibility of the drug producing mutations in germinal cells. Contraception is advisable during therapy.
7. This drug suppresses lymphocyte formation and this is a powerful immunosuppressant. This fact contraindicates concomitant, though not subsequent, immunotherapy.[1]

Precautions
1. Administer with caution in the presence of
   a. Pre-existing leukopenia
   b. Thrombocytopenia
   c. Bone marrow infiltration by tumor cells
   d. Previous x-ray therapy
   e. Previous therapy with other cytotoxic agents
   f. Impaired hepatic function
   g. Impaired renal function; these patients will require reduction in dosage to prevent oversuppression of the bone marrow.
2. Cyclophosphamide suppresses immunologic responses to infection. Dosage must be modified in the event of bacterial, fungal or viral infections. This is especially true in patients with concomitant or recent steroid therapy.

Adverse Reactions
1. Secondary malignancies have been reported in association with cyclophosphamide (bladder, myeloproliferative and lym-

phoproliferative). These have been detected up to 2 years after drug was discontinued.

2. Hematopoietic: Leukopenia is expected due to bone marrow suppression, and is used as a guide to dosage. Leukocyte count should be kept between 3000–5000. Low WBC usually occurs 9–14 days after the first dose and returns to normal 7–14 days after cessation of therapy. Thrombocytopenia and anemia may also occur. These effects are reversible when therapy is discontinued.[2] Hemolytic anemia (negative Coombs' test) has been reported.

3. Gastrointestinal: Anorexia, nausea, vomiting are common and dose-related. Hemorrhagic colitis, oral mucosal ulceration, and jaundice have also been reported. Hepatitis may occur and is indicated by hyperbilirubinemia.

4. Genitourinary: Sterile hemorrhagic cystitis can occur and has been fatal. Nonhemorrhagic cystitis has also been reported. Both forms may be prevented with ample fluid intake and frequent voiding to flush the bladder of drug metabolites.

   If either occur, therapy should be interrupted. Hematuria may disappear from 2 days to several months after cessation of therapy. Blood replacement or iron therapy may be necessary. Electrocautery, urinary diversion or cryosurgery may also be required.

   Nephrotoxicity as indicated by rising BUN and creatinine has been seen. There may be drug-induced dilutional hyponatremia. Irreversible amenorrhea and absence of sperm production have been reported. Cyclophosphamide affects prepuberal gonads. Adult females may have false-positive Pap tests.

5. Skin and soft tissue: Hair loss (50% of patients on IV therapy),[3] darkening of skin and fingernails and nonspecific dermatitis have been seen.

6. Pulmonary: Interstitial fibrosis can be seen in cases where high doses are administered over a long period of time. This may be irreversible.[4]

7. Cardiotoxicity: With doses greater than 50 mg/kg, congestive heart failure has been seen. This drug may also potentiate the cardiotoxicity of daunomycin and doxorubicin. If the agents are administered concomitantly with cyclophosphamide, their total dose should not exceed 450 mg/M^2.

   Impaired water excretion may also precipitate acute congestive heart failure in susceptible patients.[5,6]

☐ **Nursing Implications**

1. The patient receiving this medication will be experiencing the emotional and physical effects of the malignancy. Knowledge of the patient's feelings about his disease and its implications will assist in helping him tolerate the chemotherapy. The incidence of uncomfortable side effects and adverse reactions is high. It is within the nurse's role to assist the patient in coping with the discomforts of the disease and its treatment, and to help him work through depression and anger toward acceptance of the disease at his own pace. Despite the unpleasantness this drug may bring, it can be a source of hope for the patient.

2. Many patients experience fewer injection side effects when they are placed in a prone or reclining position during the administration of this drug.

3. Management of hematologic effects:
   a. Be aware of the patient's white blood cell and platelet counts prior to each injection.
   b. If the WBC falls to 2000/cu mm, take measures to protect the patient from infection such as protective

cyclophosphamide
(continued)

(reverse) isolation, avoidance of invasive procedures, maintenance of bodily (especially perineal) cleanliness, carrying out strict urinary catheter care when appropriate, etc. Monitor for infection by recording temperatures every 4 hours, examining for rashes, swellings, drainage and pain. Explain these measures to the patient.

c. If the platelet count falls below 100,000/cu mm, monitor for thrombocytopenic bleeding: petechiae, purpura, hematuria, melena, blood in stools, gum bleeding, vaginal bleeding, epistaxis, hematemesis, etc. Avoid trauma. Transfusions may be ordered.

d. Instruct the patient and family on the importance of follow-up blood studies if the drug is being administered on an outpatient basis.

e. Patients who develop anemia are often given iron and B vitamin supplements. Decreased exercise tolerance and fatigue are frequently seen in cancer patients, as is anemia (not secondary to drugs). This can be depressing. Assist the patient in developing a daily plan of rest and activity, encourage adequate diet, and allow time for him to discuss frustration.

4. Management of nausea and vomiting:

a. Usually occurs 1–3 hours after injection. Vomiting may subside after 8 hours, but nausea can persist for 24 hours.

b. Administer this drug at night if possible to correlate with normal sleep pattern, accompanied by sedation and an antiemetic drug to combat these side effects.

c. To be effective, antiemetics should be administered 1 hour prior to the injection of the drug.

d. Small frequent meals, timed with periods when the patient feels his best, are advisable. Bland foods are usually tolerated. Carbohydrate and protein content should be high.

e. If the patient is anorexic, encourage high nutrient liquids and water to maintain hydration.

f. Keep accurate measurements of emesis volume and total intake and output to guide the physician in ordering parenteral fluids when necessary.

g. Administer antacids as ordered. Monitor for onset of diarrhea and gastrointestinal bleeding.

5. Thrombophlebitis can occur at the injection site. Notify the physician at onset. Apply warm compresses as ordered; elevate the extremity. Protect the area from trauma. Avoid extravasation; if it occurs, apply warm compresses until symptoms (burning pain) subside. Monitor the area for tissue sloughing. See Appendix.

6. Management of hair loss:

a. Use scalp tourniquet during injection if ordered to help prevent hair loss.

b. Counsel the patient on the possibility of hair loss to enable him to prepare for this disfigurement.

c. Reassure him of regrowth of hair following discontinuation of the drug.

d. Provide privacy and time for the patient to discuss his feelings.

7. Management of stomatitis:

a. Administer preventive oral care every 4 hours and/or after meals.

b. For preventive care use a very soft toothbrush (child's) and toothpaste; avoid trauma to tissues.

c. Examine oral membranes at least daily (instruct patient and/or family) to detect the onset of inflammation or ulceration.

d. If stomatitis occurs, notify the physician and begin therapeutic oral care.

e. Order a mechanical soft, bland diet for patients with mild inflammation. If the stomatitis is severe, the patient may be placed on a liquid diet or NPO status by the physician.

f. For patients who can tolerate oral intake, administer Xylocaine Viscous or acetaminophen elixir as a mouthwash prior to meals to decrease pain (do not use aspirin rinses), as ordered by the physician.

g. Patients with severe stomatitis may require parenteral analgesia.

8. Monitor for jaundice; notify the physician at onset.

9. See Adverse Reaction No. 7, cardiotoxicity. If the patient is receiving a dose greater than 50 mg/kg or has pre-existing heart disease, monitor for the onset of congestive heart failure: decreased exercise tolerance, fatigue, shortness of breath, dyspnea, increased respiratory rate, rales, increased resting heart rate, peripheral pitting edema. Notify the physician of these findings when they are noted.

10. Assist in preventing cystitis by ensuring a high fluid intake (preferably water), to keep the bladder flushed of drug metabolites. For the anorexic or vomiting patient, administer antiemetics as described in No. 4. Intravenous infusions may be necessary for the patient who cannot maintain a high fluid intake. Encourage voiding every 2—3 hours to keep the bladder empty. Inform the patient as to the rationale for this intervention. The symptoms of chemi- cally induced cystitis include frequency, urgency, pain on urination and hematuria.

11. Pulmonary fibrosis can occur in patients receiving long-term or high-dose therapy. The time of onset varies but can be long after the drug has been discontinued. Symptoms include cough, shortness of breath and changes in the chest x-ray. Report the onset of any one of these to the physician. Instruct the patient and/or family to do the same if the patient is at home.

References

1. Marsh, John C., and Mitchell, Malcom S.: Chemotherapy of Cancer, II.: Drugs in Current use. In *Drug Therapy*, (Hospital Edition), October 1976, p. 43.
2. Silver, Richard T., Lauper, R. David, and Jarwoski, Charles: *A Synopsis of Cancer Chemotherapy*, The York Medical Group, New York, Dun-Donnelly Publishing Company, 1977, p. 17.
3. Ibid.
4. Rosenow, E. C.: The Spectrum of Drug-Induced Pulmonary Disease. *Annals of Internal Medicine*, 77(6):978, December 1972.
5. Chabner, Bruce A., et al.: The Clinical Pharmacology of Antineoplastic Agents. *New England Journal of Medicine*, 292(22):1167, May 29, 1975.
6. Marsh and Mitchell, p. 43.

Suggested Readings

Bolin, Rose Homan, and Auld, Margaret E.: Hodgkin's Disease. *American Journal of Nursing*, 74(11):1982–1986, November 1974.

Bruya, Margaret Auld, and Madeira, Nancy Powell: Stomatitis After Chemotherapy. *American Journal of Nursing*, 75(8):1349–1352, August 1975 (references).

Donely, Diana L.: Nursing the Patient Who is Immunosuppressed. *American Journal of Nursing*, 76(10):1619–1625, October 1976 (references).

Laatsch, Nancy: Nursing the Woman

cyclophosphamide
(continued)

Receiving Adjuvant Chemotherapy of Breast Cancer. *Nursing Clinics of North America*, 13(2):337–349, June 1978.

LeBlanc, Donna Harris: People with Hodgkin's Disease: The Nursing Challenge. *Nursing Clinics of North America*, 13(2):281–300, June 1978.

Schumann, Delores, and Patterson, Phyllis: Multiple Myeloma. *American Journal of Nursing*, 75(1):78–81, January 1975 (references).

Showfety, Mary Patricia: The Ordeal of Hodgkin's Disease. *American Journal of Nursing*, 74(11):1987–1991, November 1974.

Sovik, Corinne: The Nursing Care of Lung Cancer Patients (Emphasizing Chemotherapy). *Nursing Clinics of North America*, 13(2):301–317, June 1978.

cytarabine ■
(Cytosine Arabinoside, Ara-C, Cytosar U)

Actions/Indications
Antineoplastic agent of the antimetabolite (cell-cycle specific) type with cytotoxic effects limited to those tissues with high rates of cellular proliferation, e.g., bone marrow.

Currently used for induction and maintenance of remission in patients with acute and chronic leukemias, myeloblastic and lymphoblastic forms. Primary use is in acute myelocytic leukemia in adults and children.

Some response has also been seen in patients with lymphomas and Hodgkin's disease.

It may be used alone or in combination with other antineoplastic agents, the latter often producing the best results.

Dosage
The dosage schedule and method of administration are highly variable according to the type of leukemia and program of therapy being used. Some dosages are based on the patient's weight and others on body surface area. A common dosage schedule is as follows:

Adults and Children:
Initial rapid injection—2 mg/kg/day for 10 days. Continue until blood count shows antileukemic effect or toxicity (see Adverse Reactions).

If after 10 days there is no effect, increase dose to 4 mg/kg/day, maintain until antileukemic or toxic effect is seen.

Alternate method of administration: Infusion—0.5–1.0 mg/kg/day in 1-, 4-, 12- or 24-hour infusions. Continue for 10 days. If no response, increase to 2.0 mg/kg/day and treat until toxicity or remission is evident.

Maintenance—All remissions must be maintained with periodic injections—1 mg/kg weekly or semiweekly. (This drug is sometimes combined with thioguanine or daunomycin HCl.)

See Precaution No. 1.

Safety for use in infants has not been established.

Preparation and Storage
Available in multidose vials containing 100 mg and 500 mg of drug.

To reconstitute from powder add *bacteriostatic water for injection* in the following amounts:

100-mg vial: 5 ml diluent (resulting solution is 20 mg/ml).

500-mg vial: 10 ml diluent (resulting solution is 50 mg/ml).

Store at room temperature and discard after 48 hours or if solution develops a haze.

Drug Incompatibilities
Do not mix with any other medication in any manner.

Modes of IV Administration

Injection
Yes
Reconstituted solutions can be injected without further dilution. Inject over 2–3 min. See Dosage section.

Flush vein with NS (10–20 ml) after injection.

Intermittent Infusion
Yes
1-hr infusions are most convenient means of administration. Use D5W or NS in any convenient volume.
  Flush vein with NS (10–20 ml) after infusion.

Continuous Infusion
Yes
Add 24-hr dose to 1000 ml D5W or NS and infuse over 24 hours.
  Flush vein with NS (10–20 ml) after infusion.

Contraindications; Warnings; Precautions; Adverse Reactions

Contraindications
Hypersensitivity to the drug

Warnings
1. This drug is a potent bone marrow suppressant. Therapy should be started cautiously in patients with pre-existing drug-induced bone marrow depression. Leukocyte and platelet counts and bone marrow examinations should be performed frequently during therapy.
2. Cytarabine has potential for producing fetal abnormalities when given during pregnancy, especially the first trimester. This drug should not be used in pregnancy unless the expected benefits outweigh potential risks to the mother and fetus.
3. Anaphylaxis has been reported.

Precautions
1. Therapy should be suspended, or modified, when drug-induced marrow depression results in a platelet count under 50,000/cu mm or a white cell count under 1000/cu mm. Cell counts may continue to fall and may reach lowest level 12–24 days after discontinuation. Restart therapy when there are signs of marrow recovery and above cell counts are reached and exceeded. **Do not wait for cell counts to return to normal.**

2. Nausea and vomiting frequently occurs several hours post-injection. These symptoms may be less severe if drug is given by infusion rather than injection.
3. Use with caution and at reduced dosage in the presence of hepatic impairment. (This drug is detoxified by the liver.) May cause further hepatic impairment. If liver enzyme levels are significantly elevated, the drug should be discontinued.
4. Monitor renal function during therapy.
5. Safety for use in infants has not been established.
6. Hyperuricemia may occur secondary to lysis of neoplastic cells.

Adverse Reactions
A. *Expected*
  Blood dyscrasias secondary to bone marrow suppression including: leukopenia, anemia, thrombocytopenia, megaloblastosis and reduced reticulocytes (see Precaution No. 1)
B. *Most Frequent Reactions*
  1. Nausea and vomiting (most frequent after rapid injection; very common in children)
  2. Diarrhea
  3. Inflammation or ulceration of oral and anal membranes
  4. Hepatic dysfunction: elevated liver enzymes
  5. Fever, rash
  6. Thrombophlebitis at injection site
  7. Bleeding (all sites)
C. *Less Frequent Reactions*
  1. Sepsis
  2. Pneumonia
  3. Cellulitis at injection site
  4. Skin ulceration
  5. Urinary retention, renal dysfunction
  6. Sore throat, esophageal inflammation or ulceration
  7. Chest or abdominal pain
  8. Freckling
  9. Jaundice
  10. Conjunctivitis

cytarabine
(continued)
11. Dizziness
12. Alopecia (hair loss)
13. Anaphylaxis

☐ **Nursing Implications**
1. The patient receiving this medication will be experiencing the emotional and physical effects of the malignancy. Knowledge of the patient's feelings about his disease and its implications will assist in helping him tolerate the chemotherapy. The incidence of uncomfortable side effects and adverse reactions is high. It is within the nurse's role to assist the patient in coping with the discomforts of the disease and its treatment, and to help him work through depression and anger toward acceptance of the disease at his own pace. Despite the unpleasantness this drug may bring, it can be a source of hope for the patient.
2. Take all precautions to prevent extravasation; see Appendix.
3. Management of nausea and vomiting:
   a. Administer this drug by slow (1–8 hours or continuous) infusion to decrease these side effects, unless this method is deemed undesirable by the physician.
   b. If nausea and vomiting occur, administer antiemetics at frequency ordered and time doses for 1 hour prior to meals.
   c. Small frequent meals, timed with periods when the patient feels his best, are advisable. Bland foods are usually tolerated more readily by a patient who is anorexic or nauseated. Carbohydrate and protein content should be high.
   d. If the patient is totally anorexic, encourage high nutrient liquids and water to maintain hydration and to avoid complications of hyperuricemia.
   e. Keep accurate measurements of emesis volume and total intake and output to guide the physician in ordering parenteral fluids when necessary.
4. Management of hematologic effects:
   a. See Precaution No. 1.
   b. Be aware of the patient's white blood cell and platelet count prior to each injection.
   c. If WBC falls to 2000/cu mm, take measures to protect the patient from infection such as protective (reverse) isolation, avoid invasive procedures, maintain bodily (especially perineal) cleanliness, carry out strict urinary catheter care when appropriate. Monitor for infection by recording temperatures every 4 hours, examining for rashes, swellings, drainage and pain. Explain these measures to the patient.
   d. If platelet count falls below 100,000/cu mm, monitor for thrombocytopenic bleeding: petechiae, purpura, hematuria, melena, blood in stools, gum bleeding, oozing from an incision, vaginal bleeding, epistaxis, hematemesis, etc. Avoid trauma. Transfusions may be ordered.
   e. Instruct patient and family of importance of follow-up blood work and the reporting of the signs and symptoms listed above in "c" and "d" if the drug is being administered on an outpatient basis.
5. Thrombophlebitis can occur at the injection site. Notify the physician at onset; apply warm compresses as ordered and elevate the extremity. Protect the area from trauma.
6. Management of hair loss:

a. Use a scalp tourniquet during rapid injection or short-term infusion, if ordered, to help prevent hair loss.

b. Counsel the patient on the possibility of hair loss to enable him to prepare for this disfigurement.

c. Reassure him as to the possibility of regrowth of hair following discontinuation of the drug.

d. Provide privacy and time for the patient to discuss his feelings.

7. Management of stomatitis and esophagitis:

a. Monitor for symptoms of esophagitis, e.g., burning chest pain, pain in the throat, pain on swallowing. Administer antacids as ordered. A bland, mechanical soft diet is advisable. Avoid irritating liquids such as fruit juice.

b. Administer preventive oral care every 4 hours and after meals.

c. For preventive care use a soft toothbrush (child's) and toothpaste; avoid trauma to tissues.

d. Examine oral membranes at least daily (instruct family) to detect onset of inflammation and erythema.

e. If stomatitis occurs, notify the physician and carry out therapeutic oral care.

f. For stomatitis, order a bland, mechanical soft diet. If inflammation is severe and accompanied by ulceration of oral membranes, the patient may be placed on NPO status by the physician.

g. For patients who can tolerate oral intake, administer Xylocaine Viscous or acetaminophen elixir as a mouthwash prior to meals to decrease pain (do not use aspirin rinses), as ordered by the physician.

h. Patients with severe stomatitis may require parenteral analgesia.

Suggested Readings

Bolin, Rose Homan, and Auld, Margaret E.: Hodgkin's Disease. *American Journal of Nursing*, November 1974, pp. 1982–1986.

Bruya, Margaret Auld, and Madeira, Nancy Powell: Stomatitis After Chemotherapy. *American Journal of Nursing*, 75(8):1349–1352, August 1975.

Foley, Genevieve V., and McCarthy, Ann Marie: The Child with Leukemia in a Special Hematology Clinic. *American Journal of Nursing*, July 1976, pp. 1115–1119.

———The Disease (Hodgkin's) and Its Treatment, *American Journal of Nursing*. July 1976, pp. 1109–1114 (references).

Giadquinta, Barbara: Helping Families Face the Crisis of Cancer. *American Journal of Nursing*, October 1977, pp. 1583–1588.

Gullo, Shirley: Chemotherapy—What To Do About Special Side Effects. *R.N*, April 1977, pp. 30–32.

Hannan, Jeanne Ferguson: Talking is Treatment, Too. *American Journal of Nursing*, November 1974, pp. 1991–1992.

Martinson, Ida: The Child With Leukemia: Parents Help Each Other: *American Journal of Nursing*, July 1976, pp. 1120–1121.

Showfety, Mary Patricia: The Ordeal of Hodgkin's Disease: *American Journal of Nursing*, November 1974, pp. 1987–1991.

dacarbazine ■
(DTIC-Dome, Imidazole Carboxamide)

Actions/Indications

Antineoplastic agent, acts as an alkylating agent.

Indicated primarily in the treatment of metastatic malignant melanoma (20% response rate). Also used in Hodgkin's disease. Use in combination with other chemotherapeutic agents has often shown

dacarbazine
(continued)
an improved response over use of single agent.

Dosage
Adults:
2.0–4.5 mg/kg/day for 10 days repeated every 4 weeks, or 250 mg/M^2/day for 5 days repeated every 2–3 weeks.
(Dosage should be reduced in the presence of renal impairment.)

Preparation and Storage
Available in vials containing 100 mg or 200 mg of drug.
Reconstitute from powder with sterile water for injection or NS in the following amounts:
100-mg vial: 9.9 ml
200-mg vial: 19.7 ml
The resulting solutions contain 10 mg/ml.
If stored at room temperature, discard after 8 hours; if refrigerated discard after 72 hours.

Drug Incompatibilities
Do not mix with any other medication.

Modes of IV Administration

Injection
Yes
Prepared solution (see Preparation section) may be injected without further dilution, over 1 min.

Intermittent Infusion
Yes
Add dose to 50–100 ml D5W or NS and infuse over 30 min.

Continuous Infusion
No

Contraindications; Warnings; Precautions; Adverse Reactions

Contraindications
Hypersensitivity to dacarbazine

Warnings
1. This drug causes bone marrow suppression that results primarily in reduction in leukocytes and platelets, although mild anemia may also occur. Suppression may be serious enough to cause death.
2. Hepatic toxicity with necrosis can be rarely seen in advanced stages of malignancy when (a) other anti-neoplastic agents are given concomitantly or (b) in the presence of preexisting liver disease.
3. Anaphylaxis can occur.
4. Safety for use in pregnancy has not been established; this drug causes fetal abnormalities in animals.

Precautions
1. The hematopoietic system must be closely monitored during therapy.
2. Extravasation of this drug into the tissues may cause local tissue damage and severe pain.

Adverse Reactions
1. Bone marrow suppression: leukopenia usually occurs 10 days after the first injection, and thrombocytopenia 10–15 days after. These may continue 2–4 weeks after the last dose.
2. Nausea and vomiting: most patients experience these to some degree, usually within 1 hour of adminstration, persisting for up to 12 hours. These effects may decrease after 1–2 days of therapy. Phenobarbital and/or prochlorperazine may relieve these symptoms. Intractable nausea and vomiting may necessitate discontinuation of the drug.
3. Diarrhea: (rare) restricting oral intake 4–6 hours prior to an injection may help to avoid this problem, which usually subsides after 1–2 days of therapy.
4. Flulike syndrome: fever, muscle aches, malaise occur usually 7 days after an injection, and may persist for 7–21 days. This may recur with successive courses of the drug.
5. Abnormal kidney and liver function tests (transient and rarely seen)

6. Hair loss
7. Facial flushing
8. Mental depression (rare)
9. Erythematous and urticarial rashes
10. Photosensitivity

☐ **Nursing Implications**

1. Take anaphylaxis precautions. See Appendix.
2. The patient receiving this medication will be experiencing the emotional and physical effects of the malignancy. Knowledge of the patient's feelings about his disease and its implications will assist in helping him tolerate the chemotherapy. The incidence of uncomfortable side effects and adverse reactions is high. It is within the nurse's role to assist the patient in coping with the discomforts of the disease and its treatment, and to help him work through depression and anger toward acceptance of the disease at his own pace. Despite the unpleasantness this drug may bring, it can be a source of hope for the patient.
3. Be aware of the patient's WBC (leukocyte count). If it falls below 2000/cu mm, the drug may be discontinued. Protective (reverse) isolation may be advisable at this time to help prevent infection. Avoid procedures that produce breaks in the skin or mucous membranes, such as intramuscular injections, catheterizations, etc. These could be a source of infection. Monitor for signs and symptoms of infection until white cell count returns to normal.
4. Be aware of the patient's platelet count. Bleeding may occur if the count falls below 50,000/cu mm (normal is 200,000 to 400,000/cu mm). Examine for purpura (purple blotches in the skin that do not blanch on pressure). Monitor for all other signs of bleeding, e.g. melena, hematemesis, hematuria, oozing from an incision, epistaxis, etc.,

and notify the physician of these lesions or other signs. The patient will probably be given transfusions of fresh whole blood or platelets to alleviate the thrombocytopenia. The drug is usually withheld if the platelet count reaches 50,000/cu mm, and restarted when the level returns to a normal range.
5. Antiemetics can be given prior to the injection of the drug to help control nausea and vomiting (phenobarbital, prochlorperazine, or chlorpromazine). These agents are not effective in some patients. Antiemetics can also be given prior to meals if necessary. Assist in maintaining adequate fluid intake, orally if possible, or intravenously if oral intake is limited. The drug is usually discontinued if vomiting is uncontrollable. In some patients, nausea and vomiting improve after several doses of dacarbazine.
6. If diarrhea occurs following the injection, restrict oral intake for 4–6 hours prior to the next infusion. Lomotil may be used if necessary. Maintain hydration with oral or intravenous fluids. Hypokalemia may occur if diarrhea is severe. This side effect may also subside after 1–2 days of therapy.
7. Prevent extravasation; see Appendix. If it occurs, apply warm compresses for 2 hours initially, and for 20–30 minutes every 4 hours until pain and redness subside. Protect the tissue from damage. Necrosis and sloughing may occur.
8. Management of hair loss:
   a. Use scalp tourniquet during injection, if ordered, to help prevent hair loss.
   b. Counsel the patient on the possibility of hair loss to enable him to prepare for this disfigurement.
   c. Reassure him of regrowth of hair following discontinuation of the drug.

dacarbazine
(continued)
  d. Provide privacy and time for the patient to discuss his feelings.

Suggested Readings
Donley, Diana L.: Nursing the Patient Who Is Immunosuppressed. *American Journal of Nursing*, 76(10):1619–1925, October 1976 (references).
Schumann, Delores: Multiple Myeloma. *American Journal of Nursing*, 75(1):78–81, January 1975 (references).

dactinomycin ■
(Cosmegen, ACT-D, Actinomycin-D, DACT)

Actions/Indications
An actinomycin antibiotic, antineoplastic agent, cell-cycle specific.

Recommended *only* in the treatment of hospitalized patients with Wilms' tumor (a malignant tumor of the kidney region with metastases to the lungs and lymph), rhabdomyosarcoma, carcinoma of the testes and uterus, Ewing's sarcoma in adults, choriocarcinoma that is methotrexate-resistant, Kaposi's sarcoma, and other soft tissue sarcomas.

Often used in combination with other antineoplastic agents and x-ray therapy.

The toxic properties of this drug preclude its use as an antibiotic in the treatment of infectious diseases.

Dosage
Dosage varies with patient's tolerance, size and location of the tumor and use of other therapy.
Adults:
Usual dose is 500 mcg. (0.5 mg) daily for maximum of 5 days.
Children:
15 mcg/kg (0.015 mg/kg) for 5 days or total dose of 2500 mcg (2.5 mg)/M^2 body surface over one week.

Dosage for adults and children should not exceed 15 mcg/kg or 400–600 mcg/M^2 of body surface daily for 5 days.

Dosage for obese or edematous patients should be calculated by surface area in order to relate dosage to lean body mass.

A second course may be given after 3 weeks if all signs of toxicity have passed.

May be given by isolation-perfusion technique (arterial infusion to an extremity or region of the body). This allows use of much higher doses while minimizing toxic effects. Dosages: 50 mcg (0.05 mg)/kg for lower extremity or pelvis, 35 mcg (0.035 mg)/kg for upper extremity.

Preparation and Storage
Supplied as powder in vials containing 500 mcg (0.5 mg) of drug.

Reconstitute by adding 1.1 ml of sterile water for injection (use no other diluent). This yields a solution of 500 mcg/ml.

Since the drug does not contain preservative, care must be taken during preparation to maintain sterility. Discard any unused portion.

Solution is normally yellow-gold in color.

Drug Incompatibilities
Do not mix with any other medication in syringe or IV line.

Modes of IV Administration

Injection
Yes
No further dilution needed. Inject into the tubing of a running IV.

Intermittent Infusion
Yes
Use D5W or NS, 100–200 ml, infuse over 30–60 min.

When an in-line micropore filter is used, inject or infuse the drug via the injection port *below* the filter since certain types will remove some of the drug.

Continuous Infusion
No

Contraindications; Warnings; Precautions; Adverse Reactions

Contraindications

If administered at the time of infection with chickenpox or herpes zoster a severe generalized disease may occur, which may result in death.

Warnings

1. Use for other than treatment of the conditions listed under Actions/Indications is experimental.
2. DRUG IS EXTREMELY CORROSIVE TO SOFT TISSUE. EXTRAVASATION WILL CAUSE SEVERE TISSUE DAMAGE.

Precautions

1. This is a toxic drug, frequent observation of the patient is essential, especially when multiple chemotherapy is employed. If stomatitis, diarrhea or severe bone marrow depression occur during therapy, the drug should be discontinued until the patient recovers.
2. Anaphylaxis can occur.
3. Abnormalities in renal, hepatic and bone marrow function have been produced by this drug; all three systems should be closely monitored.
4. Evidence suggests that this drug potentiates the effects of x-ray therapy and vice versa. Increased incidence of gastrointestinal toxicity and bone marrow suppression have been reported with such combined therapy and may be more likely if high doses of both are used or in particularly sensitive patients.
5. This drug is known to produce fetal abnormalities in animals. It should not be used in pregnancy unless the expected benefits outweigh the potential risks to the fetus.
6. It is recommended that breastfeeding be stopped before beginning treatment with this drug.
7. Use of this drug in infants under 6–12 months of age is not recommended.
8. Administer with caution after recent irradiation for right-sided Wilm's tumor.
9. Second primary tumors have been reported following treatment with anti-neoplastic agents and radiation.

Adverse Reactions

1. Gastrointestinal: nausea and vomiting occur within a few hours after administration and may be alleviated with antiemetics; anorexia, abdominal pain, diarrhea, GI ulceration.
2. Oral: esophagitis, pharyngitis, ulcerative stomatitis, dysphagia.
3. Blood: bone marrow depression producing anemia, aplastic anemia, agranulocytosis, leukopenia, thrombocytopenia, pancytopenia, reticulopenia. Monitor platelet and white cell counts daily; if either markedly decreases, withhold drug until marrow recovers.
4. Dermatologic: alopecia, acne, increased redness or pigmentation of previously irradiated tissues.
5. Other: malaise, fatigue, lethargy, fever, myalgia, proctitis, hypocalcemia.

Except for nausea and vomiting, other reactions appear 2–4 days *after* course of therapy is stopped. Deaths have occurred, but most reactions are reversible on discontinuation of therapy.

☐ Nursing Implications

1. The patient receiving this medication will be experiencing the emotional and physical effects of the malignancy. Knowledge of the patient's feelings about his disease and its implications will assist in helping him tolerate the chemotherapy. The incidence of uncomfortable side effects and adverse reactions is high. It is within the nurse's role to assist the patient in coping with the discomforts of the

dactinomycin
(continued)

disease and its treatment, and to help him work through depression and anger toward acceptance of the disease at his own pace. Despite the unpleasantness this drug may bring, it can be a source of hope for the patient.

2. Assist in obtaining an accurate history for recent exposure to, or infection with, chickenpox.
3. Take all precautions to avoid extravasation; see Appendix.
4. Management of nausea, vomiting and diarrhea:
   a. See Adverse Reaction No. 1
   b. It is likely that the patient will experience these effects while at home. Instruct the patient and/or family on the timing of antiemetic agents, the maintenance of hydration and nutrition, and the signs and symptoms of dehydration, proctitis and esophagitis, and what to do if they occur.
5. Management of hematologic effects:
   a. Be aware of the patient's complete blood count and platelet count prior to each injection. Anemia, leukopenia and thrombocytopenia are the dose-limiting side effects.
   b. If the white blood count falls to 2000/cu mm, take measures to protect the patient from infection, such as protective (reverse) isolation, avoidance of invasive procedures, maintaining bodily (especially perineal) cleanliness, carrying out strict urinary catheter care when appropriate, etc. Monitor for infection by recording temperature every 4 hours, examining for rashes, swellings, drainage and pain. Explain these measures to the patient.
   c. If the platelet count falls below 100,000/cu mm, monitor for thrombocytopenic bleeding: petechiae, purpura, hematuria, melena, blood in stools, gum bleeding, vaginal bleeding, epistaxis, hematemesis, etc. Avoid trauma. Transfusions may be ordered.
   d. Instruct the patient and family on the importance of follow-up blood studies if the drug is being administered on an outpatient basis. Also instruct on the importance of reporting possible infections or unusual bleeding.
6. Management of hair loss:
   a. Use the scalp tourniquet during injection, if ordered, to help prevent hair loss. This may be ineffective in preventing hair loss because of the prolonged presence of this drug in the blood.
   b. Counsel the patient on the possibility of hair loss to enable him to prepare for this disfigurement.
   c. Reassure him of the possibility of regrowth of hair following discontinuation of the drug.
   d. Provide privacy and time for the patient to discuss his feelings.
7. Management of stomatitis:
   a. Administer preventive oral care every 4 hours and/or after meals.
   b. For preventive care, use a very soft toothbrush (child's) and toothpaste; avoid trauma to the tissues.
   c. Examine oral membranes at least daily (instruct patient and/or family) to detect the onset of inflammation or ulceration.
   d. If stomatitis occurs, notify the physician and begin therapeutic oral care.
   e. Order a bland, mechanical soft diet for patients with mild inflammation. If the

stomatitis is severe, the patient may be placed on NPO status by the physician.

f. For patients who can tolerate oral intake, administer Xylocaine Viscous or acetaminophen elixer as a mouthwash prior to meals to decrease pain (do not use aspirin rinses), as ordered by the physician.

g. Patients with severe stomatitis may require parenteral analgesia.

8. Monitor for fever every 4–6 hours. This reaction is usually treated symptomatically with antipyretics.

Suggested Readings

Bruya, Margaret Auld, and Madeira, Nancy Powell: Stomatitis After Chemotherapy. *American Journal of Nursing,* 75(8):1349–1352, August 1975.

Giadquinta, Barbara: Helping Families Face the Crisis of Cancer. *American Journal of Nursing,* 77:1583–1588, October 1977.

Vietti, Teresa J., and Valeriote, Frederick: Conceptual Basis for the Use of Chemotherapeutic Agents and Their Pharmacology. *Pediatric Clinics of North America,* 23:67–92, February 1976.

dantrolene sodium ■
(Dantrium)

Actions/Indications
Skeletal muscle relaxant used to manage the fulminant hypermetabolism by skeletal muscle in malignant hyperthermia crisis caused by certain anesthetic agents.

Dosage
Adults and Children:
Administer as soon as the malignant hyperthermia reaction is diagnosed. Discontinue all anesthetic agents. Beginning dose—1 mg/kg by rapid, intravenous injection; continue administration until symptoms subside or until the maximum cumulative

dose of 10 mg/kg has been reached. Repeat if symptoms reappear. Effective dose is directly dependent on the patient's degree of susceptibility to the disorder, the amount and time of exposure to the triggering agent (anesthetic or barbiturate) and the time elapsed between onset of the crisis and initiation of treatment.

Preparation and Storage
Supplied in vials of 20 mg of drug powder. Reconstitute by adding 60 ml of sterile water for injection (*without* bacteriostatic agent). Shake until solution is clear. Protect from light and temperature over 86°; use within 6 hours.

Drug Incompatibilities
Do not mix with any other medication in any manner.

Modes of IV Administration

Injection
Yes
Reconstituted solution can be given undiluted.

Intermittent Infusion
No

Continuous Infusion
No

Contraindications; Warnings; Precautions; Adverse Reactions

Contraindications
None currently known.

Warnings
Supportive measures for the treatment of malignant hyperthermia must also be initiated with the dantrolene infusion; i.e., discontinuation of triggering agent, administration of oxygen, management of metabolic acidosis, body cooling, monitoring of urinary output and electrolyte balance.

Precautions
1. Avoid extravasation; solution is highly alkaline.

dantrolene sodium
(continued)

2. Safety for use in pregnancy has not been established; use when the potential benefits to the mother have been weighed against possible risks to the mother and child.

Adverse Reactions
Reactions have only been seen in chronic oral administration; none during short-term intravenous therapy.

☐ **Nursing Implications**
1. Assist in supportive management of the hyperthermia crisis:
   a. Monitor body temperature; continuously if equipment is available.
   b. Apply cooling blanket as ordered; monitor effect on body temperature.
   c. Monitor urine output; report if less than 30 ml/hour for 2 consecutive hours.
   d. Maintain open vein for fluids and electrolytes.
2. Avoid extravasation. If it occurs, elevate the extremity after discontinuing injections and report to the physician. Prompt local care is imperative to prevent tissue damage. Monitor site carefully for the next 24 hours. See Appendix.
3. Patients who have experienced a hyperthermia episode should be informed about the precipitating agent. He should wear a Medic Alert appliance.

deslanoside ▨
(Cedilanid-D)

Actions/Indications
A digitalis cardiac glycoside, which:
• Increases the force of myocardial contraction (positive inotropic effect)
• Slows the discharge rate of the sinus node
• Slows conduction through the A-V node to decrease the ventricular rate

Onset of action is 5 minutes after IV injection, peaks in 2–4 hours, lasts 2–5 days.
Used:
• To treat congestive heart failure of all degrees
• To slow the ventricular rate in atrial fibrillation
• To convert atrial flutter to normal sinus rhythm
• To control paroxysmal atrial tachycardia
In cardiogenic shock, the value of digitalis has not been established, but the drug is frequently used, especially when the condition is accompanied by pulmonary edema.

Dosage
Adults:
IV route used only when rapid digitalization is urgent. This can be obtained in 12 hrs by giving 1.6 mg (8 ml) in one dose, or in portions of 0.8 mg (4 ml) each.
Premature and Full-Term Newborns, and Infants With Reduced Renal Function or Myocarditis:
For digitalization—0.022 mg/kg (0.3 mg/M^2) in 2–3 doses[1]
Children 2 Weeks to 3 Years:
0.025 mg/kg (0.75 mg/M^2) in 2–3 doses.
Children 3 Years and Older:
0.0225 mg/kg (0.75 mg/M^2) in 2–3 doses.
Oral digitalization can be cautiously carried out with digoxin, 12–24 hrs. after the last dose of deslanoside has been given.

Preparation and Storage
Available in 2-ml ampuls (0.2 mg/ml).
Store at room temperature. Discard unused portions.
Do not add to IV fluids; this drug is unstable when diluted.

Drug Incompatibilities
Do not add to an IV line containing:
Any calcium preparation
Protein hydrolysate

Modes of IV Administration

Injection
Yes
At a rate of 0.2 mg/min. Should be given as close to cannula as possible, either into the cannula hub or through the lowest Y injection site, to avoid mixing the drug with IV fluid.

Intermittent Infusion
No
Do not dilute in solution.

Continuous Infusion
No
Do not dilute in solution.

Contraindications; Warnings; Precautions; Adverse Reactions

Contraindications
1. Digitalis toxicity
2. In the presence of ventricular tachycardia unless congestive heart failure occurs after a protracted episode of tachycardia not caused by digitalis
3. Ventricular fibrillation
4. Hypersensitivity

Warnings
1. The arrhythmias that digitalis preparations are indicated for can also be those caused by digitalis toxicity. Digitalis toxicity should be ruled out before administering this drug.
2. Patients in congestive heart failure may complain of nausea, anorexia, and vomiting. These symptoms can also be associated with digitalis toxicity, which should be ruled out prior to administration of the drug.

Precautions
1. Toxicity can develop in the presence of hypokalemia, even at usual dosage. Hypokalemia also reduces the positive inotropic effect of the drug. Patients on diuretics, hemodialysis, corticosteroid therapy, or with diarrhea are prone to hypokalemia.

Monitor and correct serum potassium levels when indicated.
2. Concomitant conditions may sensitize the myocardium to the effects of digitalis and to toxicity:
   a. Acute myocardial infarction
   b. Advanced congestive heart failure
   c. Fibrotic heart diseases
   d. Severe pulmonary diseases
3. Calcium preparations can produce serious arrhythmias in patients receiving digitalis.
4. Patients with myxedema require lower dosage of this drug.
5. Administer with caution in the presence of any degree of A-V block. Because of its effects on A-V conduction, digitalis may increase the degree of block, slowly.
6. Patients with chronic constrictive pericarditis will react unfavorably to digitalis.
7. This drug, or any digitalis preparation, is usually not given to patients with idiopathic hypertrophic subaortic stenosis.
8. Renal impairment delays excretion of this drug and requires modification of maintenance dosage of digitalis preparations.
9. Electrical conversion of arrhythmias may require adjustment of dosage.

Overdosage, Toxic Effects
1. Early symptoms of toxicity are anorexia, nausea, vomiting, and diarrhea in adults, but are rarely present in infants. There may also be weakness, and visual disturbances, such as yellow vision, and headache.
2. Arrhythmias of all types can be seen in toxicity. Premature ventricular contractions are most common except in infants and young children. Junctional rhythms, A-V dissociation and paroxysmal atrial rhythms are also common.
3. Slowing of the sinus rate and A-V block, which may proceed to complete heart block, are advanced signs of toxicity.

deslanoside
(continued)

4. Treatment:
   a. Discontinue the drug until all signs of toxicity have passed.
   b. Give potassium as indicated; monitor for hyperkalemia with ECG. (Do not use in presence of advanced heart block).[2]
   c. EDTA may be given to bind serum calcium and counteract arrhythmias.
   d. Give other antiarrhythmics as needed; phenytoin (drug of choice), quinidine, procainamide and propanolol. (If propranolol is used, monitor atrioventricular conduction; this drug may increase heart block.) Atropine can be used to treat bradyarrythmias. See entries for each drug for further details on their use.
5. If profound bradycardia and/or complete A-V block occur, transvenous temporary pacing may be necessary until toxicity resolves.

☐ **Nursing Implications**
1. Patients receiving this medication intravenously should, in most instances, be observed for arrhythmias via continuous ECG monitoring. Observe for improvement if the drug is given to treat an arrhythmia, and observe for arrhythmias which may be produced by the drug. Some of the more common arrhythmias produced by toxic levels of deslanoside are: sinus bradycardia, premature ventricular and atrial contractions, atrioventricular block of all degrees, paroxysmal atrial tachycardia. Notify the physician of improvement in arrhythmia being treated, and document with an ECG tracing. If arrhythmias of toxicity appear, notify the physician, document with an ECG tracing, and hold the next dose of deslanoside until the physician decides

what course of action is appropriate.
2. Be prepared to administer immediate care in the event of arrhythmias due to toxicity. (See Overdosage, No. 4, above.) Atropine 0.5–1.0 mg can be given for a heart rate less than 50–60/minute. (In units where registered nurses are expected to administer drugs in such an event, the unit physician should decide at what heart rate the atropine should be administered and in what amount.) See page 24 for details on atropine. For premature ventricular tachycardia, lidocaine 50–100 mg can be given by intravenous injection. Again, unit policy should dictate when and how much drug is given. See page 186 for details on lidocaine.
3. Observe for noncardiac symptoms of digitalis toxicity: anorexia; nausea; vomiting and diarrhea; visual disturbances, e.g., rainbow vision or yellow vision (rare); in children, poor feeding and irritability; headache (rare); confusion; severe fatigue.[3]
4. Monitor for signs of improvement if the patient is being treated for congestive heart failure:
   a. Reduction in weight (weigh the patient daily)
   b. Reduction in peripheral edema
   c. Increased urine output (measure every 8 hours)
   d. Decreased resting heart rate to normal limits (record every 4–8 hours)
   e. Decreased respiratory rate, disappearance of rales
   f. Increased exercise tolerance
   Note that worsening congestive failure despite digitalis administration may be a sign of digitalis toxicity.
5. Be aware of the patient's serum potassium. Hypokalemia can precipitate digitalis toxicity. Administer potassium supplements as ordered. These may produce

nausea and vomiting (liquid preparations especially) usually soon after administration. The nurse's observations will be needed to differentiate between potassium-induced nausea and vomiting and that due to digitalis toxicity. Potassium supplements, both oral and intravenous, can produce hyperkalemia—monitor serum potassium for elevations. (Normal serum potassium: 3.5–5.5 mEq/liter.) The signs and symptoms of hyperkalemia are: (a) peaked T-waves on ECG, (b) muscular weakness, (c) nausea, abdominal pains, diarrhea, (d) paresthesias of hands, feet, and face.

6. Rarely, elderly patients experience hallucinations, anxiety, and delusions secondary to toxic levels of digitalis preparations. Monitor for onset of this complication, notify the physician, and initiate safety measures, e.g., side rails, restraints as indicated, close observation, reassurance.

7. Patients who will require a digitalis preparation on a chronic basis must be instructed on safe self-administration.

References

1. Shirkey, Harry C.: *Pediatric Drug Handbook*. Philadelphia: W. B. Saunders Company, 1977, p. 133.
2. Davis, Richard H., and Risch, Charles: Potassium and Arrhythmias. *Geriatrics*, November 1970, p. 110.
3. Lely, A. H., and van Enter, C. H. J.: Noncardiac Symptoms of Digitalis Intoxication. *American Heart Journal*, 83(2):150, February 1972.

Suggested Readings

Amsterdam, Ezra A., et al.: Systemic Approach to the Management of Cardiac Arrhythmias. *Heart and Lung*, 2(5):747–753, September–October 1973 (references).

Arbeit, Sidney, et al.: Recognizing Digitalis Toxicity. *American Journal*

of Nursing, 77(12):1936–1945, December 1977 (references).

James, Frederick W., and Love, Ervena: Congestive Heart Failure in Infants. *Heart and Lung*, 3(3):396–400, May–June, 1974 (references).

Lely, A. H., and van Enter, C. H. J.: Noncardiac Symptoms of Digitalis Intoxication. *American Heart Journal*, 83(2):149–152, February 1972.

Rosen, Michael R., Wit, Andrew, and Hoffman, Brian F.: Electrophysiology and Pharmacology of Cardiac Arrhythmias. IV Cardiac Antiarrhythmic and Toxic Effects of Digitalis. *American Heart Journal*, 89(3):391–399, March 1975 Pages 391–339 (References).

———: Treatment of Cardiac Arrhythmias. *Medical Letter on Drugs and Therapeutics*, 16(25):101–108, December 6, 1974.

dexamethasone sodium phosphate ■
(Decadron Phosphate, Dexacen-4, Hexadrol Phosphate)

Actions/Indications
Adrenocorticosteroid, synthetic. Has rapid onset but short duration of action. Used in:
- Endocrine disorders, especially adrenocortical insufficiency
- Rheumatic disorders, with inflammation
- Collagen diseases
- Dermatologic diseases
- Allergy
- Ophthalmic disorders with inflammation
- Gastrointestinal diseases (e.g., ulcerative colitis and regional ileitis)
- Respiratory diseases (including sarcoidosis and aspiration pneumonia)
- Hematologic diseases
- Neoplastic diseases
- Nephrotic syndrome
- Tuberculous meningitis
- Trichinosis with neurologic or myocardial involvement
- Diagnostic testing of adrenocortical hyperfunction

dexamethasone sodium phosphate
(continued)
• Cerebral edema
• Shock unresponsive to conventional therapy if adrenalcortical insufficiency exists.

Adrenocortical steroids have antiinflammatory effects and affect electrolyte balance.

Dosage
Adults and Children:
DOSAGE REQUIREMENTS ARE VARIABLE AND MUST BE INDIVIDUALIZED ACCORDING TO THE DISEASE, THE CONDITION OF THE PATIENT AND THE RESPONSE PRODUCED BY THE INITIAL DOSES. Dosage may vary from day to day. Use the lowest dose possible.

Initial dose—0.5–20 mg/day, given in divided doses every 12 hrs.

In shock, as high as 2–6 mg/kg as a single injection has been given.

Maintenance—Initial dosage can be maintained if a favorable response is seen in a reasonable amount of time. After a response is obtained, the dosage should be decreased in small decrements until the lowest dosage is reached that produces the desired results.

Preparation and Storage
Available as 4 mg/ml solution in 1.0- and 2.5-ml syringes, and 1.0-, 5- and 25-ml vials; as a 10 mg/ml solution in a 10-ml vial and 1-ml syringe; a 20 mg/ml solution in a 5-ml vial and 1-ml syringe; and a 24 mg/ml solution in 5- and 10-ml vials.

Store at room temperature.

Drug Incompatibilities
Infusions completed within 12 hours *are stable* with vitamins B and C, sodium bicarbonate, heparin, and tetracycline.

Consider all other medications *incompatible.*

Modes of IV Administration

Injection
Yes

Inject over at least one to several minutes. No further dilution required. Rapid injection can produce premature ventricular contractions.

Intermittent Infusion
Yes
Use D5W or NS in any volume.

Continuous Infusion
Yes
Use D5W or NS in any volume.

Use this mode when constant maximal effect is desired.

Contraindications; Warnings; Precautions; Adverse Reactions

Contraindications
1. Hypersensitivity
2. Systemic fungal infections

Warnings
1. Dosage should be increased prior to any unusual stress (surgery) and for a short time following.
2. Steroids mask some signs of infection. There may also be decreased resistance and inability to localize infection.
3. Large doses cause elevation of blood pressure, salt and water retention, and increased excretion of potassium and calcium. Salt restriction and potassium supplements may be required.
4. Immunization procedures should not be carried out, especially for smallpox.
5. Use in active tuberculosis should be limited to fulminating or disseminated types. Latent tuberculosis may be reactivated; chemoprophylaxis should be given during prolonged therapy.
6. Anaphylaxis has occurred.
7. Use in pregnancy and lactation requires that benefits to the mother be weighed against risks to the fetus or nursing infant.
8. Following prolonged therapy with steroids, too-rapid withdrawal may induce secondary adrenocortical insufficiency;

gradual reduction in dosage may minimize this effect.

9. This drug may activate latent amebiasis; that should be ruled out whenever possible before initiating therapy.

Precautions

1. There is an enhanced effect of corticosteroids in patients with hypothyroidism and cirrhosis; these patients will require lower dosage.
2. Psychic derangements may appear, ranging from euphoria, insomnia, personality changes, depression, to psychosis. Pre-existing problems may be aggravated.
3. Use aspirin with caution in patients with hypoprothrombinemia and in all patients taking corticosteroids, to avoid gastric ulceration.
4. When large doses of this drug are given, antiulcer therapy should be instituted.
5. Steroids should be used with caution in nonspecific ulcerative colitis if there is a possibility of impending perforation or abscess, diverticulitis, fresh intestinal anastomoses, active or latent peptic ulcer, renal insufficiency, hypertension, osteoporosis, or myasthenia gravis.
6. Concomitant administration of phenytoin, phenobarbital, ephedrine and rifampin may decrease the activity of this drug, requiring adjusted dosage.
7. Evidence suggests that corticosteroids alter the response to coumarin anticoagulants. Monitor the prothrombin time closely in patients receiving both drugs.
8. Concomitant administration of potassium-depleting diuretics requires close observation for hypokalemia.
9. Use with caution in patients with ocular herpes simplex; corneal perforation can occur.
10. This drug can decrease the number and motility of spermatozoa.

Adverse Reactions Seen in Short-Term Intravenous Therapy

1. Fluid and electrolyte imbalances: sodium and water retention with possible secondary hypertension, hypokalemia, hypocalcemia.
2. Gastrointestinal: peptic ulcer with possible perforation, pancreatitis, ulcerative esophagitis.
3. Dermatologic: impaired wound healing, burning or tingling (especially in perineal area), cutaneous reactions (allergic dermatitis, urticaria, angioneurotic edema).
4. Neurologic: increased intracranial pressure, seizures (increasing frequency in patients with pre-existing seizure disorder), vertigo, headaches, mental confusion, euphoria, exacerbation of psychosis.
5. Endocrine: decreased glucose tolerance, increased need for insulin and oral hypoglycemics in diabetics.
6. Eye: increased intraocular pressure.
7. Metabolic: negative nitrogen balance secondary to rapid muscle catabolism.
8. Other: anaphylaxis, thromboembolism, nausea, malaise.

☐ Nursing Implications

1. Take precautions to prevent infections in wounds by using strict aseptic technique in dressing changes, etc. Avoid invasive procedures such as catheterizations. The skin may become more fragile because of the steroid therapy. Patients on bed rest and those with general body weakening secondary to an acute illness should be turned hourly (except during sleep, then every 2–3 hours) to prevent skin breakdown. Initiate the use of supportive measures such as flotation pads, water mattress, etc. Administer skin care to prevent infection.
2. Monitor blood pressure every 2–4 hours, or as the patient's condition dictates. Monitor

dexamethasone sodium phosphate
(continued)

blood pressure before, during and immediately after intravenous injection; hypotension can occur. In patients with cardiac disorders, monitor for premature ventricular contractions during and after injection. See Warning No. 3.

3. Weigh the patient daily to detect water and sodium retention. Dietary restriction in sodium may be prescribed by the physician. Examine daily for peripheral edema.

4. There may be delayed healing of wounds; take precautions to prevent dehiscence. Sutures may be left in longer than usual for this reason.

5. Monitor urine glucose in patients on high-dose therapy and with diabetes. Diabetic individuals may require a larger dosage of insulin or oral agent.

6. Administer antiulcer therapy as ordered to assist in preventing peptic ulcer. Monitor for signs of the development of an ulcer and/or acute intestinal bleeding: melena, positive stool guaiac, hematemesis, epigastric pain and/or distention, anemia or falling hematocrit.

7. Monitor for signs and symptoms of hypokalemia:[1] weakness, irritability, abdominal distention, poor feeding in infants, muscle cramps. Dietary or pharmacologic potassium supplements may be ordered, guided by serum potassium levels.

8. Monitor for signs and symptoms of hypocalcemia (serum calcium less than 6 mg%):[2] irritability, change in mental status, seizures, nausea, vomiting, diarrhea, muscle cramps, late effects —cardiac arrhythmias, laryngeal spasm and apnea. Dietary or pharmacologic supplements may be ordered, guided by serum calcium levels.

9. Patients with a history of seizure activity may have an increasing number of seizures while on steroid therapy. Apply appropriate safety precautions.

10. Monitor for behavioral changes, which may range from simple euphoria to depression and psychosis. Apply appropriate safety precautions. A change in dosage may relieve such symptoms.

11. Tuberculin testing should be carried out prior to initiation of steroid therapy, if possible. The patient's reactivity to the tuberculin is altered by the drug, giving a false result.

12. Ambulate the patient with caution if vertigo occurs, and initiate the use of side rails to prevent patient injury. Report the onset to the physician.

13. Be alert to the signs of increasing intraocular pressure:[3] eye pain, rainbow vision, blurred vision, nausea and vomiting. Notify the physician immediately.

References

1. Beeson, Paul B., and McDermott, Walsh (editors): *Textbook of Medicine* (14th ed.), Philadelphia: W. B. Saunders Company, 1975, p. 1587.
2. Ibid., p. 1815.
3. Newell, Frank W., and Ernest, J. Terry: *Opthalmology—Principles and Concepts* (3rd ed.), St. Louis: C. V. Mosby Company, 1974, p. 329.

Suggested Readings

Glasser, Ronald J.: How the Body Works Against Itself: Autoimmune Diseases. *Nursing '77*, September 1977, pp. 34–38.
Melick, Mary Evans: Nursing Intervention for Patients Receiving Corticosteroid Therapy. In *Advanced Concepts in Clinical Nursing* (2nd ed.), K. C. Kintzel, ed., Philadelphia: J. B. Lippincott Company, 1977, pp. 606–617.
Newton, David W., Nichols, Arlene and Newton, Marion: You Can Minimize the Hazards of Corticosteroids: *Nursing '77*, June 1977, pp. 26–33.
Reichgott, Michael J., and Melmon, Kenneth L.: The Role of Cortico-

steroids in Shock. In *Steroid Therapy*, Daniel Azarnoff, ed., Philadelphia, W. B. Saunders Company, 1975 pp. 118–133.

dextran-40 ■

(Rheomacrodex, L.M.D.—Low Molecular Weight Dextran)

Actions/Indications

A polymer of glucose that can simulate the colloidal properties of albumin, that is, draw fluid from the cellular and intercellular spaces into the blood to expand blood volume and thus increase blood pressure.

Used as a *temporary* blood substitute in hemorrhagic and traumatic shock or shock due to burns until whole blood and plasma can be given. May be used for priming of extracorporeal circulation.[1]

Also used in certain clinical situations to enhance microcirculation and to decrease platelet aggregation.

Dosage

Must be individualized based on amount of fluid lost, and resultant hemoconcentration. This preparation of dextran can expand plasma volume to almost twice the volume infused. This expansion decreases in 3–4 hrs.

Adults and Children:
Do not exceed 20 ml/kg of a 10% solution in the first 24 hrs. Subsequent doses on following days should not exceed 10 ml/kg. Do not extend infusions beyond 5 days.
Usual dose—500 ml.
For extracorporeal priming—10–20 ml/kg. Do not exceed 20 ml/kg.

Preparation and Storage

Supplied in 500-ml bottles, a 10% solution in NS or D5W.

Solution may crystallize over time or when stored at a temperature greater than 25°C (77°F).

If flakes are seen in solution heat to 100°C (210°F) until dissolution occurs. Cool to body or room temperature before use. Store at a constant temperature, not over 25°C.

Use only if seal is intact, solution is clear and vacuum is detectable.

Drug Incompatibilities

Do not mix with any other medication.

Do not add medications to the solution bottle.

Modes of IV Administration

Injection
No

Intermittent Infusion
Yes
First 500 ml can be infused rapidly; subsequent doses more slowly (20 ml/min).

Continuous Infusion
Yes
Titrated with blood pressure or according to clinical need and dosage guidelines.

Contraindications; Warnings; Precautions; Adverse Reactions

Contraindications
1. Known hypersensitivity
2. Bleeding disorders due to qualitative or quantitative defects in clotting factors
3. Renal disease with oliguria or anuria
4. Oliguria secondary to hemorrhagic shock that does not improve after the first dose
5. Severe congestive heart failure

Warnings
1. Anaphylaxis and other allergic reactions can occur but are less frequent than with the use of dextran-70; usually seen within first 15–20 minutes of infusion.
2. Administer nonosmotically active fluids to prevent dehydration and to maintain adequate urine output.
3. The renal excretion of dextran increases urine viscosity and specific gravity (minor elevation).
4. To assess the state of the patient's hydration, use serum or

dextran-40
(continued)

urine osmolarity. Administer additional fluids accordingly.

5. Mannitol may be used to maintain an adequate urine flow.
6. Renal failure occurring during use of dextran-40 has been reported.
7. Abnormal renal and hepatic function values can sometimes be seen following the use of dextran. The cause of this is unknown.
8. Administer with caution in the presence of hemorrhage. Increased blood pressure and microperfusion may increase bleeding.
9. Safety for use in pregnancy has not been established.

Precautions

1. Dosages of this drug at 15 ml/kg of body weight will cause a prolonged bleeding time, a decreased blood factor VIII, decreased fibrinogen, factor V, and factor IX to a greater extent than with hemodilution alone.
2. Dextran may also facilitate lysis of fibrin by plasmin.
3. Watch for early signs of abnormal bleeding.
4. Infusion of this solution can cause circulatory overload. This is especially likely in patients with decreased renal clearance of the dextran. Use with caution in these patients and in patients who are susceptible to, or have pre-existing, congestive heart failure.
5. Falsely high blood glucose results may be seen when the laboratory uses a technique involving high concentrations of acids (sulfuric or acetic).
6. Dextran may interfere with blood-typing procedures. Obtain blood samples for typing before infusion. If this is not possible, inform the laboratory that the patient has been given dextran.
7. Prevent depression of the he-

matocrit below 30, by administering whole blood or packed RBCs.

Adverse Reactions

1. Allergic reactions ranging from urticaria to anaphylaxis.
2. Nausea, vomiting, fever, joint pains.
3. Renal failure (rare).

☐ **Nursing Implications**

1. Monitor for anaphylaxis and discontinue infusion at the earliest signs; see Appendix for anaphylaxis precautions and treatment. Notify physician.
2. Monitor the following parameters for effectiveness of infusion when used in the treatment of shock:
   a. Blood pressure (direct arterial or indirect), frequency depending on the clinical situation
   b. Heart and respiratory rate (should decrease as blood pressure rises)
   c. If available, pulmonary artery pressure (preferable) or CVP to assess the expansion of blood volume, and the heart's ability to pump
   d. Urine output (at least hourly). Output should increase with the blood pressure (to at least 30 ml/hour). If it has not after the first 500 ml of dextran has infused, notify the physician and do not infuse dextran without further orders
   e. Specific gravity of urine; if specific gravity does not decrease with increased urine output, or if a high value (greater than 1.030) is accompanied by oliguria, discontinue infusion and notify physician. Keep the patient hydrated with nonosmotically active fluids (D5W, RL, NS)
3. Monitor for onset of cardiac failure:
   a. Fall in blood pressure
   b. Rise in pulse rate

c. Rise in central venous pressure or pulmonary artery (wedge) pressure
d. Rises in respiratory rate and effort
e. Onset of rales in the lungs
f. Fall in PaO$_2$ (arterial blood oxygen content)
Slow infusion and notify the physician immediately
4. Monitor for bleeding disorders:
   a. Oozing at incision lines
   b. Oozing at venipuncture sites
   c. Bleeding from any orifice or drainage system
   d. Fall in blood pressure, rise in pulse rate, diaphoresis, and other signs and symptoms of shock

Reference
1. Buchanan, E. Clyde: Blood and Blood Substitutes for Treating Hemorrhagic Shock. *American Journal of Hospital Pharmacy*, 34:634, June 1977.

dextran-70 ■
(Macrodex)

Actions/Indications
Polymer of glucose that can simulate the colloidal properties of albumin, that is, draw fluid from the cellular and intercellular spaces into the blood to expand blood volume and thus increase blood pressure.

Used as a *temporary* blood substitute in hemorrhagic shock, shock due to burns or trauma, until whole blood or plasma can be given. This form of dextran increases plasma volume by slightly more than the volume infused, depending on fluid available to be drawn into the vascular space, and the rate of dextran clearance in the kidney.[1]

This agent is also known to enhance microcirculation and to decrease platelet aggregation.

Dosage
Must be individualized, based on the amount of fluid lost and the resultant hemoconcentration.

Adults:
Do not exceed 20 ml/kg in the first 24 hrs, and 10 ml/kg thereafter.
Usual dose—500 ml.
Children:
Do not exceed 20 ml/kg in the first 24 hrs or 10 ml/kg thereafter each 24 hrs.

Preparation and Storage
Supplied in 500-ml bottles, a 6% solution, in NS or D5W.

This solution may crystallize if stored for long periods. If flakes are present, heat to 100°C (210°F) until dissolution occurs. Cool to body temperature before using.

Store away from extremes of temperature. Use only if seal is intact, solution is clear, and vacuum detectable.

Drug Incompatibilities
Do not mix with any other medication.

Do not add any medication to solution bottle.

Modes of IV Administration

Injection
No

Intermittent Infusion
Yes
At a rate of 20–40 ml/min, depending on dosage, titrated with blood pressure or other clinically appropriate parameters.

Continuous Infusion
Yes
At a rate of 20–40 ml/min, depending on dosage, titrated with blood pressure or other clinically appropriate parameters.

Contraindications; Warnings; Precautions; Adverse Reactions

Contraindications
1. Known hypersensitivity
2. Bleeding disorders due to qualitative or quantitative defects in clotting factors
3. Renal disease with oliguria or anuria

dextran-70
(continued)
4. Oliguria secondary to hemorrhagic shock that does not improve after the first dose
5. Severe congestive heart failure

Warnings
1. Anaphylaxis can occur, usually during the first 15–20 minutes of the infusion.
2. May interfere with platelet adhesiveness, resulting in a transient prolonged bleeding time, especially in doses greater than 1000 ml.
3. Prevent depression of the hematocrit below 30 secondary to hemodilution by administering whole blood or packed RBC's.
4. When large volumes are given, plasma protein levels will be decreased.
5. Safety for use in pregnancy has not been established.

Precautions
1. Dosages of this drug at 15 ml/kg of body weight will cause a prolonged bleeding time, a decreased blood factor VIII, decreased fibrinogen, factor V and factor IX, to a greater extent than with hemodilution alone.
2. Dextran may also facilitate lysis of fibrin by plasmin.
3. Watch for early signs of abnormal bleeding.
4. Infusion of this solution can cause circulatory overload. This is especially likely in patients with decreased renal clearance of the dextran. Use with caution in these patients and in patients who are susceptible to or have pre-existing congestive heart failure.
5. Falsely high blood glucose results may be seen when the laboratory uses a technique involving high concentrations of acids (sulfuric or acetic).
6. Dextran may interfere with blood-typing procedures. Obtain blood samples for typing before infusion. If this is not possible, inform the laboratory

that the patient has been given dextran.

Adverse Reactions
1. Allergic reactions ranging from urticaria to anaphylaxis; antihistamines may relieve mild allergic reactions
2. Nausea, vomiting, fever, joint pain

□ **Nursing Implications**
1. Monitor for anaphylaxis and discontinue infusion at the earliest signs; see Appendix for anaphylaxis precautions and treatment. Notify physician.
2. Monitor for effectiveness of infusion when used in the treatment of shock:
   a. Blood pressure (direct arterial or indirect), frequency depending on the clinical situation
   b. Heart and respiratory rate (should decrease as blood pressure rises)
   c. If available, pulmonary artery pressure (preferable) or CVP to assess the expansion of blood volume, and the heart's ability to pump
   d. Urine output (at least hourly). Output should increase with the blood pressure (to at least 30 ml/hour). If it has not after the first 500 ml of dextran has infused, notify the physician and do not infuse dextran without further orders.
   e. Specific gravity of urine; if specific gravity does not decrease with increased urine output, or if a high value (greater than 1.030) is accompanied by oliguria, discontinue infusion and notify physician. Keep the patient hydrated with nonosmotically active fluids (D5W, RL, NS)
3. Monitor for onset of cardiac failure that can be precipitated by volume expansion:
   a. Fall in blood pressure
   b. Rise in pulse
   c. Rise in central venous pres-

sure or pulmonary artery (wedge) pressure
d. Rise in respiratory rate and effort
e. Rales in the lungs
f. Fall in PaO$_2$ (arterial blood oxygen)
Slow infusion and notify the physician immediately.
4. Monitor for bleeding disorders:
a. Oozing at incision lines
b. Oozing at venipuncture sites
c. Bleeding from any orifice or drainage system
d. Worsening signs and symptoms of shock.

Reference
1. Buchanan, E. Clyde: Blood and Blood Substitutes for Treating Hemorrhagic Shock. *American Journal of Hospital Pharmacy*, 34:634, June 1977.

diazepam ▓
(Valium)

Actions/Indications
Short-acting CNS depressant, tranquilizer, anticonvulsant, skeletal muscle relaxant.
Used in short-term symptomatic relief of tension and anxiety states, psychoneurotic states.
In acute alcohol withdrawal, it may be useful in relieving agitation, tremor, impending or overt delirium tremens and hallucinations.
For endoscopic or operative procedures and cardioversion to decrease anxiety and recall.
Adjunct to the treatment of status epilepticus and recurrent seizures. For the relief of skeletal muscle spasm caused by local pathology, motor-neuron disorders, athetosis and tetanus.

Dosage
Dosage must be individualized according to age and the condition being treated.
Adults and Older Children (Over 12):
2–20 mg every 3–4 hrs. Use lower

doses (2–5 mg) in the elderly or when other sedatives are used. Maximum of 30 mg in 8 hrs.
Children 5 Years or Older:
Tetanus—5–10 mg every 3–4 hrs. as needed to control spasms.
Status epilepticus and recurrent seizures —1 mg every 2–5 min. up to a maximum of 10 mg. slowly, every 2–4 hrs.
Infants Over 30 Days of Age and Children Up to 5 Years:
Tetanus—1–2 mg, repeated every 3–4 hrs, as needed to control spasms.
Status epilepticus and recurrent seizures —0.2–0.5 mg slowly, every 2–5 min. up to a maximum of 5 mg.

Preparation and Storage
Available in 2 ml ampuls, 2 ml disposable syringes and 10 ml vials each containing 5 mg/ml.
Do not mix with IV solutions; the drug precipitates. It is not currently known what effect the crystalized drug may have in the body. Protect vials from light in manufacturer's box.

Drug Incompatibilities
Do not mix with any other medication.

Modes of IV Administration

Injection
Yes
Only acceptable mode of administration.
Inject, undiluted, directly into the vein, cannula or into an IV tubing injection site that is *immediately* above the junction between the cannula and the tubing. This prevents the drug from mixing with fluid. After injection flush vein and tubing with NS to prevent thrombophlebitis.
Inject *slowly*, no more rapidly than 5 mg/min.
In children, inject dose over a 3 min. period.

Intermittent Infusion
No
Drug will precipitate upon dilution in *any* solution.

diazepam
(continued)
Continuous Infusion
No
Drug will precipitate upon dilution in *any* solution.

Contraindications; Warnings; Precautions; Adverse Reactions

Contraindications
1. Known hypersensitivity
2. Acute narrow-angle glaucoma; and open-angle glaucoma unless controlled by appropriate therapy
3. Parenterally in children under 30 days of age
4. In the presence of jaundice in children

Warnings
1. The following procedures must be applied to prevent venous thrombosis, tissue and vascular damage:
   a. Inject slowly; 1 minute for each 5 mg
   b. Use large veins
   c. Avoid intra-arterial administration
   d. Prevent extravasation
   e. Flush vein with NS following injection
2. Do not mix with any intravenous solutions, or with other drugs.
3. **Extreme caution** must be exercised when administering to patients with limited pulmonary reserve, the elderly or the very ill to prevent apnea and cardiac arrest.
4. Concomitant use of barbiturates or other central nervous system depressants increases the risk of apnea. Respiratory support equipment must be readily available.
5. Do not administer to patients in shock, coma, or in acute alcoholic intoxication with depression of vital signs.
6. USE IN PREGNANCY: THERE IS AN INCREASED RISK OF CONGENITAL MALFORMATION ASSOCIATED WITH THE USE OF THIS DRUG DURING THE FIRST TRIMESTER. USE MUST BE AVOIDED.
7. This drug enters cord blood. Obstetrical use is not recommended.
8. Use in children: Safety for use in infants less than 30 days of age has not been established. Use in neonates has been associated with prolonged central nervous system depression due to an inability to metabolize the drug.
9. Apnea and hypotension can result from rapid injection.
10. When diazepam is administered with a narcotic analgesic, the dosage of either drug must be reduced and administered with caution.
11. Tonic status epilepticus has been precipitated in patients treated with IV diazepam for petit mal status or petit mal variant status.

Precautions
1. Do not use for *maintenance* control of seizures.
2. Use cautiously with other drugs that may potentiate the action of this drug, such as phenothiazines, narcotics, barbiturates, MAO inhibitors and antidepressants. Hypotension and severe muscle weakness may occur.
3. In highly anxious patients with accompanying depression, **protective measures should be taken** to prevent suicidal behavior.
4. Patients with impaired liver or renal function as well as elderly and debilitated patients will require reduced dosage and monitoring for signs of toxicity for longer periods of time.
5. There may be an increase in the cough reflex and a greater likelihood of laryngospasm in peroral endoscopic procedures. Topical anesthetics should be used and countermeasures available.
6. Abrupt withdrawal after several

days administration can precipitate convulsions, delirium, abdominal and muscle cramps, vomiting and sweating.

Adverse Reactions
1. Thrombophlebitis at IV injection site
2. Central nervous system disturbances; drowsiness, fatigue, ataxia, depression, slurred speech, syncope, vertigo, confusion, headache, tremor.
3. Genitourinary: incontinence, urinary retention
4. Respiratory depression with large doses, can lead to apnea
5. Cardiovascular: bradycardia, hypotension, shock (most often with rapid injection)
6. Blurred vision, diplopia, and nystagmus
7. Skin rash and urticaria
8. Psychological: paradoxical reactions such as hyperexcited states, anxiety, confusion, insomnia, hallucinations, sleep disturbances. If any of these occur the drug should be discontinued.
9. In peroral endoscopic procedures, coughing, depressed respiration, dyspnea, hyperventilation, laryngospasm and pain in the throat or chest have been reported.

☐ Nursing Implications
1. Respiratory depression is the greatest hazard associated with intravenous administration of this drug. The respiratory status of all patients must be monitored frequently during the first few hours after injection:
   a. Count the respiratory rate every 2–5 minutes for the first 30 minutes and then every 15 minutes for the next hour and one-half.
   b. Observe for pallor or cyanosis of the mucous membranes and nail beds during this time.
   c. Be prepared to provide respiratory support. Have oxygen, suction equipment, an airway and manual breathing bag at the bedside ready for use. Endotracheal tubes and laryngoscope should also be readily available.
   d. Do not leave the patient unattended during the first hour after injection.
   e. Respiratory depression is more likely to occur in the following types of patients: those with pre-existing cardiac, pulmonary, renal, hepatic or neuromuscular disease (myasthenia gravis); patients with chest trauma or deformities; patients who have received other respiratory depressing drugs (see Precaution No. 2); and the elderly or very young.
2. If respiratory depression occurs, i.e., if the respiratory rate falls below 8/minute in an adult or normal rate in children, take the following actions:
   a. If the patient can be aroused, verbally instruct him to breathe; repeat command to produce a respiratory rate of 10–12/minute.
   b. Stay with the patient until depressant effects have subsided.
   c. If the patient cannot be aroused, maintain an open airway and ventilate the patient with the manual breathing bag at a rate of 10–12/minute. The physician will determine whether the patient requires intubation. If cyanosis is present, begin administration of oxygen via the breathing bag.
3. Monitor blood pressure every 15–30 minutes during the first 2 hours following injection. If hypotension occurs, notify the physician and place the patient in a Trendelenburg position if it is not contraindicated. Vasopressors may be prescribed.
4. The patient should be kept at bed rest for the first 2 hours after injection. Ambulate with caution thereafter.

diazepam
(continued)

5. Monitor for urinary retention in susceptible patients (those with a history of prostatic hypertrophy or urethral stricture). Palpate bladder size every 4 hours and monitor urinary output.

6. Monitor psychiatric patients for exacerbation of depression or anxiety, take suicide precautions as indicated.

7. If this drug is used to control ventilation in the patient on a respirator:

   a. Because the patient will be respirator-dependent following a ventilation-controlling dose, check respirator connections frequently; they must be tight.

   b. Set all available respirator alarm systems (apnea and pressure-sensitive) and keep them in continual operation.

   c. Check arterial blood gases frequently for adequacy of ventilation

   d. Some hospital policies require constant attendance of a registered nurse for such patients

diazoxide ■
(Hyperstat IV)

Actions/Indications
Rapid-acting antihypertensive agent. Produces prompt reduction in blood pressure by relaxing the smooth muscles in the peripheral arterioles. Cardiac output increases; coronary and cerebral blood flow are maintained. Renal blood flow is increased. Pressure falls within one minute. Effect lasts less than 12 hours. Is indicated in the emergency reduction of blood pressure in malignant hypertension in hospitalized patients, when prompt reduction is needed.

Dosage
Administer only into *peripheral* veins, with patient recumbent.

Adults:
Inject 1–3 mg/kg to a maximum of 150 mg. Repeat at 5–15 min. intervals until pressure has been adequately reduced. Such minibolus administration is as effective and more safe than a single dose of 300 mg. Response to successive doses is often better than to the initial injection. Repeated doses at intervals of 4–24 hours usually will maintain blood pressure below pretreatment levels until oral antihypertensive becomes effective. Duration of treatment with diazoxide should be limited to a few days.

Children, Very Large or Very Small Adults:
5 mg/kg.[1] Follow directions above for administration.

Preparation and Storage
Supplied in 20-ml ampuls (300 mg), 15 mg/ml.

Protect from light. Store away from heat or extreme cold. Do not use darkened solutions.

Drug Incompatibilities
Do not mix with any other medication.

Modes of IV Administration

Injection
Yes
Only effective when injected rapidly (over less than 30 sec). Administer undiluted.

Intermittent Infusion
No
The drug must be injected rapidly. Slow rates and dilution are less effective in reducing blood pressure.

Continuous Infusion
No
The drug must be injected rapidly. Slow rates and dilution are less effective in reducing blood pressure.

Contraindications; Warnings; Precautions; Adverse Reactions

Contraindications
1. Do not use in the treatment of compensatory hypertension as-

sociated with coarctation of the aorta or arteriovenous shunt.
2. Do not use in patients hypersensitive to diazoxide or other thiazide derivatives, unless possible benefits outweigh the risks.
3. Dissecting aortic aneurysm.

Warnings
1. Safety for use in pregnancy has not been established.
2. Information is not available concerning the passage of diazoxide in breast milk. The drug does cross the placental barrier to appear in cord blood and can produce fetal or neonatal hyperbilirubinemia, thrombocytopenia, altered carbohydrate metabolism and possibly other adverse effects. When given for eclampsia, this drug may stop labor; oxytocin may be used in this event.
3. Safety for use in children has not been established (see Dosage section).
4. Hypotension may (rarely) result from administration of this drug. If it occurs and requires therapy, it usually responds to sympathomimetic agents (norepinephrine).
5. Hyperglycemia occurs in the majority of patients but usually requires treatment only in patients with diabetes mellitus. It responds to insulin.
6. Cataracts have been reported after repeated daily doses.
7. Use with caution in preexisting renal or heart failure. This drug causes sodium retention. Repeated doses may cause edema and precipitate congestive heart failure. This responds to diuretics when renal function is adequate.
8. Concurrently administered thiazide diuretics may potentiate the antihypertensive, hyperglycemic and hyperuricemic effects of diazoxide.
9. When diazoxide is administered with propranolol or to a patient recently treated with propranolol or guanethidine, its dose

must be lower than usual to prevent possible excessive hypotension.[2]
10. Effectiveness of diazoxide will be improved if extracellular fluid is shifted into the vascular compartment and eliminated with the use of a diuretic such as furosemide.
11. Patients concomitantly on coumarin or its derivatives may require a reduction in the anticoagulant dose.
12. Hypertensive crises due to pheochromocytoma or monoamine oxidase inhibitor therapy should not be treated by diazoxide; these conditions respond more specifically to an alpha-adrenergic receptor blocking drug such as phentolamine.[3]
13. Administer with caution to patients concomitantly on: methyldopa, reserpine, hydralazine, nitrites or papaverine-like compounds.

Precautions
1. Close monitoring of the patient's blood pressure must be carried out. Hypotension may occur and may require treatment (see Warning No. 4).
2. Use only peripheral veins for injection; avoid extravasation. If extravasation occurs, treat conservatively.
3. Rapid injection (over less than 30 seconds) is required for an effective, sustained antihypertensive response.
4. Use with caution in patients with impaired cerebral or cardiac circulation. Any abrupt reduction in blood pressure may cause ischemia.
5. Patients with impaired renal function usually do not require a reduction in dosage.
6. Hemo- and peritoneal dialysis will remove some diazoxide from the blood. More than one injection may be needed.

Adverse Reactions
Frequently seen:

diazoxide
(continued)
1. Sodium and water retention after repeated injections
2. Hyperglycemia

Infrequently seen:
1. Hypotension to shock levels
2. Transient myocardial ischemia which may lead to infarction, manifested by angina, atrial and ventricular arrhythmias, and ST segment changes
3. Cerebral ischemia, usually transient, but possibly leading to thrombosis, manifested by unconsciousness, seizures, paralysis, confusion or focal neurologic deficits
4. Increased BUN
5. Hypersensitivity reactions such as rashes, leukopenia, fever
6. Acute pancreatitis (rare)

Other reactions:
1. Postural hypotension and other signs of vasodilation.
2. Transient neurological findings (headache, dizziness, sleepiness)
3. Bradycardia, tachycardia
4. Warmth or pain along injected vein; cellulitis or phlebitis at extravasation site.
5. Nonanginal chest discomfort
6. Nausea and vomiting
7. Many other somatic sensations

☐ **Nursing Implications**
1. Of primary importance is the frequent monitoring of the blood pressure. Generally, blood pressure starts to decrease within 1 minute. The lowest blood pressure will be reached within 2–5 minutes. The pressure will rise rapidly over the next 10–30 minutes, and then more slowly over the following 2–12 hours, reaching but rarely exceeding pretreatment levels.
2. During the first 10 minutes, record the blood pressure at least once every 1–2 minutes; then every 5 minutes for one hour; then hourly for the next 2 hours; then every 2 hours for the next 2 hours and finally every 4 hours for the next 12 hours. This cycle should be interrupted *only* for additional injections, at which time the cycle should be repeated.
3. The patient should be kept recumbent during and for at least 1 hour after an injection. Check the lying and standing pressures before allowing a patient to become ambulatory. If there is a significant fall of pressure on standing, keep the patient at bed rest for an additional hour. Recheck lying and standing pressures again. Warn the patient against standing rapidly from bed or chair. (See No. 11).
4. Monitor for signs and symptoms of fluid and sodium retention in patients with a history of congestive heart failure or renal impairment:
   a. Increased weight (weigh daily)
   b. Rise in heart rate (take pulse every 4 hours)
   c. Dyspnea, orthopnea, rales, onset of third and/or fourth heart sound
   d. Rising jugular venous distension
   e. Peripheral pitting edema
   f. Decreased urinary output (record every 4–8 hours). Diuretics (*furosemide*) may be ordered to prevent this.
5. Nausea and vomiting occur frequently. Be prepared to prevent aspiration.
6. Do not leave the patient alone during the first hour, and then only when vital signs have stabilized.
7. Be prepared to treat hypotension:
   a. Trendelenburg position
   b. A vasopressor should be on hand
   c. Fluids
8. Prevent extravasation. See Appendix.
9. Monitor urine fractionals in diabetic patients during the first 24 hours. Insulin coverage may be ordered.
10. Monitor for the onset of cardiac arrhythmias. Instruct the patient to report chest pain of any type,

or palpitations. Patients with a history of arrhythmias or previous myocardial infarction should be observed continously via a bedside ECG monitor. Be prepared to treat arrhythmias:
a. Drugs: lidocaine, atropine, oxygen
b. An open intravenous line
c. Defibrillator
11. Patients in hypertensive crisis should be kept at rest in bed. Monitor for the consequences of an acute and extreme elevation of blood pressure:
a. Encephalopathy: confusion, stupor
b. Cerebrovascular accident
c. Myocardial ischemia and/or infarction: chest pain, arrhythmias, sudden fall in blood pressure not related to medication administration
d. Left ventricular failure: shortness of breath, orthopnea, elevated central venous pressure, tachycardia, onset of third and/or fourth heart sounds, rales
e. Renal failure: oliguria, rising BUN.[4]
These complications can also occur if the blood pressure is overly reduced by medication.
12. After the hypertension emergency has passed, the patient will require intensive hypertension education and follow-up to prevent subsequent crises and complications.

References
1. Koch-Weser, Jan: Diazoxide. *New England Journal of Medicine*, 294(23):1272, June 3, 1976.
2. Ibid.
3. Ibid.
4. Romankiewicz, J. A.: Pharmacology and Clinical Use of Drugs in Hypertensive Emergencies. *American Journal of Hospital Pharmacy*, 34(2):185, February 1977.

Suggested Readings
American Medical Association Committee on Hypertension: The Treatment of Malignant Hypertension and Hypertensive Emergencies, *JAMA*, 228:1673–1679, 1974.
Dhar, Sisir K., and Freeman, Philip: Clinical Management of Hypertensive Emergencies. *Heart and Lung*, 5(4):571–575, July–August 1976 (references).
Fleischmann, L. E.: Management of Hypertensive Crises in Children. *Pediatric Annals*, 6(6):410–414, June 1977.
Jones, L. N.: Symposium on Teaching and Rehabilitation of the Cardiac Patient. Hypertension: Medical and Nursing Implications. *Nursing Clinics of North America*, 11:283–295, June 1976.
Keith, Thomas: Hypertension Crisis, Recognition and Management. *JAMA*, 237(15):1570–1577, April 11, 1977.
Koch-Weser, Jan: Diazoxide. *New England Journal of Medicine*, 294(23):1271–1274, June 3, 1976 (references).
———: Hypertensive Emergencies. *New England Journal of Medicine*, 290:211, 1974.
Long, M. L., et al.: Hypertension: What the Patient Needs to Know. *American Journal of Nursing*, 76: 765–770, May 1976.
McDonald, W. J., et al.: Intravenous Diazoxide Therapy in Hypertensive Crisis. *American Journal of Cardiology*, 40(3):409–415, September 1977.
Romankiewicz, J. A.: Pharmacology and Clinical Use of Drugs in Hypertensive Emergencies. *American Journal of Hospital Pharmacy*, 34(2):185–193, February 1977 (references).
Tanner, Gloria: Heart Failure in the MI Patient. *American Journal of Nursing*, 77:230–234, February 1977 (discusses signs and symptoms of the onset of congestive heart failure).

diethylstilbestrol diphosphate ■
(Stilphostrol)

Actions/Indications
Synthetic estrogen. A potent, long-lasting nonsteroidal estrogen. Used

diethylstilbestrol diphosphate
(continued)
for palliative treatment of inoperable cancer of the prostate.

Dosage
Adults Only:
500 mg on first day, followed by 1 gm daily for 5 days.
   Maintenance—250–500 mg, 1–2 times weekly.

Preparation and Storage
Available in 5-ml ampuls containing 250 mg of drug.
   Add only to D5W or NS for infusion.

Drug Incompatibilities
Do not mix with any other medication.

Modes of IV Administration

Injection
No

Intermittent Infusion
Yes
Usually 0.5 gm in 300 ml NS or D5W at a rate of 20–30 macro-drops/min (2–3 ml/min) during the first 10–15 min, and then at a rate so that the entire amount is given in 1 hour.

Continuous Infusion
No

Contraindications; Warnings; Precautions; Adverse Reactions

Contraindications
1. Markedly impaired liver function
2. Thrombophlebitis, thromboembolic disorders, cerebral thrombosis or embolism, or past history of any one of these disorders

Warnings
1. **A statistically significant association has been shown between use of estrogen-containing drugs and thrombophlebitis, pulmonary embo-** lism and cerebral thrombosis.[1,2] Evidence is also suggestive of an association with retinal thrombosis and optic neuritis. Recent data suggests that the risks are in part dose-related.
2. The patient must be observed closely for earliest signs of thrombotic disorders; should any occur or be suspected, the drug must be discontinued.
3. Sudden onset of proptosis, diplopia or migraine requires withholding the drug pending examination. If papilledema or retinal vascular lesions are found, discontinue the drug.

Precautions
1. Use with caution in patients with epilepsy, migraine, asthma, cardiac or renal disease since the drug induces salt and water retention.
2. Carefully observe patients with a history of psychic depression; should serious depression recur, discontinue the drug.
3. There may be a decrease in glucose tolerance; monitor diabetic patients carefully.
4. Use with caution in patients with metabolic bone diseases that are associated with hypercalcemia or patients with renal insufficiency.
5. The pathologist should be advised that the patient is on estrogen therapy when relevant specimens are submitted.
6. Certain liver and endocrine function tests may be affected by treatment with estrogen. If such tests are abnormal in a patient taking this drug, it is recommended that they be repeated after the drug has been withdrawn for 2 months.

Adverse Reactions
1. This drug may increase the incidence of thromboembolic disease (see Warnings 1 and 2).
2. Gastrointestinal: anorexia, nausea, vomiting, diarrhea, cholestatic jaundice, abdominal cramps.

3. Central nervous system: headache, malaise, depression, anxiety, dizziness
4. Breast engorgement (male and female) and tenderness, loss of libido
5. Hypersensitivity reactions including anaphylaxis, rash
6. Renal: salt and water retention, edema, rise in BUN
7. Skin: acne, purpura, hair loss, erythema nodosum, itching, hemorrhagic eruption, erythema multiforme

☐ **Nursing Implications**
1. Monitor for signs and symptoms of:
   a. Thrombophlebitis—pain, swelling, positive Homans' sign in the legs
   b. Cerebral thrombosis—change in mental status, weakness and numbness of the face or extremities, seizures
   c. Pulmonary embolism
   d. Coronary thrombosis—chest pain, diaphoresis, fall in blood pressure
   e. Neuro-ocular lesions—changes in vision
   Report findings immediately to the physician; hold the next dose of the drug until further instructions from the physician.
2. There may be an increase in seizure activity; take seizure precautions when appropriate.
3. Monitor vulnerable patients for exacerbation of congestive heart failure secondary to fluid retention in susceptible patients:
   a. Increased weight
   b. Peripheral edema
   c. Increased respiratory rate, dyspnea, orthopnea
   d. Rales
   e. Increased heart rate
   f. Increased distention of the jugular veins
4. Monitor patients with renal insufficiency for signs of worsening of the condition:
   a. Weigh daily
   b. Record intake and output every 8 hours. Compare

findings with pretherapy values; report changes to the physician
   c. Be aware of the patient's pretherapy BUN and changes during therapy
5. Notify the physician immediately at the onset of proptosis (downward displacement of the eyeball, double vision, migraine headache, head pain accompanied by visual changes, nausea, vomiting). The drug should be discontinued.

References
1. Vessey, MP, Doll, R: Investigation of relation between use of oral contraceptives and thromboembolic disease. A further report. *British Medical Journal* 2:651–657, 1969.
2. Sartwell, PE et. al: Thromboembolism and oral contraceptives: An epidemiological case control study. *American Journal of Epidemiology.* 90:365–380, 1969.

digoxin ■
(Lanoxin Injection, Lanoxin Injection—Pediatric)

Actions/Indications
Cardiac glycoside. Acts directly on cardiac muscle to increase the force of myocardial contraction. The indirect actions mediated by the autonomic nervous system include slowing of the discharge of the sinus node, and thus slowing of heart rate and slowing of conduction through the A-V node. Initial effect occurs within 5–10 minutes with maximal effect in 1–2 hours.

Used in the treatment of all degrees of congestive heart failure; to control heart rate in atrial tachycardia, flutter, and fibrillation by slowing impulse formation and A-V conduction; and in cardiogenic shock when accompanied by pulmonary edema to improve myocardial contractility.

Dosage
Recommended doses are practical, average figures; dosage must be de-

digoxin
(continued)
termined by the patient's sensitivity
to the drug (See Warnings and Precautions), disease being treated,
body size, renal function, age and
other diseases or drugs likely to alter response to the drug.
*Adults and Children Over 10 Years
of Age:*
Full digitalization may require 1.0
mg total dosage. Maintenance dosage is 0.125–0.5 mg daily. Therapeutic serum levels—0.5–2.5
ng*/ml. Dosage should be decreased in the presence of renal failure.
*Nanograms

Children Under Age 10:
Premature and newborn
   Total digitalizing dose—0.025–
0.040 mg/kg. 1/2 dose stat; 1/4
dose in 4–8 hours; 1/4 dose in 4–8
hours.
   Maintenance—1/10–1/5 of digitalizing dose every 12 hours.
Two weeks to 2 years
   Total digitalizing dose—0.035–
0.050 mg/kg divided into 3–6 doses
with 6 or more hrs between each
dose.
   Maintenance—1/5 of digitalizing
dose divided into 2 doses daily.
Over 2 years–10 years
   Total digitalizing dose—0.025–
0.040 mg/kg divided into 3–6 doses
with 6 or more hrs between each
dose.
   Maintenance—1/5 of digitalizing
dose.

Preparation and Storage
Supplied in 2-ml ampuls, 0.25
mg/ml. Store at room temperature.
   (Pediatric Injection: 0.1 mg/ml
ampuls)

Drug Incompatibilities
Do not mix with any other medication in any manner.

Modes of IV Administration

Injection
Yes
Give undiluted, or diluted with 10
ml sterile water for injection, NS or
5% Dextrose. (If less than a 4-fold
dilution is used, precipitation of the
drug can occur). *Once diluted use immediately.*
   Inject slowly, over 5 minutes or
longer. Rapid injection can cause
systemic and coronary arteriolar
constriction; *caution is advised.*
   If given undiluted, inject as close
to the IV cannula as possible, either
into the cannula hub or into the
lowest Y injection site. In pulmonary
edema, give dose over 10–15 min.

Intermittent Infusion
No

Continuous Infusion
No

Contraindications; Warnings; Pre-cautions; Adverse Reactions

Contraindications
1. Digitalis toxicity
2. Hypersensitivity to cardiac glycosides
3. Ventricular fibrillation

Warnings
1. Titrate dosage carefully,
   monitoring heart rate, ECG,
   and serum levels to avoid intoxication.
2. Newborns vary in their tolerance to digitalis depending on
   their maturity. Premature and
   immature infants are very sensitive to this drug. Dosage must
   be individualized.
3. Many arrhythmias for which digitalis is prescribed can also be
   the result of digitalis intoxication. Rule out intoxication prior
   to continuing administration.
4. Patients in congestive heart failure may complain of nausea and
   vomiting. Exclude the possibility
   of digitalis intoxication before
   continuing with drug administration.
5. Patients with renal insufficiency
   will require lower dosage due to
   drug accumulation in the body.
   Creatinine clearance can be

used to help estimate the rate of digoxin excretion by the kidneys, and thus dosage in the presence of renal failure.

6. Use solely for the treatment of obesity is unwarranted and dangerous.

Precautions

1. Atrial arrhythmias associated with hyperthyroidism and febrile states are resistant to digoxin. When high doses are needed, guard against toxicity; monitor ECG and serum levels carefully. (See Dosage section.)
2. The following clinical situations make the myocardium more prone to toxicity and require careful dosage management:
   a. Hypokalemia, even at usual digitalis dosage levels. (Use caution with potassium depleting drugs such as corticosteroids or diuretics given concurrently.)
   b. Hypercalcemia
   c. Hypomagnesemia
   d. Long-standing cardiac disease (extensive myocardial fibrosis)
   e. Acute myocardial infarction
   f. Severe pulmonary disease (chronic obstructive or fibrotic disease)
   g. Rheumatic carditis or viral myocarditis
   h. Concurrent quinidine administration
3. The following clinical situations require reduction and careful titration of dosage in adults and children:
   a. Renal insufficiency
   b. Myxedema
   c. Following electrical conversion of arrhythmias
   d. Congestive heart failure accompanying acute glomerulonephritis (antihypertensives such as reserpine should be given at the same time)
4. Administer with extreme caution in the following clinical situations:
   a. Advanced or complete heart block (cardiac pacing may be needed)
   b. Ventricular tachycardia
   c. If the patient has received digitalis within the last 2–3 weeks
   d. Sinus node disease (sick sinus syndrome)
   e. Wolff–Parkinson–White syndrome and atrial fibrillation (extremely rapid ventricular rate or ventricular fibrillation can result)
5. Do not administer in the presence of idiopathic hypertrophic subaortic stenosis or constrictive pericarditis; a fall in cardiac output may result.
6. Avoid administering intravenous calcium to patients on digitalis drugs; fatal arrhythmias have resulted.
7. If used during pregnancy the risk of fetal harm appears remote yet such use should be limited to those clearly needing it.
8. This drug enters breast milk. Though levels are below usual infant maintenance dose, give cautiously to nursing mothers.

Adverse Reactions

1. Hypersensitivity: rash, urticaria, anaphylaxis (rare)
2. Gynecomastia
3. Toxic effects in children: supraventricular tachycardias (atrial and junctional) and A-V block are most common. Sinus bradycardia, premature ventricular contractions or almost any arrhythmia can be seen; also vomiting, poor feeding.
4. Toxic effects in adults:
   a. Gastrointestinal—anorexia, nausea, vomiting, diarrhea
   b. Central nervous system—headache, weakness, apathy, blurred vision, yellow vision, rainbow vision, confusion
   c. Arrhythmias—the most commonly seen are premature ventricular contractions (usually bigeminal or trigeminal) and sinus bradycardia;

digoxin
(continued)

however, almost any arrhythmia may be produced by digitalis toxicity

Treatment of Digitalis Toxicity

1. Discontinue the drug at the first suspicion of toxicity and do not reinitiate until signs and symptoms of toxicity subside.
2. Initiate continuous ECG monitoring if not already present.
3. Maintain a normal serum potassium (3.5–5.5 mEq/liter), but do *not* administer potassium in the presence of advanced or complete heart block secondary to digitalis toxicity; the block may increase.[1]
4. Pharmacologic treatment of toxicity should by guided by the arrhythmia produced. Phenytoin (Dilantin) is usually the drug of choice. Lidocaine, procainamide, and propranolol can also be used depending on the clinical situation. (If propranolol is used, monitor atrioventricular conduction closely. This drug may cause increasing A-V block.) Atropine can be used to treat bradyarrhythmias. See entries for each drug for further details on their use.
5. If profound bradycardia and/or complete A-V block occur, transvenous temporary pacing may be necessary until toxicity resolves.

☐ **Nursing Implications**

1. Patients receiving this medication intravenously should, in most instances, be observed for arrhthymias via continuous ECG monitoring. Observe for improvement if the drug is given to treat an arrhythmia, and observe for arrhythmias which may be produced by the drug. Some of the more common arrhythmias produced by toxic levels of digoxin: sinus bradycardia, premature ventricular and atrial contractions, atrioventricular block of all degrees, paroxysmal

atrial tachycardia. Notify the physician of improvement in arrhythmia being treated, and document with an ECG tracing. If arrhythmias of toxicity appear, notify the physician, document with an ECG tracing, and hold the next dose of digoxin until the physician decides what course of action is appropriate.
2. Be prepared to administer immediate care in the event of arrhythmias due to toxicity. See Treatment of Digitalis Toxicity above. Atropine 0.5–1.0 mg can be given for a heart rate less than 50–60/minute. (In units where registered nurses are expected to administer drugs in such an event, the unit physician should decide at what heart rate the atropine should be administered and in what amount.) See page 24 for details on atropine.
   For premature ventricular contractions or ventricular tachycardia, lidocaine 50–100 mg can be given by intravenous injection. Again, unit policy should dictate when and how much drug is given. See page 186 for details on lidocaine.
3. Observe for noncardiac symptoms of digitalis toxicity: anorexia; nausea; vomiting and diarrhea; visual disturbances, e.g., rainbow vision or yellow vision (rare); in children, poor feeding and irritability; headache (rare); confusion; severe fatigue.[2]
4. Monitor for signs of improvement if the patient is being treated for congestive heart failure:
   a. Reduction in weight (weigh the patient daily)
   b. Reduction in peripheral edema
   c. Increased urine output (measure every 8 hours)
   d. Decreased resting heart rate to normal limits (record every 4 to 8 hours)
   e. Decreased respiratory rate; disappearance of rales

f. Increased exercise tolerance
Note that worsening congestive
failure, despite digitalis administration, may be a sign of digitalis toxicity.
5. Be aware of the patient's serum
potassium. Hypokalemia can
precipitate digitalis toxicity. Administer potassium supplements
as ordered. These may produce
nausea and vomiting (liquid
preparations especially), usually
soon after administration. The
nurse's observations will be
needed to differentiate between
potassium-induced nausea and
vomiting and that due to digitalis toxicity. (Normal serum potassium: 3.5–5.5 mEq/liter.)
6. Rarely, elderly patients experience hallucinations, anxiety,
and delusions secondary to toxic levels of digitalis preparations. Monitor for onset of this
complication, notify the physician, and initiate safety measures, such as side rails, restraints (as necessary), close
observation, reorientation, and
reassurance.
7. Patients who will require this
drug on a chronic basis must be
instructed on safe self-administration of the digitalis.

References

1. Davis, Richard H., and Fisch,
Charles: Potassium and Arrhythmias. *Geriatrics*, November 1970,
p. 110.
2. Lely, A. H., and van Enter, C.
H. J.: Noncardiac Symptoms of
Digitalis Intoxication. *American
Heart Journal*, 83(2):150, February 1972.

Suggested Readings

Amsterdam, Ezra A., et al.: Systemic
Approach to the Management of
Cardiac Arrhythmias. *Heart and
Lung*, 2(5):747–753, September–
October 1973 (references).
Arbeit, Sidney, et al.: Recognizing
Digitalis Toxicity. *American Journal
of Nursing*, 77(12):1936–1945, De-
cember 1977 (references).
Isacson, Lauren Marie, and Schultz,

Klaus: Treating Pulmonary Edema. *Nursing '78*, February 1978,
pp. 42–46.
James, Frederick W., and Love,
Ervena: Congestive Heart Failure
in Infants and Children, *Heart and
Lung*. 3(3):396–400, May–June
1974.
Lely, A. H., and van Enter, C. H. J.:
Noncardiac Symptoms of Digitalis
Intoxication. *American Heart Journal*, 83(2):149–152, February
1972.
Rosen, Michael R., Wit, Andrew,
and Hoffman, Brian F.: Electrophysiology and Pharmacology of
Cardiac Arrhythmias. IV: Cardiac
Antiarrhythmic and Toxic Effects
of Digitalis. *American Heart Journal*,
89(3):391–399, March 1975 (ref-
erences).
———Treatment of Cardiac Arrhythmias. *Medical Letter on Drugs
and Therapeutics*, 16(25):101–108,
December 6, 1974.
Tanner, Gloria: Heart Failure in the
MI Patient. *American Journal of
Nursing*, 77:230–234, February
1977.

diphenhydramine hydrochloride ■
(Benadryl)

Actions/Indications

Potent antihistaminic, anticholinergic
(antispasmotic), antiemetic and sedative agent. Used for:
• Prevention and treatment of allergic reactions to blood and plasma
• Anaphylaxis along with other
measures
• Uncomplicated allergic reactions
when oral route cannot be used
• Motion sickness
• Parkinsonism, including drug-induced extra-pyramidal reactions

Dosage

Adults:
10–50 mg (maximum daily dose is
400 mg; maximum single dose is
100 mg), for all indications.
Children:
5 mg/kg/24 hrs or 150 mg/M^2/24
hrs; divided into 4 doses. Maximum

diphenhydramine hydrochloride
(continued)
dose is 300 mg in 24 hours for all indications.

Preparation and Storage
Available in 10 ml and 30 ml vials containing 10 mg/ml of drug and 1 ml ampuls and disposable syringes and 10 ml vials containing 50 mg/ml.

Drug Incompatibilities
Do not mix with:
Amobarbital
Amphotericin B
Cephalothin
Hydrocortisone
Iodipamide meglumine
Pentobarbital
Phenobarbital
Potassium iodide
Secobarbital
Thiopental

Modes of IV Administration

Injection
Yes
Slowly.

Intermittent Infusion
Yes
Use any fluid, 50–100 ml. Drip rate should be set according to hourly dose prescribed and patient response.

Continuous Infusion
Yes
Use any fluid in any volume. Drip rate should be set according to hourly dose prescribed and patient response.

Contraindications; Warnings; Precautions; Adverse Reactions

Contraindications
1. Do not use in premature or newborn infants.
2. Nursing mothers.
3. Asthma attacks or other lower respiratory tract symptoms.
4. Hypersensitivity to this drug or chemically-related antihistamines.

5. Patients receiving monoamine oxidase (MAO) inhibitors.

Warnings
1. Use with extreme caution in patients with:
   a. narrow angle glaucoma
   b. stenosing peptic ulcer
   c. pyloroduodenal obstruction
   d. symptomatic prostatic hypertrophy
   e. bladder neck obstruction
2. Overdosage may produce convulsions and death, especially in infants and children. Correct dosage can produce excitation or diminish mental alertness in young children.
3. Drowsiness, sedation and hypotension can occur, especially in the elderly. Take precautions when ambulating the patient.
4. Administer with caution during pregnancy; there exists potential for harm to the fetus.
5. Anaphylaxis can occur.
6. This drug has additive effects when given with other CNS depressants.

Precautions
1. Avoid extravasation.
2. This drug has anticholinergic effects such as tachycardia, dry mouth, blurring of vision, and urinary retention.
3. Use with caution in patients with a history of asthma, increased intraocular pressure, hyperthyroidism, cardiovascular disease, hypertension. (See Contraindication No. 3 and Warning No. 1.)

Adverse Reactions
1. General: urticaria, rash, anaphylaxis, photosensitivity, chills, dryness of mucous membranes.
2. Cardiovascular: hypotension, headache, palpitations, tachycardia.
3. Nervous system: sedation, dizziness, disturbed coordination, confusion, insomnia, blurred vision, convulsions.
4. Hematologic: hemolytic anemia, thrombocytopenia, agranulocytosis.

5. Gastrointestinal: epigastric distress, nausea, vomiting, diarrhea, constipation.
6. Genitourinary: urinary retention, frequency, dysuria, early menses.
7. Respiratory: thickened bronchial secretions, wheezing, tightness in the chest.

☐ **Nursing Implications**
1. Ambulate patients with care following injection to prevent injury; the patient may be dizzy as well as drowsy.
2. Be prepared to manage confusion. Keep side rails up for elderly patients or those who develop confusion or excitement, e.g. children. These patients may require one-to-one care until the adverse effects subside. Reassurance, reorientation and mild restraints should be used as necessary.
3. Monitor all patients for urinary retention, i.e., urinary output and bladder size every 2–4 hours.
4. Notify the physician of the onset of any adverse reactions.
5. Administer supportive care to patients being treated for allergic reactions. See Appendix on anaphylaxis.
6. Be prepared to manage vomiting in a drowsy patient, to prevent aspiration.
7. Take precautions to prevent extravasation; see Appendix.

dobutamine hydrochloride ■
(Dobutrex)

Actions/Indications
Inotropic agent (synthetic catecholamine), directly stimulates beta-1 receptors in the heart. As a result, the force of myocardial contraction and stroke volume are increased. Mild chronotropic, hypertensive, arrhythmogenic and vasodilative effects are also seen at higher doses. Onset of action is within 1–2 minutes, peak effect after 10 minutes. Plasma half-life is 2 minutes. This drug is metabolized in the liver and excreted through the kidneys.

Used in *short-term* treatment of adults with cardiac decompensation due to depressed contractility resulting from organic heart disease or cardiac surgery.

Dosage
Adults:
2.5 to 10 mcg/kg/min, rarely infusion rates up to 40 mcg/kg/min have been required. Adjust to patient response (heart rate, presence of PVCs, blood pressure, urine flow, CVP, pulmonary capillary wedge pressure, cardiac output). See table below.
Children:
No recommendations available.

Preparation and Storage
Supplied in vials containing 250 mg.
Reconstitute with sterile water for

Rates of Infusion for Concentrations of 250, 500 & 1000 mcg/ml

Desired Drug Delivery Rate (mcg/kg/min)	Infusion Delivery Rate		
	250 mcg/ml[1] (ml/kg/min)	500 mcg/ml[2] (ml/kg/min)	1000 mcg/ml[3] (ml/kg/min)
2.5	0.01	0.005	0.0025
5.0	0.02	0.010	0.005
7.5	0.03	0.015	0.0075
10.0	0.04	0.020	0.0100
12.5	0.05	0.025	0.0125
15.0	0.06	0.030	0.015

(Courtesy of Eli Lilly and Company)

[1]250 mg per liter of diluent
[2]500 mg per liter or 250 mg per 500 ml of diluent
[3]1000 mg per liter, 500 mg/500 ml of diluent, or 250 mg per 250 ml of diluent

dobutamine hydrochloride
(continued)

injection or D5W. Add 10 ml, agitate; add another 10 ml if material does not completely dissolve. Store in refrigerator; discard after 48 hours. This reconstituted form must then be diluted in at least 50 ml prior to administration. Use D5W, NS or sodium lactate. Use solution within 24 hours. Solution may be slightly colored; coloration may increase over time—this is normal. See Dosage section for solution concentrations.

Drug Incompatibilities
Do not add to alkaline solutions such as sodium bicarbonate.

Modes of IV Administration

Injection
No

Intermittent Infusion
No
Administered by titration

Continuous Infusion
Yes
Use an infusion pump

Contraindications; Warnings; Precautions; Adverse Reactions

Contraindications
Idiopathic hypertrophic subaortic stenosis.

Warnings
1. This agent may cause a marked rise in systolic blood pressure and heart rate. Reduction in dose reverses these effects promptly.
2. There is enhanced A-V node conduction, which in the presence of atrial fibrillation or flutter can cause a rapid ventricular response. Digitalis should be administered if possible before initiating dobutamine therapy
3. Patients with preexisting hypertension are at greater risk of developing an exaggerated pressor response.
4. There may be precipitation or exaggeration of PVCs. Ventricular tachycardia is rare.

Precautions
1. Infusion rate must be governed by pulmonary wedge pressure, cardiac output, ECG, and blood pressure.
2. Hypovolemia should be corrected with volume expanders prior to treatment with this agent.
3. Studies suggest that this drug may be less effective in patients who have recently received a beta-blocking drug. In this case peripheral vascular resistance may increase.
4. Lack of improvement in clinical status may be seen in patients with cardiac mechanical obstruction such as severe aortic valvular stenosis.
5. Safety for use in myocardial infarction is unknown. There is concern that with increased contractile force the size of the infarction may increase by intensifying ischemia.
6. Safety for use in pregnancy has not been established; use only when expected benefits to the mother outweigh possible risks to the fetus.
7. Use of this drug in children has not been studied.
8. Drug interaction studies have shown no evidence of deleterious interactions between dobutamine and other drugs including digitalis, furosemide, spironolactone, lidocaine, glyceryl trinitrate, isosorbide dinitrate, morphine, atropine, heparin, protamine, potassium chloride, folic acid, and acetaminophen. Concomitant use of dobutamine and nitroprusside results in a higher cardiac output and usually a lower pulmonary wedge pressure than when either drug is used alone.

Adverse Reactions
1. Tachycardia, increased blood pressure, PVCs. These effects are dose-related.

2. Uncommon effects: nausea, headache, anginal pain, nonspecific chest pain, palpitations, shortness of breath.
3. Infusions of up to 72 hours have revealed no adverse reactions other than those listed above.

Management of Overdosage
Overdosage is evidenced by excessive rise in blood pressure or tachycardia. Reduction in the infusion rate will quickly remedy these problems; usually no additional measures are necessary.

☐ **Nursing Implications**
1. The following suggested monitoring regimen is designed to guide dosage, to detect presence or absence of drug effectiveness, and to avoid overdosage. Monitor the following parameters:
   a. Cardiac output—drug should cause an increase.
   b. Arterial blood pressure—direct measurement is recommended along with indirect. This should rise but not to hypertensive levels. Decrease infusion rate if an inordinate rise is seen (see Overdosage above).
   c. Pulmonary capillary wedge pressure and/or C.V.P.—as cardiac output improves (increases) the P.C.W.P. or C.V.P. will decrease to more normal levels (except in the presence of primary pulmonary hypertension).
   d. Urine output—should increase with increase in cardiac output. Report if output is less than 30 ml/hour over 8 hours time.
   e. Heart rate and rhythm—rate may rise with infusion; decrease infusion rate to eliminate this. May be an increase in P.V.C.'s. These can also be controlled with reduced dosage. Monitor for rapid ventricular rates in patients with atrial fibrillation. Re-

port rates over 100/minute; digitalize as ordered. Report lack of response to drug; e.g., failure of cardiac output to rise with normal dosage.
2. Report onset of anginal pain or shortness of breath to the physician.

dopamine hydrochloride ■
(Intropin)

Actions/Indications
A sympathomimetic amine, precursor of norepinephrine. Increases cardiac output by direct inotropic effect on the heart muscle; and indirectly by stimulating the release of norepinephrine.[1]

Onset of action is rapid, within 5 min. The duration is about 10 min. Specific actions are dose-dependent:
Low Dose
(1–2 mcg/kg/min) Dilatation of renal and mesenteric vessels, no change in heart rate, blood pressure or cardiac output.
Intermediate Dose
(2–10 mcg/kg/min)
Increased cardiac output, increased systolic blood pressure, increased perfusion of the abdominal viscera, and kidneys with secondary increase in glomerular filtration and sodium excretion, and minimal increase in myocardial oxygen requirements.
High Dose
(greater than 20 mcg/kg/min)
Pronounced peripheral, renal and mesenteric vasoconstriction.
Indicated in the management of:
- Septic shock unresponsive to fluid challenge and steroids
- Acute myocardial infarction or immediate postoperative cardiac surgery with shock unresponsive to volume expanders
- Chronic congestive heart failure unresponsive to diuretics and digitalis, with or without vasodilator therapy
- Severe cirrhosis with renal insufficiency (this is a possible indication)

dopamine hydrochloride
(continued)
Dosage
Adults (starting doses):
Septic shock—2–5 mcg/kg/min.
Titrate to maintain an adequate tissue perfusion and systolic blood pressure (direct arterial), pulmonary capillary wedge pressure, CVP and urinary output (see Nursing Implications).
Acute myocardial infarction—2–6 mcg/kg/min.
Titrate as described above.
Chronic congestive heart failure—1–2 mcg/kg/min.
Titrate to produce an adequate urine output (at least 30–50 ml/hr) and tissue perfusion.
Renal perfusion alone—0.5–2.0 mcg/kg/min.
Titrate to obtain desired urine output without undesirable changes in heart rate and blood pressure.
For more seriously ill patients—start with 5 mcg/kg/min. Increase gradually using 5–10 mcg/kg/min increments up to 20–50 mcg/kg/min.
At any dosage level, once the desired response is obtained, maintain the infusion rate at the lowest level that produces optimal results.
Children:
Not currently recommended for use in children.

Preparation and Storage
Available in 5 ml ampuls, 5 ml vials and 5 ml additive syringes, each containing 200 mg (40 mg/ml), and in 5 ml vials and 5 ml additive syringes containing 400 mg (80 mg/ml), 800-mg vial (160 mg/ml); pre-mixed IV solutions in D5W: 200 mg in 250 ml, 400 mg in 500 ml, 400 mg in 250 ml, 800 mg in 500 ml. *See Table Below.*
Preparation of Dopamine Solutions

Fluid Volume (ml)	Ampuls Of Dopamine (200 mg/ ampul)	Resultant Concentration (mcg/ml)	mcg/Microdrop
500	2 (400 mg)	800	13

Fluid Volume (ml)	Ampuls Of Dopamine (200 mg/ ampul)	Resultant Concentration (mcg/ml)	mcg/Microdrop
500	4 (800 mg)	1600	26
500	6 (1200 mg)	2400	40
500	8 (1600 mg)	3200	53

This drug must be mixed THOROUGHLY with the solution to avoid inadvertent administration of a bolus of the drug.
Solutions utilizing the fluids listed in the Continuous Infusion section are stable for 48 hours.[4]
Do not use solutions that are discolored.
As with all drugs that must be titrated, dopamine must not be mixed with other drugs in the same solution bottle; infuse it as a secondary IV line.

Drug Incompatibilities
Do not add any other medication to a solution bottle containing dopamine.
Do NOT mix in any manner with:
Amphotericin B[5]
Sodium bicarbonate
Any alkaline solution
The following drugs CAN be piggy-backed into IV lines containing dopamine.[6]
Calcium chloride
Calcium gluconate
Carbenicillin
Cephalothin
Chloramphenicol
Gentamicin
Heparin
Hydrocortisone
Kanamycin
Lidocaine
Methylprednisolone
Oxacillin
Potassium chloride
Potassium penicillin
Procainamide
Tetracycline
Vitamins

Modes of IV Administration

Injection
No
IT MUST BE HIGHLY DILUTED
BEFORE ADMINISTRATION

Intermittent Infusion
No

Continuous Infusion
Yes
Use any of the following fluids:
NS
D5W
D5/NS
D5/0.45 saline
D5/RL
Sodium Lactate, 1/6 Molar
RL
20% Mannitol
 Use no other fluids.
 See Preparation section for solution preparation.
Use an Infusion Pump.

Contraindications; Warnings; Precautions; Adverse Reactions

Contraindications
1. Pheochromocytoma
2. Uncorrected tachyarrhythmias or ventricular fibrillation

Warnings
1. This is a potent drug that must be highly diluted before use.
2. Use with caution and in reduced dosage in patients who are on, or have received within the last 14 days, MAO inhibitor drugs. The manufacturer suggests a dose 1/10 of the normal calculated dose.
3. Use in pregnancy requires that the expected benefits to the mother be weighed against possible risks to the fetus.
4. Safety for use in children has not been established.
5. The shorter the time period between onset of signs and symptoms and the initiation of dopamine therapy, the better the prognosis. Patients respond best when such parameters as

urinary output, blood pressure and cardiac function have not undergone profound deterioration.

Precautions
1. If possible, before beginning treatment, correct any hypovolemia with either whole blood or plasma.
2. In the presence of shock, the pulmonary artery wedge pressure should be in the 14–18 mmHg range (or CVP between 10–15) prior to the administration of this drug.
3. Decrease the infusion rate if the diastolic blood pressure rises disproportionately to the systolic pressure (i.e., a decrease in pulse pressure). This indicates the presence of predominate vasoconstriction, and can be undesirable in certain clinical situations.
4. Avoid extravasation, which can lead to tissue necrosis and sloughing. Do not use small veins for infusion if at all possible. If extravasation occurs, *immediately* infiltrate the area with 10–15 ml of a solution of normal saline containing 5–10 mg of phentolamine (Regitine). Using a syringe with a 25 or 26 gauge needle, infiltrate liberally. The area will become red secondary to the vasodilatation produced by the phentolamine. Protect the area from subsequent trauma and monitor for signs of necrosis (see Appendix).
5. In patients with a history of occlusive vascular disease (arteriosclerosis, arterial embolism, Raynaud's disease, cold injury, diabetic endarteritis, Buerger's disease, etc.) monitor closely for changes in circulation to the extremities. (See Nursing Implications.)
6. Use with extreme caution in patients receiving cyclopropane or halogenated hydrocarbon anesthetics. There may be in-

dopamine hydrochloride
(continued)

creased myocardial irritability and resultant arrhythmias.

7. Close monitoring of urine flow, cardiac output and blood pressure is essential during infusion of dopamine.

Adverse Reactions

1. Arrhythmias—premature ventricular contractions and ventricular tachycardia (both responsive to lidocaine), bradycardia
2. Angina pectoris
3. Nausea and vomiting
4. Headache
5. Dyspnea
6. Hypotension and hypertension
7. Decreased urine output (usually seen in high dosage), increased BUN

Treatment of Overdosage (Evidenced by excessive blood pressure elevation)

1. Slow or stop the infusion and stay with the patient.
2. Monitor blood pressure every 1–2 minutes.
3. Usually additional measures are not necessary due to the short duration of action.
4. If the patient does not stabilize, a short-acting alpha adrenergic blocking agent (phentolamine) can be administered as an intravenous infusion. See page 273.
5. If the patient is able, instruct him, prior to the initiation of the infusion, to report chest pain of any kind. If it occurs, slow the infusion and monitor heart rate and blood pressure carefully. Observe for arrhythmias.
6. See Nursing Implications section for further details.

☐ **Nursing Implications**

1. Before beginning therapy, weigh the patient, if possible, for dosage determination.
2. Use an infusion pump at all times during the administration of this drug, to prevent over- or underdosage. If a pump is not available, microdrop intravenous infusion tubing must be used. (Always monitor ml's, or *volume* delivered, therefore mcg's delivered, *not* drops of fluid, to keep dosage accurate.)

Whether using a pump or microdrop tubing, monitor the infusion rate frequently. With microdrop tubing the drip rate should be counted with each blood pressure determination. Prevent changes in drip rate secondary to patient movement, arm position, etc. with restraints and armboards. When the frequency of blood pressure determinations decreases with stabilization of the patient's condition, count the drip rate again at least every 15 to 30 minutes.

Extreme caution must be exercised when using highly concentrated solutions of dopamine. Small changes in the infusion rate can change the dosage of the drug drastically.

3. Monitoring the patient's condition and drug effectiveness:
   a. It is recommended that the following parameters be continually evaluated and used to guide the dosage of dopamine during therapy:[7,8]
      1. Continuous direct arterial blood pressure via arterial cannulation (rather than by the less accurate, and at times deceptive, sphygmomanometry)
      2. Central venous pressure
      3. Pulmonary artery wedge pressure (especially in patients with, or who are likely to develop, left ventricular failure)
      4. Arterial blood gases and acid-base balance
      5. Urine output and specific gravity
      6. In some instances, cardiac output
      7. Heart rate and rhythm

When using these parameters it is helpful to have pretreatment values for comparison.

b. Initial dosage and titration routine must be ordered by the physician. The dosage must be prescribed in mcg/kg/min terms, based on the response desired (see Actions/Indications section). Arterial blood pressure and other parameter goals of therapy must also be set by the physician. Ideal levels must be determined for each patient depending on the clinical situation. However, an adequate arterial systolic pressure is considered to be approximately 80 to 90 mm Hg[9], the CVP 12 to 14 mm Hg, the pulmonary artery wedge pressure 14 to 18 mm Hg[10] (see Precaution No. 1), and a urine output of at least 30 ml per hour.

c. Begin titration with the prescribed initial dosage. The onset of action will be within 5 minutes, the duration up to 10 minutes. Increase the dose of dopamine by 0.5 mcg/kg/min increments every 5 minutes until the arterial pressure and other parameter goals are reached. It is recommended to use the lowest dosage of dopamine that can maintain the desired response (see Dosage section).

d. Obtain arterial pressures every 2 to 5 minutes during the initial titration phase, whenever the patient becomes unstable, or during the weaning phase of administration. Keep blood pressure monitor alarms set at appropriate levels. During the maintenance phase of administration, when the patient's parameters are stable at adequate levels, monitor blood pressure every 15 to 30 minutes. The patient may require dopamine therapy for several days; careful titration and monitoring will be required throughout this therapy.

As the patient's condition improves to the point at which the dosage of dopamine can be decreased, the arterial pressure may fall as the low-dose range is reached (see Actions/Indicatons section). It may be advisable to stop the infusion at this point. The pressure may then rise back to a more desirable level. Continue to monitor pressures frequently for the next several hours to evaluate the patient's response. Be prepared to restart the infusion.

e. Monitor heart rate with each blood pressure determination. The ECG should be monitored throughout therapy for the onset of arrhythmias.

f. The central venous pressure and pulmonary artery wedge pressure should be obtained as frequently as the patient's condition dictates, usually hourly during the initial phase of therapy.

g. Measure urine output via a Foley catheter every hour during the initial titration phase, when the patient is unstable, if the patient is being treated for acute tubular necrosis, has pre-existing renal disease, and during the weaning phase of drug titration. As the cardiac output and arterial blood pressure increase, the urine output will also increase. In low-dose therapy, this drug causes dilatation of the renal arteries, increasing glomerular filtration, thus increasing the urine output (see Actions/Indications section).

Monitor urine specific gravity at least every 4 hours and report changes to the physician. The value should

dopamine hydrochloride
(continued)

stay within normal limits in most patients.

h. Monitor arterial blood gases every 2 to 4 hours via the arterial cannula, as the patient's condition dictates. Improvement in circulation with the rise in cardiac output and blood pressure should bring the pH and pCO_2 values within normal limits where they had previously indicated an acidotic state secondary to shock.

i. Monitor cardiac output as necessary under physician order.

4. Management of adverse reactions:

a. Excessive elevation in arterial pressure (greater than the target pressure prescribed by the physician):
Decrease the infusion rate by 0.5 mcg/kg/min increments every 5 minutes and monitor the arterial pressure every 1 to 2 minutes. Continue the downward titration until a desirable pressure is reached. Note the dosage of dopamine that produced the rise in pressure, notify the physician.

b. Hypotension:
High doses of this drug (greater than 20 mcg/kg/minute) can cause hypotension. If this occurs with such a dosage, reduce the infusion rate by 0.5 mcg/kg/min increments until the arterial pressure begins to rise. If a rise is not seen, notify the physician. Note the dosage of dopamine that produced this effect. Low-dose therapy can also produce hypotension in some patients; see Nursing Implications No. 3d above.
Hypotension can also be the result of deterioration in the patient's condition, due to hypovolemia, sepsis, increasing cardiac decompensation, etc. Changing the dosage (increasing or decreasing, depending on the situation) may remedy this; if not, notify the physician.

c. Chest pain (angina), nausea, headache, dyspnea:
Instruct the patient to report the onset of any of these symptoms, if he is able. The patient who is unable to complain of the symptoms may become restless, or show an increase in heart or respiratory rate. In either case, stay with the patient; reassure him that the situation can be controlled. Decrease the infusion rate by 0.5 mcg/kg increments every 5 minutes and monitor the arterial pressure. If these symptoms were due to the dopamine, they will usually subside within 10 minutes. If they do not subside with a decrease in dosage, notify the physician at once. Be prepared to manage vomiting to prevent aspiration.

d. Arrhythmias: Dopamine can produce sinus and ventricular tachycardia and premature ventricular contractions. These arrhythmias can also be caused by the patient's underlying pathology or by fever, hypoxemia, pain, fear or physical exertion (struggling against a respirator, restlessness). If these other causes have been ruled out, reduce the infusion rate of dopamine by 0.5 mcg/kg/min (or 5 drops/min) increments, monitor the arterial pressure and notify the physician. Ventricular irritability (premature ventricular contractions and ventricular tachycardia) can be controlled by lidocaine. Be prepared to administer a bolus of lidocaine if either one of these arrhythmias occurs. Document the arrhythmia, the amount of lidocaine given, and notify the physician (follow hospital policy on the administration of lidocaine). If these arrhythmias continue to occur, a lidocaine infusion may be ordered (see page 186).

e. Peripheral vasoconstriction: This can occur during high-dose therapy, see Actions/Indications section. A disproportionate rise in diastolic blood pressure will occur with a reduction in pulse pressure. The blood pressure via sphygmomanometry will be reduced. Other signs will be mottling of the skin, reduction in skin temperature, cyanosis of the nail beds, pallor, and diaphoresis (see Precaution No. 5).
If these signs appear, reduce the dosage of dopamine by 0.5 mcg/kg/min increments every 5 minutes. Observe the arterial pressure frequently and watch for changes in the presenting signs. If an improvement is not seen, notify the physician (see Precaution No. 3).

f. Oliguria: High-dose therapy (greater than 20 mcg/kg/minute) can produce renal artery constriction with a resultant fall in renal perfusion and urine output.[11] Deterioration in the patient's condition can also reduce the urine output. If output decreases below 30 ml/minute, notify the physician and continue careful monitoring. The physician may order a change in the dosage of dopamine, the administration of a diuretic, mannitol or fluids as needed.

5. Take all precautions to prevent extravasation; see Appendix. Keep phentolamine readily available; see Precaution No. 3. If extravasation is even suspected (blanching of the skin around the intravenous cannula, swelling, etc.) notify the physician at once. Infiltration of the affected area with phentolamine must be carried out as soon as possible to help prevent tissue necrosis. After treatment, protect the area from further trauma and observe for sloughing of the tissue.

6. If this drug is administered during advanced life support (CPR), take all precautions to avoid mixing the dopamine with sodium bicarbonate. Flush the intravenous line with plain fluid before injecting the sodium bicarbonate and after, before restarting the dopamine infusion. If possible, use a separate intravenous line for the administration of the bicarbonate. These drugs are incompatible (see Drug Incompatibility section).

References

1. Lee, W. C., and Yoo, C. S.: Mechanism of Cardiac Activities of Sympathomimetic Amines on Isolated Auricles of Rabbits. *Archives International, of Pharmacodynamics* (French), 151:93, 1964.
2. Horwitz, David, Fox, Samuel, and Goldberg, Leon I.: Effects of Dopamine in Man. *Circulation Research*, 10:239, February 1962.
3. Meyer, M. B., McNay, John L., and Goldberg, Leon I.: Effects of Dopamine on Renal Function and Hemodynamics in the Dog. *Journal of Pharmacology and Experimental Therapeutics*, 156(1):187, 1967.
4. Gardella, L. A., et al.: Intropin (Dopamine Hydrochloride) Intravenous Admixture Compatibility. *American Journal of Hospital Pharmacy*, 36(6):577, June 1978.
5. Gardella, L. A., et al.: Intropin (Dopamine Hydrochloride) Intravenous Admixture Compatibility, Part 3: Stability With Miscellaneous Additives, *Ameri-*

dopamine hydrochloride
(continued)

can *Journal of Hospital Pharmacy,*
35(5):582, May 1978.
6. Ibid, p. 578.
7. Jahre, Jeffery A., et al.: Medical
Approach to the Hypotensive
Patient and the Patient in
Shock. *Heart and Lung,* 4(4):578,
July–August 1975.
8. Ayers, Stephen M., et al.: *Care of
the Critically Ill* (2nd ed.), New
York: Appleton-Century-Crofts,
1974, p. 259.
9. Tarazi, Robert C.: Sympathomimetic Agents in the Treatment
of Shock. *Annals of Internal Medicine,* 81, September, 1974.
10. Ayers, p. 262.
11. Ibid.

Suggested Readings

Amsterdam, Ezra, A., et al.: Evaluation and Management of Cardiogenic Shock, Part I: Approach to
the Patient. *Heart and Lung,*
1(3):402–408, May–June 1972
(references).
————: Evaluation and Management
of Cardiogenic Shock, Part II:
Drug Therapy. *Heart and Lung,*
1(5):663–671, September–October
1972 (references).
Goldberg, Leon I., and Hsieh, Y.:
Clinical Use of Dopamine. *Ratio-
nal Drug Therapy,* 11:1–5, November 1977 (references).
Jahre, Jeffery, et al.: Medical
Approach to the Hypotensive Patient and the Patient in Shock.
Heart and Lung, 4(4):577–587 (references).
Tarazi, Robert C.: Sympathomimetic
Agents in the Treatment of
Shock. *Annals of Internal Medicine,*
81:364–371, September 1974.
Woods, Susan L.: Monitoring Pulmonary Artery Pressure. *American
Journal of Nursing,* 76(11):1765–
1771, November 1976 (references).
Dopamine for the Treatment of
Shock. *The Medical Letter,* 17:13–
14, 1975 (references).
Intravenous Infusion of Vasopressors—Programmed Instruction.
American Journal of Nursing,
65(11):129–152, November 1965
(useful information on theories
behind drug titration).

doxapram hydrochloride ■
(Dopram Injectable)

Actions/Indications
Respiratory stimulant, through direct effects on central respiratory
centers. Produces an increased tidal
volume and slightly increased respiratory rate. Onset of action: 20–40
seconds; peak: 1–2 minutes; duration: 5–12 minutes.

Used as *adjunct* to therapy for:
• Postanesthesia respiratory apnea
  or depression other than that due
  to muscle relaxant drugs
• Stimulating deep breathing postoperatively
• Hastening return of pharyngeal
  reflexes secondary to drug overdose
• Drug-overdose respiratory
  depression
• Chronic pulmonary disease associated with acute hypercapnia (as a
  temporary measure), in hospitalized patients.

Dosage
Do not exceed maximum total dosage. To minimize side effects use
minimum effective dosage.
Postanesthesia:
Injection—0.5–1 mg/kg, repeat if
necessary at 5-min intervals.
Infusion—initiate a 1 mg/ml solution
at 5 mg/min until desired response
is seen. Maintain infusion rate of 1–
3 mg/min. Recommended total dosage is 4 mg/kg, not to exceed 3 gm.
Drug Induced CNS Depression
Injection—Give a priming dose of 2
mg/kg; repeat in 5 min. Repeat
same dose every 1–2 hrs until patient awakens. Watch for relapse
into unconsciousness, or development of respiratory depression.

If a relapse occurs, resume 1- to
2-hr doses until arousal is sustained
or maximum dosage (3 gm) is
reached. If maximum dosage is
reached, maintain respiration mechanically.

Do not repeat doses to patients who do not respond to the first dose; evaluate CNS for the cause of sustained depression.

Infusion—Give a priming dose of 1 mg/kg.

If patient awakens, watch for relapse. If there is no response, continue mechanical ventilation and repeat priming dose in 1–2 hrs.

If some respiratory response is seen, begin infusion of the 1 mg/ml solution, at a rate of 1–3 mg/min, 1–2 mg/min if depression is mild, 2–3 mg/min in moderate CNS depression. Discontinue if patient awakens, or at the end of 2 hrs. Then, continue supportive therapy for 1/2–2 hrs and repeat above infusion. Do not exceed a total daily dose of 3 gm.

Chronic Obstructive Pulmonary Disease Associated With Hypercapnia:

Obtain baseline arterial blood gases. Using a 2 mg/ml solution, begin an infusion at a rate of 1–2 mg/min. If necessary, increase dose to a maximum of 3 mg/min.

Monitor blood gases every 1/2 hr during infusion to detect the onset of carbon dioxide retention and acidosis. Titrate oxygen administration and drug with arterial blood gases. If patient's respiratory condition deteriorates despite above regimen, discontinue drug infusion.

DO NOT GIVE ADDITIONAL INFUSIONS BEYOND THE SINGLE MAXIMUM 2-HOUR ADMINISTRATION PERIOD

Safety for use in children under 12 years of age has not been established.

Preparation and Storage

Supplied in 20 ml vials containing 400 mg of drug (20 mg/ml).

Do not add to any infusion fluid other than those listed.

Suggested method of preparation of infusion:

Add 250 mg of doxapram (12.5 ml) to 250 ml infusion fluid. Concentration produced is 1 mg/ml.

To make a 2 mg/ml solution, add 400 mg of drug to 180 ml of fluid.

Drug Incompatibilities

Do not mix with any other medication.

Admixture with alkaline solutions such as thiopental or sodium bicarbonate will result in precipitation.

Modes of IV Administration

Injection
Yes
Slowly, no further dilution necessary.

Intermittent Infusion
Yes
Use one of the following infusion fluids:
NS
D5W
D10W
D5/NS
D10/NS
Follow recommended infusion rates; rapid infusion can cause hemolysis.
Use an infusion pump.

Continuous Infusion
Yes
Use one of the following infusion fluids:
NS
D5W
D10W
D5/NS
D10/NS
Follow recommended infusion rates; rapid infusion can cause hemolysis.
Use an infusion pump.

Contraindications; Warnings; Precautions; Adverse Reactions

Contraindications;
1. Convulsive states
2. Respiratory failure due to muscle weakness, flail chest, pneumothorax, airway obstruction or asthma, dyspnea (extreme).
3. Severe hypertension
4. Acute CVA
5. Hypersensitivity
6. Evidence of a head injury

doxapram hydrochloride
(continued)
7. Suspected or confirmed pulmonary embolus
8. Coronary artery disease
9. Frank decompensated congestive heart failure
10. Pulmonary fibrosis

Warnings
1. This drug is not antagonistic to muscle relaxants nor a specific antagonist to narcotics.
2. Insure adequate airway and oxygenation before administration
3. Since narcosis can recur in postop patients after stimulation with this drug, observe closely for 1/2–1 hour after patient becomes alert.
4. Administer with great caution to patients with: cerebral edema, bronchial asthma, severe tachycardia or other arrhythmias, severe cardiac disease, hyperthyroidism or pheochromocytoma.
5. Safe use in pregnancy has not been established.
6. Not recommended for use in children under 12 years of age.

Precautions
1. Monitor blood pressure and deep-tendon reflexes to prevent overdosage.
2. Excessive dosage produces hyperventilation which leads to respiratory alkalosis, hypocapnia with tetany, and eventually apnea.
3. Avoid extravasation or repeated use of single injection site.
4. Have oxygen, short-acting barbiturates and resuscitative equipment on hand to manage overdosage (evidenced by excessive CNS stimulation).
5. Administer with caution if patient has received sympathomimetics or MAO inhibitors. The combination may produce hypertension.
6. Discontinue if hypotension or dyspnea develops.
7. This drug may mask the residual effects of muscle relaxants.

8. Delay administration for 10 minutes after discontinuing halothane or cyclopropane anesthetics.
9. When used in acute respiratory insufficiency secondary to chronic obstructive pulmonary disease, use only for a short time (2 hours) as an aid to prevent elevation of arterial pCO_2 when oxygen is being given. Monitor arterial blood gases initially, then every half hour. Do not use with mechanical ventilation. Do not exceed suggested infusion rate to increase pCO_2 reduction; this drug increases the work of breathing and will cause fatigue.

Adverse Reactions
1. CNS: headache, dizziness, apprehension, disorientation, dilated pupils, hyperactivity, convulsions, muscle spasticity, increased reflexes, fever.
2. Respiratory: cough, dyspnea, laryngospasm, bronchospasm, rebound hypoventilation, tachypnea, hiccough.
3. Cardiovascular: mild to moderate increase blood pressure, sinus tachycardia, bradycardia, PVC's, lowered T-waves, tightness in chest, chest pain, phlebitis
4. GI: Nausea, vomiting, diarrhea
5. GU: Spontaneous voiding, urinary retention, albuminuria
6. Hematologic: decreased hematocrit, hemoglobin and red cell count, further decreased WBC count, elevated BUN.

Symptoms and Treatment of Overdosage
Signs: hypertension, tachycardia, skeletal muscle hyperactivity, increased deep tendon reflexes.
   Duration of effects is short; monitor and support until signs disappear. Do not administer follow-up dose until at least 15 minutes after signs return to normal. Short-acting barbiturates may relieve these effects. Be prepared to assist ventilation mechanically.

☐ Nursing Implications

1. Monitor blood pressure before the injection or infusion and at least every 2–3 minutes for one-half hour following. Overdosage causes marked elevation in blood pressure; see Symptoms and Treatment of Overdosage above. Report elevations to the physician.
2. The respiratory stimulant action produced by this drug is an increase in tidal volume and respiratory rate. Monitor the respiratory rate with each blood pressure determination. Also examine for the presence or absence of cyanosis. Maintain a patent airway and oxygen administration according to arterial blood gases. It is suggested that blood gases be obtained every 30 minutes to determine changes in pCO_2, pO_2, pH, and $pHCO_3$. Report abnormalities to the physician. Usually a marked rise in pCO_2 or fall in pO_2 is treated with mechanical ventilation. Doxapram should be discontinued at this time.
3. Patients with a history of cardiac disease and/or arrhythmias should be observed on a continuous ECG monitor. Be prepared to treat tachy- and bradyarrhythmias.
4. Maintain seizure precautions.
5. Be prepared to manage vomiting to prevent aspiration.
6. Monitor for the neurologic signs of overdosage, i.e., skeletal muscle hyperactivity and increased deep tendon reflexes. Notify the physician of the onset.
7. Take precautions to prevent injury, e.g., side rails, close observation, restraints as needed.
8. Monitor for urinary retention for the first 8–10 hours after the drug has been given. Palpate bladder size and record urine output every 2–4 hours. This is especially likely to occur in elderly males and any patient with a history of obstructive uropathy.
9. Extravasation can cause local tissue irritation. Take measures to prevent this; see Appendix. If it occurs, conservative treatment with warm compresses may be indicated.
10. Adhere strictly to suggested infusion rate. An infusion pump is advisable to control the flow rate.
11. Patients with chronic pulmonary disease being treated with this drug are usually apprehensive. Provide close observation and reassurance. Be prepared at all times to assist breathing mechanically. Keep airways, suction, and a manual breathing bag at the bedside.

doxorubicin hydrochloride ▦
(Adriamycin)

Actions/Indications
Cytotoxic antibiotic, cell-cycle specific. Use in the management of:
- Acute leukemias (lymphocytic and myelogenous)
- Lymphomas (Hodgkin's and non-Hodgkin's)
- Sarcomas (Ewing's, osteogenic and soft tissue)
- Breast cancer
- Bladder and bronchogenic carcinomas (especially oat cell)
- Wilms' tumor
- Neuroblastoma
- Ovarian carcinoma

Dosage
Adults:
60–75 mg/M^2 at 21-day intervals. (Alternate schedule: 30 mg/M^2 for 3 successive days repeated every 4 weeks.) Total dose limit: 550 mg/M^2.
Children:
30–35 mg/M^2, same frequency as listed above for adults. Total dose limit: 400 mg/M^2.

In the presence of liver impairment, see Warning No. 5.

When this drug is used concomitantly with cyclophosphamide or in patients with a history of radiotherapy to the heart, the total dose limit should be 450 mg/M^2 (adults).[1]

doxorubicin hydrochloride
(continued)

Preparation and Storage
Available in vials containing 10 mg and 50 mg of drug.

To reconstitute from powder, use NS or sterile water for injection. To the 10-mg vial add 5 ml of diluent; to the 50-mg vial, add 25 ml. *Shake Until Dissolution Is Seen.* Resulting solution provides concentration of 2 mg/ml. Discard after 24 hours if stored unrefrigerated or after 48 hours if refrigerated.

Skin reactions can occur. Take precautions to avoid skin contact with this drug during preparation; *Use Of Gloves Is Recommended.* If the drug comes in contact with the skin, **immediately** wash with soap and water.

Drug Incompatibilities
Do not mix with heparin. If using a heparin lock device, flush system with saline both before and after injecting.

Do not mix with any other medication in any manner.

Modes of IV Administration

Injection
Yes
Inject the reconstituted solution, into the tubing of a running IV of NS or D5W.

The IV cannula should be a winged-needle unit inserted into a large vein. Avoid veins over joints or extremities with impaired venous or lymphatic drainage.

The specific administration rate depends on the dosage and size of vein but the injection should be given over at least 3–5 minutes time. A more rapid rate can cause facial flushing and streaking along the vein.

Intermittent Infusion
Yes
Add reconstituted solution dose to 50–150 ml D5W or NS; infuse over 15–30 minutes.

Continuous Infusion
No

Contraindications; Warnings; Precautions; Adverse Reactions

Contraindications
1. Bone marrow depression secondary to other drugs or radiation
2. Pre-existing heart disease
3. History of previous cumulative doses of this drug or daunorubicin that have reached or exceeded total dose limits

Warnings
1. *This drug can cause serious irreversible myocardial toxicity with delayed congestive failure that does not respond to usual therapies unless caught in its early stages.* This usually occurs in patients who have received doses exceeding total dose limits (550 mg/M^2), but may occur at lower doses (400 mg/M^2) in patients who have received mediastinal radiotherapy or other cardiotoxic drugs. Therapy should be discontinued at the earliest sign of toxicity. The ECG sign of cardiac toxicity is reduced voltage of the QRS complex. Cardiac toxicity can occur up to 6 months post-treatment.
2. **Acute life-threatening arrhythmias have been reported** during or within a few hours after administration.
3. Transient, nonsignificant ECG changes may also occur. These changes include supraventricular tachyarrhythmias, premature ventricular contractions and ST-T wave changes. These are seen in 10–30% of patients receiving therapy and occur during the first few days of administration.
4. Bone marrow suppression is seen in all patients achieving objective tumor remission. Leukopenia (WBC as low as 1000/cu mm) and thrombocytopenia occur maximally during the second week of administra-

tion and return to normal by the third week. Significant suppression (WBC *less* than 1000/cu mm) should prompt a dosage reduction or discontinuation of the drug.

5. Dosage should be reduced in the presence of liver impairment since biliary excretion is the major excretion route:

Serum Bilirubin	or	BSP (Bromsulphalein) Retention	Dosage
1.2–3.0 mg%		9–15%	1/2 normal dose
> 3.0 mg%		> 15%	1/4 normal dose

6. Dosage reduction is required in patients with bone marrow impairment secondary to tumor infiltration.
7. This drug may potentiate the toxicity of other anticancer therapies.
8. This drug causes fetal abnormalities in animals, and has mutagenic and carcinogenic properties. Use in pregnancy must weigh expected benefits to potential toxicity to the fetus. Possible effects on male and female fertility have not been excluded.
9. Extravasation can occur with or without stinging or burning sensation during administration even if blood return is good from needle aspiration. Injection or infusion should be immediately terminated if extravasation is suspected. SEVERE LOCAL TISSUE NECROSIS WILL RESULT.

Precautions
1. Hospitalization of the patient during the first phase of therapy is recommended.
2. Hyperuricemia may be produced by this agent secondary to lysis of tumor cells. Monitor serum uric acid levels. Pharmacologic agents may be necessary to control this effect.

3. Urine will be discolored red for 1–2 days after administration.
4. This is not an antimicrobial agent.

Adverse Reactions
1. Dose-limiting toxicities: bone marrow suppression (leukopenia), myocardial failure.
2. Skin: hair loss in 80% of all patients (reversible, occurs 3–4 weeks after first dose); increased pigmentation of palms, soles of feet and proximal nailbeds in black patients (rare); increase in skin changes produced by radiation if the two therapies are administered concomitantly.
3. Gastrointestinal: nausea, vomiting and diarrhea in 50% of all patients; stomatitis and esophagitis with severe ulcerations (80% of all patients), begins with a burning sensation with erythema leading to ulceration within 2–3 days.
4. Vascular: sclerosis of small veins used for injection; facial flushing with too rapid an injection.
5. Hypersensitivity, ranging from fever, chills and urticaria to anaphylaxis can occur. Cross-sensitivity to lincomycin has been reported.

☐ **Nursing Implications**
1. Take anaplylaxis precautions. See Appendix.
2. The patient receiving this medication will be experiencing the emotional and physical effects of the malignancy. Knowledge of the patient's feelings about his disease and its implications will assist in helping him tolerate the chemotherapy. The incidence of uncomfortable side effects and adverse reactions is high. It is within the nurse's role to assist the patient in coping with the discomforts of the disease and its treatment, and to help him work through depression and anger toward acceptance of the disease at his own pace. Despite the unpleasantness this drug may bring, it

doxorubicin hydrochloride
(continued)
can be a source of hope for the patient.

3. Monitor for signs and symptoms of acute left ventricular failure: increased respiratory rate, dyspnea, tachycardia, orthopnea, appearance of third and fourth heart sounds, bilateral basilar rales, elevation of jugular venous pulse, and frank pulmonary edema. Notify physician with the appearance of any one of these signs and symptoms. Place patient at rest in a semi-Fowler's position. Monitor vital signs and above signs and symptoms for deterioration in patient's condition. The doxorubicin will be discontinued with the onset of this complication.

4. Avoid extravasation; see Appendix. If a stinging or burning sensation is felt during administration, stop the injection, relocate the needle and complete the dosage. Notify physician if extravasation occurs or is suspected. Sclerosis may occur in small veins used for injection.

5. *Management of gastrointestinal effects*:
   a. Administer antiemetics at appropriate times to prevent nausea and vomiting, before injection and/or before meals.
   b. Small frequent meals, timed with periods when the patient feels his best, are advisable. Bland foods are usually better tolerated. Carbohydrate and protein content should be high.
   c. If the patient is anorexic, encourage high nutrient liquids and water to maintain hydration.
   d. Keep accurate measurements of emesis volume and total intake and output to guide the physician in ordering parenteral fluids when necessary.
   e. Monitor onset of diarrhea;

notify the physician. Administer antiperistaltics as ordered. Maintain hydration and monitor for signs of hypokalemia (if diarrhea is severe), e.g., muscle cramps and weakness.

6. *Management of hematologic effects*:
   a. This is a dose-limiting toxic effect. The drug is usually discontinued or reduced as the white cell count falls toward 2000/cu mm, and should be restarted as the white count rises. The lowest white cell count is usually seen on the 14th day after the administration and returns to normal by the 21st day.
   b. Be aware of the patient's white blood cell count prior to each dose.
   c. If the WBC falls below 2000/cu mm, take measures to protect the patient from infection, such as protective (reverse) isolation, avoidance of invasive procedures, maintaining bodily (especially perineal) cleanliness, carrying out strict urinary catheter care when appropriate, etc. Monitor for infection by recording temperatures every 4 hours; examine for rashes, swellings, drainage and pain. Explain these procedures to the patient.
   d. Instruct the patient and/or family on the importance of follow-up blood studies if the drug is being administered on an outpatient basis.

7. *Management of hair loss*:
   a. Use a scalp tourniquet during the injection, if ordered, to help prevent hair loss.
   b. Counsel the patient on the possibility of hair loss to enable him to prepare for this disfigurement.
   c. Reassure him of probable regrowth of hair following discontinuation of the drug.
   d. Provide privacy, and time for

the patient to discuss his feelings.
8. *Management of stomatitis*:
   a. Administer preventive oral care every 4 hours and/or after meals.
   b. For preventive care, use a very soft toothbrush (child's) and toothpaste; avoid trauma to tissues.
   c. Examine oral membranes at least once daily (instruct patient and/or family) to detect the onset of inflammation or ulceration.
   d. If stomatitis occurs, notify the physician and begin therapeutic oral care.
   e. Order a bland, mechanical diet for patients with mild inflammation. If stomatitis is severe, the patient may be placed on NPO status by the physician.
   f. For patients who can tolerate oral intake, administer Xylocaine Viscous or acetaminophen elixir as a mouthwash prior to meals to decrease pain (do not use aspirin rinses) as ordered by the physician.
   g. Patients with severe stomatitis may require parenteral analgesia.
9. Warn the patient that the urine will be red 1–2 days after each dose.

References
1. Minow, R.A., et al: Adriamycin Cardiomyopathy—an Overview with Determination of Risk Factors. *Cancer Chemotherapy Reports, Part III*, 6(2):195–201, 1975.

Suggested Readings
Bolin, Rose Homan, and Auld, Margaret E.: Hodgkin's Disease. *American Journal of Nursing*, 74:1982–1966, November 1974.
Bruya, Margaret Auld, and Madeira, Nancy Powell: Stomatitis After Chemotherapy. *American Journal of Nursing*, 75(8):1349–1352, August 1975.
Foley, Genevieve V., and McCarthy, Ann Marie: The Child with Leukemia In a Special Hematology Clinic. *American Journal of Nursing*, 76:1115–1119, July 1976.
Foley, Genevieve, and McCarthy, Ann Marie: The Disease (Hodgkin's) and its Treatment. *American Journal of Nursing*, 76:1109–1114, July 1976 (references).
Giadquinta, Barbara: Helping Families Face the Crisis of Cancer. *American Journal of Nursing*, 77:1583–1588, October 1977.
Gullo, Shirley: Chemotherapy—What to Do About Special Side Effects. *RN*, 40:30–32, April 1977.
Hannan, Jeanne Ferguson: Talking is Treatment, Too. *American Journal of Nursing*, 74:1991–1992, November 1974.
LeBlanc, Dona Harris: People with Hodgkin's Disease: The Nursing Challenge. *Nursing Clinics of North America*, 13(2):281–300, June 1978.
Marrow, Mary: Nursing Management of the Adolescent: The Effect of Cancer Chemotherapy on Psychosocial Development. *Nursing Clinics of North America*, 13(2):319–335, June 1978.
Martinson, Ida: The Child With Leukemia: Parents Help Each Other. *American Journal of Nursing*, 76:1120–1122, July 1976.
Showfety, Mary Patricia: The Ordeal of Hodgkin's Disease. *American Journal of Nursing*, 74:1987–1991, November 1974.
Vietti, Teresa J., and Valeriote, Frederick: Conceptual Basis for the Use of Chemotherapeutic Agents and Their Pharmacology. *Pediatric Clinics of North America*, 23:67–92, February 1976.

doxycycline hyclate ■
(Vibramycin)

Actions/Indications
Broad-spectrum tetracycline antibiotic. Primarily bacteriostatic, is thought to exert its antimicrobial effect through inhibition of protein synthesis.

doxycycline hyclate
(continued)

Indicated in the treatment of infections secondary to:
- Rickettsiae
- *Mycoplasma pneumoniae*
- Agents of psittacosis, ornithosis, lymphogranuloma venereum, relapsing fever
- *Haemophilus ducreyi*
- *Pasteurella pestis*
- *Pasteurella tularensis*
- *Bartonella bacilliformis*
- *Bacteroides*
- *Vibrio coma*
- *Vibrio fetus*
- *Brucella*

Although not the drug of choice, this drug is indicated in the treatment of the following when bacteriologic testing indicates susceptibility:
- *E. coli*
- *Enterobacter aerogenes*
- *Shigella, Mima* and *Herellea* species
- *H. influenzae*
- *Klebsiella* species
- Streptococcus species
- *Diplococcus pneumoniae*
- *Staph. aureus*

When penicillin is contraindicated this drug is an alternative drug in the treatment of infections due to:
- *Neisseria gonorrhoeae*
- *Treponema pallidum*
- *L. monocytogenes*
- *Clostridia* species
- *Bacillus anthracis*
- *Fusobacterium fusiforme*
- *Actinomyces* species

Dosage
USUAL DOSAGE OF THIS DRUG IS MUCH LOWER THAN THAT OF OTHER TETRACYCLINES. EXCEEDING THE RECOMMENDED DOSAGE CAN INCREASE RISK OF SIDE EFFECTS
Adults:
100–200 mg/24 hrs, depending on the causative organism.

Usual dose—200 mg on first day in 1 or 2 infusions, then 100 mg–200 mg/24 hrs. Treatment should be continued for 24–48 hrs after fever and symptoms have subsided.

Primary and secondary syphilis—300 mg daily for at least 10 days.

Children Over 8 Years of Age:
100 lbs or less—2 mg/lb on the first day, then 1–2 mg/lb every 24 hrs (see Contraindications).
Over 100 lbs—use adult dose.

Preparation and Storage
Available as a powder in vials containing 100 mg and 200 mg of drug.

Reconstitute with sterile water for injection in the following amounts:
100-mg vial: 10 ml
200-mg vial: 20 ml

The resulting solution will contain 10 mg/ml. Use the following fluids for infusion:
NS
D5W
Invert sugar 10%
Ringers injection
Normosol-M in D5W
Normosol-R in D5W
Plasma-Lyte 56
Plasma-Lyte 148.
RL*
D5/RL*

Infuse within 12 hours of solution preparation.

Reconstituted vials should be stored in refrigerator and discarded after 72 hours.

*If RL or D5/RL are used for infusion, infuse within 6 hours of preparation.

Drug Incompatibilities
Do not mix with any other medication

Modes of IV Administration

Injection
No

Intermittent Infusion
Yes
Add the dose to at least 100 ml of infusion fluid (see Preparation section) or make a solution of 0.5 mg/ml. Infuse over 1–4 hours. Protect the solution from direct sunlight.

Do not exceed recommended rate of infusion to avoid adverse reactions.

Continuous Infusion
Yes

A 12-hour dose can be added to a sufficient amount of fluid to make a concentration of 0.1–0.4 mg/ml. Infuse over 12 hours. Protect from sunlight.

Use an infusion pump to maintain uniform flow.

Contraindications; Warnings; Precautions; Adverse Reactions

Contraindications
Hypersensitivity to any tetracycline

Warnings
1. May cause permanent discoloration of a child's teeth when administered during the last half of pregnancy or during infancy through the first 8 years of life. Enamel hypoplasia has also been seen.
2. Has been found to cause fetal abnormalities in animals. Avoid use during any stage of pregnancy unless it is judged to be essential to mother's welfare.
3. This drug is secreted in breast milk.
4. Exposure to sunlight or ultraviolet light may produce an exaggerated sunburn reaction.

Precautions
1. Overgrowth infections due to nonsusceptible organisms can occur.
2. This drug may depress plasma prothrombin activity, thus making it necessary to decrease the dosage of a concomitantly prescribed anticoagulant.
3. Monitor hematopoietic, hepatic and renal function during therapy. (When given at recommended dosage, this drug does not accumulate in patients with renal dysfunction, nor does it cause further renal impairment.[1,2])
4. Avoid administering this drug with penicillin. The actions of penicillin can be reduced by this drug.

Adverse Reactions
1. Gastrointestinal: anorexia, nausea, vomiting, diarrhea, dysphagia, glossitis, enterocolitis (these are rarely seen)
2. Skin: *Candida albicans* infection in the mouth (thrush) or perineum (monilia), causing a red, maculopapular, itching rash; exaggerated sunburn when skin is exposed to ultraviolet light; exfoliative dermatitis (uncommon)
3. Hypersensitivity reactions of all forms ranging from rashes to anaphylaxis
4. Hematologic: Hemolytic anemia, thrombocytopenia, neutropenia, eosinophilia.
5. Thrombophlebitis at the injection site
6. Bulging fontanels in infants and intracranial hypertension in adults; usually disappear on discontinuation of the drug.
7. Increased BUN has been reported, is apparently dose-related.

☐ Nursing Implications
1. Take anaphylaxis precautions; see Appendix.
2. If gastrointestinal disturbances occur, notify the physician. If disturbances such as nausea, vomiting and diarrhea are pronounced, the drug will probably be discontinued. Antiemetics, antacids, and constipating agents can be ordered to control symptoms. Monitor intake and output to assist the physician in planning for parenteral fluid replacement. Maintain hydration orally when possible.
3. If the patient will be taking the oral form of this drug as an outpatient, instruct him on the possibility of photosensitivity and the advisability of avoiding exposure to the sun (sun-block lotions may be of help if exposure cannot be avoided).
4. Women of childbearing age and potential, and mothers of children who may receive this drug, should be informed of Warnings No. 1, 2 and 3 by the physician. Assist in the interpretation of these warnings to the patient.
5. Even though blood dyscrasias

doxycycline hyclate
(continued)

are infrequently caused by this agent, be aware of the patient's complete blood cell count during therapy. If the platelet count begins to fall, the drug will probably be discontinued. Bleeding secondary to a low platelet count usually begins only after the count falls below 100,000/cu mm.

6. Monitor for signs and symptoms of overgrowth infections:
   a. Fever (take rectal temperature at least every 4–6 hours in all patients)
   b. Increasing malaise
   c. Newly appearing localized signs and symptoms: redness, soreness, pain, swelling, drainage (increased volume or change in character of pre-existing drainage)
   d. Monilial rash in perineal area (reddened areas with itching)
   e. Cough (change in pre-existing cough or sputum production)
   f. Diarrhea
7. Report the onset of any rash to the physician. Keep the patient's environment comfortably cool and the skin clean. Diphenhydramine (Benadryl) may be ordered to relieve itching.
8. Report the onset of jaundice to the physician.
9. Report the onset of bulging fontanels, and other signs of increasing intracranial pressure, to the physician.

References
1. Barza, Michael, and Schiefe, Richard T.: Antimicrobial Spectrum, Pharmacology and Therapeutic Use of Antibiotics, Part I: Tetracyclines. *American Journal of Hospital Pharmacy*, 34:51, January 1977.
2. Appel, Gerald B., and Neu, Harold C.: The Nephrotoxicity of Antimicrobial Agents. *New England Journal of Medicine*, 296(13):722, March 31, 1977.

droperidol ■
(Inapsine; also contained in Innovar)

Actions/Indications
Tranquilizer, sedative antiemetic. Onset of action is 3–10 minutes after injection. Full effect is seen in 30 minutes, duration is 4–12 hours.
Indicated:
- To tranquilize and reduce incidence of nausea and vomiting in diagnostic and surgical procedures
- For premedication, induction and adjunct to anesthesia
- In neuroleptanalgesia in which droperidol is given with a narcotic analgesic to aid in producing tranquility, decreasing anxiety and pain

Dosage
Dosage must be individualized according to: age, weight, pathology use of other drugs, anesthesia and type of surgery.
Adults:
Sedation in diagnostic procedures—2.5–10 mg, 30–60 min before procedure, with additional dose of 1.25–2.5 mg if needed.
Premedication prior to surgery—2.5–10 mg, 30–60 min prior to surgery.
Adjunct to general anesthesia: Induction—220–275 mcg/kg (2.5 mg/20–25 lbs). Titrate to obtain desired result.
Maintenance—1.25–2.5 mg as needed.
Adjunct to regional anesthesia—2.5–5.0 mg 30–60 min prior to surgery.

Children (2–12 years of age):
Induction of anesthesia—88–165 mcg/kg
Premedication—45–55 mcg/kg (1.0–1.5 mg/20–25 lbs)

Preparation and Storage
Supplied in 2-ml and 5-ml ampuls, and 10 ml vials each containing 2.5 mg/ml.

Drug Incompatibilities
Do not mix with barbiturates or any other medication in any manner.

Modes of IV Administration

Injection
Yes
May be injected without further dilution, over 2–3 minutes.

Intermittent Infusion
No

Continuous Infusion
No

Contraindications; Warnings; Precautions; Adverse Reactions

Contraindications
Hypersensitivity to droperidol or Innovar (fentanyl-droperidol combination drug).

Warnings
1. DROPERIDOL CAN PRODUCE HYPOTENSION; MEANS OF MANAGING IT, E.G., FLUIDS AND VASOPRESSOR AGENTS, MUST BE READILY AVAILABLE.
2. When this drug is used in conjunction with a narcotic analgesic (such as fentanyl), dose of the narcotic should be reduced and respiratory support equipment and a narcotic antagonist agent (naloxone) must be readily available in the event of respiratory depression.
3. If administering droperidol–fentanyl combination (Innovar), see page 154 for complete details on fentanyl.
4. Safety for use of this drug in children under 2 years of age has not been established.
5. Safety for use in pregnancy has not been established.

Precautions
1. Reduce initial dosage in elderly, debilitated or poor risk patients.
2. This drug has potentiating effects with CNS depressants (barbiturates, tranquilizers, narcotics, general anesthetics) when administering concomitantly, dosage of each should be reduced.
3. Hypotension is more likely in patients receiving spinal or peridural anesthesia. If this occurs, treat with vasopressors and fluids and elevation of the legs (if possible).
4. Epinephrine may paradoxically *decrease* blood pressure in patients receiving this drug.
5. Administer with caution to patients with renal or hepatic impairment. The duration of action of this drug will be prolonged in these two conditions.
6. This drug may decrease pulmonary arterial pressure.
7. When used in such procedures as bronchoscopy appropriate topical anesthesia is still required.

Adverse Reactions
1. Mild to moderate hypotension
2. Tachycardia
3. Postoperative drowsiness
4. Extrapyramidal symptoms (antiparkinson agent may be needed)
5. Dizziness
6. Hallucinations
7. Chills and/or shivering
8. Laryngospasm, bronchospasm

Treatment of Overdosage (Extension of Expected Pharmacologic Actions — Hypoventilation or Apnea)
1. Support respirations with oxygen and mechanical assistance as necessary. Maintain an open airway.
2. Maintain body warmth.
3. Maintain adequate hydration.
4. Monitor blood pressure frequently. Use vasopressors as necessary. Duration of action is 4–12 hours.

☐ Nursing Implications
1. Obtain a preinjection blood pressure. Monitor blood pressure every 5–10 minutes after administration—hypotension may occur. See Treatment of Overdosage above. Vasopressor agents (dopamine, metaraminol, etc.) should be readily available.

droperidol
(continued)

2. Be prepared to support respiration.
3. Monitor heart rate with blood pressure. Tachycardia may occur. If the patient has a history of cardiac problems, observe for cardiac decompensation if tachycardia is excessive or prolonged: increasing respiratory rate, restlessness, rales, jugular venous distention. Notify the physician if any one of these appear. Continue to monitor carefully.
4. Initiate safety precautions to prevent patient injury, e.g., side rails, frequent observation, restraints as needed. Ambulate the patient with caution, after recovery from major drug effects.
5. Be prepared to manage hallucinations with safety precautions, patient reassurance and orientation.

edrophonium chloride ■
(Tensilon)

Actions/Indications
Cholinesterase inhibitor, short-and rapid-acting. Increases the activity of the parasympathetic nervous system. Onset of action is 30–60 seconds after injection; duration is 10 min.

Used in the differential diagnosis of myasthenia gravis, and also used to differentiate a myasthenic crisis from a cholinergic crisis.

Can be used when a curare antagonist is needed to reverse the neuromuscular block produced by curare, tubocurarine, gallamine triethiodide, pancuromium, or d-tubocurarine. It is *not* effective against decamethonium or succinylcholine.

Paroxysmal atrial tachycardia unresponsive to carotid massage can sometimes be terminated with this agent.

Dosage
The Tensilon test is performed to diagnose myasthenia gravis and to differentiate between increased severity of the disease and overtreatment with a cholinesterase inhibitor. Once respiratory support is adequate the drug is given according to the dosage schedule in TABLE 1. Responses to the test are listed in TABLE 2. See Nursing Implications for additional information.

See Table 1 below for dosages for other indications.

Preparation and Storage
Supplied in multiple-dose vials of 10 ml and ampuls of 1 ml (10 mg/ml)

When used to test for myasthenia gravis, withdraw 1 ml (10 mg) in a tuberculin syringe, and administer according to directions in Table 1.

Drug Incompatibilities
Do not mix with any other medication in any manner.

Modes of IV Administration

Injection
Yes
Can be injected undiluted.

Intermittent Infusion
No
Pharmacologically inappropriate.

Continuous Infusion
No
Pharmacologically inappropriate.

Contraindications; Warnings; Precautions; Adverse Reactions

Contraindications
1. Hypersensitivity to any anticholinesterase drug
2. Mechanical urinary or intestinal obstruction

Warnings
1. Keep atropine 1.0 mg at the bedside during the use of this drug to counteract severe cholinergic reactions.
2. Use with caution in patients with asthma or cardiac arrhythmias (except those being treated by this agent). Transient bradycardia can occur (treat with at-

ropine). Cardiac and respiratory arrest have occurred.

3. Safety for use in pregnancy and lactation has not been established.

Precautions
Some patients may develop anticholinesterase insensitivity for brief or prolonged periods, and may need respiratory assistance. Dosage of such drugs (physostigmine, neostigmine, etc.) should be reduced or withheld until sensitivity returns. See Nursing Implications.

Adverse Reactions
The reactions that can be seen with this drug are common to all cholinesterase inhibitors. Those that occur are of rapid onset and short dura-

tion because of the drug's activity time:

1. Cardiovascular: bradycardia, fall in cardiac output (decreased blood pressure), cardiac arrest (usually only after high doses, or in hypersensitive patients)
2. Respiratory: (in order of progression): increased tracheobronchial secretions, laryngospasm, bronchiolar constriction, respiratory muscle paralysis, central respiratory paralysis, apnea
3. Central nervous system: difficulty speaking and swallowing, seizures
4. Eye: increasing output of tears, constricted pupils, blurred vision, diplopia (double vision), intense redness of conjunctiva

Table 1. Dosage Schedule

Indications	Initial Dose	If No Response, Repeat Dose	Maximum Dose
I. Tensilon Test for Diagnosis of Myasthenia Gravis A. Adults	2 mg. over 15–30 seconds	8 mg. (If adequate, repeat in 30 min.)	—
B. Children—over 75 lbs.	2 mg	1 mg. every 30 – 45 seconds up to 10 mg	10 mg
C. Children—under 75 lbs.	1 mg	1 mg every 30–45 seconds up to 5 mg	5 mg
D. Infants	0.1 mg	Increase to a maximum of 0.5 mg	0.5 mg
II. Test to Evaluate Treatment Requirements for Myasthenia Gravis	1 mg–2 mg	—	—
III. Tensilon Test in Crisis (with severe respiratory distress)	2 mg *After Respiratory Support Given*	—	2 mg
IV. Use As A Curare Antagonist (in adults)	10 mg over 30–45 seconds	Repeat as necessary	40 mg
V. In Paroxysmal Atrial Tachycardia (PAT)	10 mg	Repeat up to 40 mg to convert to sinus rhythm	40 mg

edrophonium chloride
(continued)
5. Gastrointestinal: increased salivation, nausea, vomiting, diarrhea, abdominal cramps
6. Urinary frequency and incontinence
7. Diaphoresis, skeletal muscle weakness

Overdosage (Cholinergic Crisis)
1. Signs and symptoms: Nausea, vomiting, diarrhea, sweating, increased bronchial and oral secretions, bradycardia. Secretions can produce airway obstruction.
2. Maintain an open airway and adequate oxygenation.
3. Monitor cardiac function (blood pressure and pulse) until completely stable.
4. Administer atropine 0.4–0.5 mg IV. Repeat every 3–10 minutes until signs and symptoms are controlled.
5. Pralidoxime chloride may also be given, 50–100 mg/min with a maximum dose of 1000 mg. Titrate dose until signs and symptoms are controlled.
6. Be prepared to manage seizures.

☐ **Nursing Implications**
1. During the Tensilon test
   a. Keep atropine 1.0 mg at the

Table 2. Expected Responses and Diagnostic Findings for the Tensilon Test for Myasthenia Gravis

SIGNS AND SYMPTOMS	MYASTHENIC RESPONSE	ADEQUATE RESPONSE	CHOLINERGIC RESPONSE
	(Seen in untreated myasthenic patients; response can establish the diagnosis of myasthenia gravis, or inadequately treated myasthenia gravis.)	*(In adequately treated myasthenics, and in normal persons.)*	*(In myasthenics who are overtreated with a cholinesterase inhibitor.)*
Muscular strength (*Ptosis; diplopia, difficulty speaking, difficulty swallowing, respiratory strength, limb strength*)	Increased*	No change	Decreased†
Muscle twitching (*Facial muscles, limb muscles, eye movement*)	Absent	Present *or* absent	Present *or* absent
Adverse effects (*Nausea, vomiting, abdominal cramps, increasing tears, diaphoresis*)	Absent	Minimal	Severe

*Improvement in signs and symptoms
†Exacerbation of signs and symptoms
(Courtesy of Roche Products, Inc.)

bedside, ready to administer, to combat above listed adverse effects of this drug, especially bradycardia.

b. Be prepared to support respirations (the patient's condition and/or the drug can cause respiratory distress). Begin respiratory support, if the adult patient, with encouragement, cannot breathe at a rate greater than 8–10/minute.

c. Be prepared to manage vomiting to prevent aspiration. Tracheal suction equipment must be at the bedside, ready for use.

d. Patients with a history of cardiac arrhythmias should be monitored electrocardiographically during administration of this drug. Watch for slowing heart rate.

e. Patients diagnosed as having myasthenia will need complete instruction on self-care, e.g., signs and symptoms of crisis, medications, etc. They should wear a medical identification appliance.

Reference

1. *Harrison's Principles of Internal Medicine* (7th ed.), New York: McGraw-Hill Book Company, 1974, p. 1134.

Suggested Readings

Guyton, Arthur C.: *Textbook of Medical Physiology* (5th ed.), Philadelphia: W. B. Saunders Company, 1976, Chapter 12, Neuromuscular Transmission; Function of Smooth Muscle, pp. 148–157; Chapter 15, The Autonomic Nervous System; The Adrenal Medulla, pp. 768–781.
Jones, LeAnna: Myasthenia and Me. *RN*, June 1976, pp. 51–55.
Brunner, Lillian Sholtis, and Suddarth, Doris Smith: *The Lippincott Manual of Nursing Practice* (2nd ed.), Philadelphia: J. B. Lippincott Company, 1978, pp. 934–937.

ephedrine sulfate ◼

Actions/Indications

Adrenergic drug. Elevates blood pressure, relaxes bronchospasm, stimulates CNS.

Used in the treatment of allergic disorders; as a vasopressor; in complete heart block to increase the ventricular rate; and to elevate blood pressure during spinal anesthesia.

Dosage

Adults:
10–50 mg. Repeat 25 mg in 5 to 10 minutes if necessary every 3–4 hours. The daily dose should not exceed 150 mg.
Children:
3 mg/kg daily in 3–4 divided doses.

Preparation and Storage

Supplied in ampuls of 25 mg/ml and 50 mg/ml. Read label carefully; **use only the preparation designed for IV use without procaine.** Store at room temperature.

Drug Incompatibilities

Do not inject into an IV line containing hydrocortisone.

Modes of IV Administration

Injection
Yes
Slowly over 1 min through Y-site or 3-way stopcock.

Intermittent Infusion
No
Do not add to IV solution.

Continuous Infusion
No
Do not add to IV solution

Contraindications; Warnings; Precautions; Adverse Reactions

Contraindications
1. Hypersensitivity
2. Glaucoma (the drug can increase intraocular pressure)
3. Patients receiving cyclopropane

ephedrine sulfate
(continued)
or halothane anesthetics (arrhythmias may result)

Precautions
1. Administer with caution to patients with congestive heart failure, angina pectoris, diabetes,
hyperthyroidism, prostatic hypertrophy, or hypertension.
This drug may cause exacerbation of these conditions.
2. Administer with caution to patients on digitalis; arrhythmias
may occur.
3. Administer with caution to patients on MAO inhibitors (par-
gyline, phenelzine, tranylcypro-
mine).
4. Prolonged use or overdosage
will produce a syndrome resembling an anxiety state.
5. Do not use to increase blood
pressure in acute hemorrhage
or cardiogenic shock.

Adverse Reactions
Most adverse reactions are extreme
forms of therapeutic actions and are
due to overdosage.
1. Headache
2. Restlessness
3. Insomnia
4. Anxiety
5. Weakness
6. Dizziness
7. Confusion
8. Hallucinations
9. Chest pain
10. Nausea and vomiting
11. Repeated injection may cause
urinary retention
Numbers 1 through 10 can usually
be managed with rest.

☐ **Nursing Implications**
1. Monitor blood pressure and
heart rate before and after injection. After injection, take
readings every 5 minutes until
stabilization occurs.
2. Monitor patients with the following pre-existing conditions
for worsening of the conditions

if this drug is administered for a
prolonged period of time.
a. Congestive heart failure
(daily weights, heart rate,
central venous pressure,
urine output)
b. Angina pectoris (patient
should report any chest
pain)
c. Diabetes (monitor urine glucose)
d. Hyperthyroidism (tremulousness, increased heart rate)
e. Prostatic hypertrophy
(urinary retention)
f. Hypertension (further elevation of blood pressure)
3. Monitor ECG continuously
when administering to patients
on digitalis.
4. Read label carefully; there are
several preparations. Intravenous preparation contains no
procaine or other compounds.

**epinephrine hydro-
chloride** ■
(Adrenalin)

Actions/Indications
The principle product of the adrenal
medulla. A potent sympathomimetic
drug that imitates all of the actions
of the sympathetic nervous system
(except those on facial arteries and
sweat glands) by stimulating the alpha and beta adrenergic receptor
cells. Effects produced include:
• Increased cardiac output and
heart rate
• Increased systolic blood pressure
• Relaxation of bronchial spasm
• Mobilization of liver glycogen
stores.
Indicated in:
• Hypersensitivity reactions, including anaphylaxis
• Bronchial spasm, i.e., acute asthmatic attacks
• Cardiac asystole to assist in the
restoration of a cardiac rhythm
• Bradycardia, to increase heart rate
• Syncope due to complete heart
block or carotid sinus hypersensi-
tivity

Dosage
Adults:
Bradyarrhythmias, bronchospasm and allergic disorders (anaphylaxis)—1.0–2.5 ml of a 1:10,000 solution; repeat as necessary, via injection.

Cardiac arrest—5 ml of a 1:10,000 solution* as an intracardiac injection, use concomitantly with basic and advanced life-support measures (CPR).
Children:
Bradyarrhythmias, bronchospasm and allergic disorders (anaphylaxis)—0.01 ml/kg or 0.3 ml/M² up to 0.5 ml of a 1:10,000 solution,† repeat every 4 hours as needed.

Cardiac arrest—0.3–2.0 ml diluted to a 1:10,000 solution† (or 0.1 ml/kg)
Neonates:
For all indications—0.1–0.5 ml/kg of a 1:10,000 solution.† (In allergic disorders, bradyarrhythmias or bronchospasm, repeat above dose every 2–4 hrs as needed.)
* When this drug is given via intracardiac injection, the 1:10,000 solution must always be used.
†A 1:10,000 solution should be used for children regardless of indication or mode of administration.

Preparation and Storage
Supplied in ampuls of 1 ml, 1:1000 solution. To make a 1:10,000 solution, add 9 ml NS to 1 ml of the 1:1000 solution.

Also supplied in 5-ml prefilled syringes of a 1:10,000 solution.

Protect vials from light. Do not use a solution that is discolored or contains a precipitate. NOTE: There are several preparations of this drug, some with additives such as oil.

Use Only Epinephrine Labeled for Intravenous Use.

Drug Incompatibilities
Do not add to sodium bicarbonate or Ionosol solutions.

Do not mix with:
Novobiocin
Warfarin
Calcium-containing preparations
Lidocaine

Cephapirin
Mephentermine

Modes of IV Administration

Injection
Yes
Most commonly used mode. Inject dose over 1 minute.

Intermittent Infusion
Yes
Use D5W or NS in any amount. Use microdrop tubing or an infusion pump to control rate. Adjust rate with patient response.

Continuous Infusion
Yes
Use D5W or NS in any amount.
Use microdrop tubing or an infusion pump to control rate. Titrate rate with patient response.

Contraindications; Warnings; Precautions; Adverse Reactions

Contraindications
1. Shock (other than anaphylaxis)
2. During anesthesia with cyclopropane or halogenated hydrocarbons (arrhythmias can result).
3. Coronary insufficiency, acute myocardial infarction and cardiac dilatation. (This drug increases myocardial oxygen demands.)
4. Narrow-angle glaucoma (can further increase intraocular pressure)
5. Organic brain damage
6. Labor (this drug may delay the second stage)

Warnings
1. Use with caution in elderly patients and in those with cardiovascular disease, hypertension, diabetes or hyperthyroidism; in psychoneurotic persons and in pregnancy.
2. Use with **extreme** caution in patients with long-standing bronchial asthma and emphysema who have developed degenerative heart disease.

epinephrine hydrochloride
(continued)
3. Inadvertent rapid injection or infusion may produce a sharp rise in blood pressure which can precipitate cerebrovascular hemorrhage.
4. When this drug must be administered in the presence of congestive heart failure, the peripheral vasoconstriction and cardiac stimulation may precipitate pulmonary edema. Nitrites or alpha adrenergic blocking agents may counteract these effects.
5. Arrhythmias may occur in patients concomitantly receiving excessive doses of digitalis, mercurial diuretics, or thiazide diuretics. Angina may be induced in patients with coronary insufficiency.

Adverse Reactions
1. Central nervous system: anxiety, fear, tremulousness, headache
2. Cardiovascular: palpitations, premature atrial and ventricular contractions, supraventricular tachycardia, ventricular tachycardia, and ventricular fibrillation; pulmonary edema in susceptible patients

☐ **Nursing Implications**
1. Bedside supportive care as indicated for the condition being treated; monitor blood pressure and heart rate before and every 2–5 minutes after injection until stabilization, then every 15–30 minutes as needed.
2. Continuous ECG monitoring is advisable in all patients. Be prepared to manage arrhythmias; keep lidocaine 100 mg at the bedside.
3. Do not leave the patient unattended during the infusion.
4. Signs of overdosage: cold, diaphoretic skin, cyanosis of the nailbeds, change in mental status, tachypnea. Stop the infusion, continue to monitor vital signs, and notify the physician.

5. This is an essential drug to keep on hand in any patient care area where medications or treatments are being dispensed, to treat anaphylaxis.

Suggested Reading
Guyton, Arthur C.: *Textbook of Medical Physiology*, Philadelphia: W. B. Saunders Company, 1976, Chapter 57, The Autonomic Nervous System; The Adrenal Medulla, pp. 768–781; Chapter 7, Immunity and Allergy, pp. 77–87.

erythromycin lactobionate and erythromycin gluceptate ■
(Erythrocin Lactobionate, Ilotycin Gluceptate)

Actions/Indications
Antibiotic. Used to treat infections due to susceptible strains of the following organisms:
• Group A beta hemolytic streptococcus*
• Alpha hemolytic streptococcus*
• *Staphylococcus aureus*
• *Streptococcus pneumoniae*
• *Mycoplasma pneumoniae*
• *Hemophilus influenzae*
• *Corynebacterium diphtheriae*
• *Listeria monocytogenes*
• *Neisseria gonorrhoeae*
• The organism of Legionnaire's disease
*Penicillin is usually considered the drug of choice in the treatment of infections due to these organisms, but erythromycin is an acceptable substitute in the presence of positive sensitivity tests, for patients who are sensitive to penicillin.

Dosage
Adults and Older Children:
15–20 mg/kg/24 hrs. Up to 4/gm/day may be given in divided doses, every 6 hrs, or by continuous infusion.
Neonates:
30–50 mg/kg/24 hrs.
Adults with Acute Pelvic Inflammatory Disease Caused by N. Gonorrhoeae:
500 mg every 6 hrs for 3 days

followed by 250 mg erythromycin stearate or base (oral preparation) every 6 hrs for 7 days.
Legionnaire's Disease:
Optimal doses have not been established. Current recommendation 1–4 gm/day in divided doses.

Preparation and Storage
Available in powdered form in vials containing 250 mg, 500 mg and 1000 mg of drug and in single dose dispensing vials containing 500 mg of drug.
Reconstitute from powder using *only* sterile water for injection (Do *not* use water for injection, bacteriostatic). Add 10 ml to the 250 mg or 500-mg vial and 20 ml to the 1000-mg vial, concentration will be 25 mg/ml. (250 mg vial), 50 mg/ml (500 and 1000 mg vials)
Once reconstituted, erythromycin *lactobionate* may be stored in refrigerator for 14 days or at room temperature for 24 hours. Erythromycin *gluceptate* may be stored in refrigerator for 7 days.

Drug Incompatibilities
Do not mix with any other medication in the IV bottle.
Do not mix in auxiliary lines containing:
Aminophylline
Cefazolin
Cephaloridine
Cephalothin
Heparin
Metaraminol
Streptomycin
Tetracyclines
Vitamin B Complex with C

Modes of IV Administration

Injection
No

Intermittent Infusion
Yes
Add 1/4 daily dose to D5W or NS for infusion, 100–250 ml. Use prepared solutions within 4 hrs, infuse over 20–60 min. A more rapid infusion may cause irritation of the vein.

Continuous Infusion
Yes
The preferred mode. Usually 1 gm is added to 1000 ml of fluid.
Dilute and infuse according to the dosage and fluid volume, and the following information:
When adding erythromycin *gluceptate* to a volume of solution which must be infused over a time greater than 4 hrs, the solution should be buffered to a pH of 7 using a sodium bicarbonate 4% solution (Abbott Lab's. Neut) or a phosphate-carbonate (Travenol's Buff). Add 1 ampul of Buff or 5 ml of Neut to 500 or 1000 ml D5W or NS. Administer solution within 24 hours after dilution.
When adding erythromycin *lactobionate* to the following fluids:
D5W
D5 in Lactated Ringer's
D5/NS Normosol-M in D5W
Normosol-R in D5W,
buffering compounds must first be added to the solution. Add 1 ml of 4% sodium bicarbonate (Abbott Lab's., Neut) to each 100 ml of solution used. When using NS, Lactated Ringer's or Normosol-R without D5W, buffering is **not** required. *Infuse all solutions within 8 hours.*

Contraindications; Warnings; Precautions; Adverse Reactions

Contraindications
Hypersensitivity

Warnings
Safety for use in pregnancy has not been established; this drug crosses the placental barrier.

Precautions
1. Reduced dosage may be advisable in patients with hepatic impairment.
2. Monitor hepatic function during therapy.
3. This drug is secreted in breast milk.
4. Overgrowth infections due to nonsusceptible organisms can occur.
5. Concomitant use of this drug

erythromycin lactobionate and gluceptate
(continued)

with high doses of theophylline can increase serum theophylline levels; dosage of theophylline should be reduced.

Adverse Reactions
1. Allergic reactions ranging in severity from rashes to anaphylaxis.
2. Venous irritation.
3. Reversible hearing loss (with 4 gm or more per day).
4. Altered liver function tests following prolonged therapy with high dosage.

☐ **Nursing Implications**
1. Monitor effectiveness of drug therapy:
   a. Temperature every 4 hours (rectal if possible)
   b. Sputum production, quality and quantity
   c. The appearance of a wound
2. Take anaphylaxis precautions; see Appendix.
3. Monitor for signs and symptoms of overgrowth infections:
   a. Fever (take rectal temperature at least every 4–6 hours in all patients)
   b. Increasing malaise
   c. Newly appearing localized signs and symptoms: redness, soreness, pain, swelling, drainage (increased volume or change in character of preexisting drainage)
   d. Monilial rash in perineal area (reddened areas with itching)
   e. Cough (change in preexisting cough or sputum production)
   f. Diarrhea

ethacrynate, sodium ■
(Sodium Edecrin)

Actions/Indications
Potent diuretic, acts on the ascending limb of the loop of Henle, the proximal and distal tubules, to produce excretion of water, chloride, hydrogen, sodium, and potassium ions. Onset of action is within 5 min after injection.
Used for the treatment of:
• Edema in: congestive heart failure, cirrhosis, renal disease
• Ascites of malignancy, idiopathic edema, lymphedema
• Pulmonary edema; magnitude of diuresis depends on degree of fluid accumulation

Dosage
Adults:
50 mg (0.5–1.0 mg/kg). May be repeated. A single dose of 100 mg may be given in critical situations.
Use small doses when giving over prolonged period.
Intravenous form is not recommended for use in pediatric age group.

Preparation and Storage
Supplied in vials containing 50 mg of drug.
Reconstitute by adding 50 ml of D5W or NS. Do not use if solution is hazy or opalescent.
Discard after 24 hours.

Drug Incompatibilities
Incompatible with Normosol M or any solution or drug with a pH below 5.
Do not mix in IV line or syringe with any other medication.

Modes of IV Adminstration

Injection
Yes
May be given through Y-site. Inject *slowly* over at least 5 min. Use new injection site for each dose or flush well with IV fluid after injection to avoid vein irritation.

Intermittent Infusion
Yes
Add reconstituted form to 50 ml NS. Run over 20–30 min. Do not use if solution is hazy.

Continuous Infusion
No

Contraindications; Warnings; Precautions; Adverse Reactions

Contraindications
1. Anuria
2. Electrolyte imbalance, azotemia, and/or oliguria; if they occur during treatment of renal disease discontinue drug.
3. Severe, watery diarrhea; if occurs discontinue and do not readminister
4. Use in infants is not recommended
5. Pregnancy of any stage
6. Nursing mothers

Warnings
1. PRODUCES PROFOUND DIURESIS WITH WATER AND ELECTROLYTE DEPLETION. Dose and dose schedule must be adjusted to each patient's needs. Serum electrolytes, CO_2 and BUN should be monitored at onset of therapy and frequently throughout active diuresis.
2. When used in cirrhotic patients, hospitalization is advised; hepatic coma may be precipitated.
3. Too vigorous a diuresis can precipitate acute hypotension. In elderly patients rapid reduction of plasma volume can give rise to thromboemboli (cerebral vascular and pulmonary).
4. Loss of serum potassium may precipitate arrhythmias in patients concomitantly receiving digitalis. Replace potassium according to serum concentration but avoid giving enteric-coated potassium tablets as small bowel lesions with or without ulceration can occur.
5. Lithium should not be given concomitantly, to prevent lithium toxicity.
6. May increase the risk of gastric hemorrhage associated with corticosteroid treatment.

Precautions
1. Liberalization of sodium intake may be necessary during therapy.

2. Metabolic alkalosis may occur in patients with cirrhosis.
3. Safety and efficacy in hypertension have not been established.
4. Orthostatic hypotension may occur in patients receiving other antihypertensive agents concomitantly.
5. Transient increase in BUN may occur. This reverses after discontinuation of the drug.
6. Monitor hearing when administering to critically ill patients or those receiving other ototoxic drugs (gentamicin, kanamycin, streptomycin, neomycin, cephaloridine). Avoid concurrent use when possible.
7. Reduction in anticoagulant dosage may be required.
8. In renal edema, hypoproteinemia may reduce responsiveness to this drug. Use of salt-poor albumin should be considered.

Adverse Reactions
1. Gastrointestinal: anorexia, nausea, vomiting, dysphagia, diarrhea
2. Renal: reversible hyperuricemia and acute gout
3. Carbohydrate metabolism—hyperglycemia in patients with cirrhosis; can potentiate oral hypoglycemic agents
4. Hematologic: agranulocytosis or severe neutropenia
5. Hepatic: jaundice, altered liver function (rarely)
6. Ear: vertigo, deafness, and tinnitus have occurred usually in renal patients; usually reversible within 24 hours; rarely is damage permanent (see Precaution No. 6.)
7. Other: (Infrequently) skin rash, chills, fever, headache, hematuria, blurred vision, fatigue, apprehension, confusion, local irritation and pain.

☐ Nursing Implications
1. Monitor for onset of diarrhea, notify physician. Drug is usually discontinued if this occurs.
2. Monitor for signs of:
   a. Sodium depletion—mental

ethacrynate, sodium
(continued)

confusion, weakness, abdominal cramps, stupor, hypotension

b. Potassium depletion—muscle cramps, weakness

c. Dehydration—weight loss greater than 2 lbs/day, dry mucous membranes, decreased skin turgor (tenting), weakness, lethargy, decreasing venous pressure, decreased urine output.

d. Hepatic encephalopathy—confusion, muscle tremors.

3. Patients also receiving digitalis should be observed via continuous ECG monitoring for onset of digitalis toxicity arrhythmias (sinus bradycardia and premature ventricular contractions most frequently seen). (See page 117 on digoxin for more detailed information on digitalis toxicity.)

4. Monitor blood pressure before and immediately after injection and every 5 minutes for the next hour. Fluids and vasopressors may be ordered to treat hypotension.

5. Ambulate with caution if patient is on any other antihypertensive agent; there may be postural hypotension.

6. Monitor for loss of hearing, tinnitus, and vertigo. Notify physician.

Suggested Readings

Kemp, Ginny, and Kemp, Doug: Diuretics. *American Journal of Nursing,* June 1978, pp. 1007–1010.

Plumb, Vance J., and James, Thomas N.: Clinical Hazards of Powerful Diuretics, Furosemide and Ethacrynic Acid. *Modern Concepts of Cardiovascular Disease,* July 1978, pp. 91–94.

fentanyl citrate ■
(Sublimaze; also contained in Innovar)

Actions/Indications

Narcotic, analgesic. Actions similar to morphine and meperidine.

Indications:

• For short-term analgesia during anesthetic periods (premedication, induction, maintenance, and immediate postoperative periods)

• As a narcotic analgesic supplement in general or regional anesthesia

• Administration with a neuroleptic (such as droperidol) as premedication, induction or adjunct in maintenance of general or regional anesthesia.

A dose of 0.1 mg is approximately equivalent in analgesic activity to 10 mg of morphine or 75 mg of meperidine.

Onset of action is almost immediate after IV injection. Maximal analgesic and respiratory depressant effects are seen after 5–15 min. The usual duration of the analgesic effect is 30–60 min.

Dosage

Dosage must be individualized by age, weight, pathology, other drugs, anesthesia to be used and type of surgery.
Adults:
Premedication—0.05–0.1 mg
  Adjunct to general anesthesia: Induction—0.05–0.1 mg repeated at 2- to 3-min intervals; for elderly and poor-risk patients—0.025–0.05 mg.
  Maintenance of anesthesia—0.025–0.05 mg as needed; *Regional anesthesia*—0.05–0.1 mg; *Postop*—0.05–0.1 mg every 2 hrs
Children: (2–12 Years)
Induction and maintenance of anesthesia—0.02–0.03 mg per 20–25 pounds.

When Innovar (fentanyl/droperidol combination) is given along with fentanyl, the dose of fentanyl contained in the Innovar must be considered in calculating the total dosage of fentanyl.

Preparation and Storage

Available in 2 ml and 5 ml ampuls containing 0.05 mg/ml.

Store at room temperature. Keep in packaging to protect from light.

This is a Schedule II drug under the Controlled Substances Act of

1970. Maintain hospital or institutional regulations guiding its use.

Drug Incompatibilities
Do not mix with:
Methohexital
Pentobarbital
Thiopental or with any other medication.

Modes of IV Administration
Injection
Yes
Slowly, over 2–3 min.

Intermittent Infusion
No

Continuous Infusion
No

Contraindications; Warnings; Precautions; Adverse Reactions

Contraindications
Hypersensitivity

Warnings
1. Resuscitative equipment and a narcotic antagonist must be readily available, to manage apnea.
2. Patients receiving this drug must not be left alone.
3. Hypotension can occur especially when drug is administered in conjunction with a tranquilizer such as droperidol (or in the combined form of Innovar). Fluids and vasopressors must be readily available.
4. When administering Innovar, see page 142 for complete details on droperidol.
5. Respiratory depressant effect lasts longer than the analgesic effects. Large doses can cause apnea. When other narcotics are required, administer 1/4 to 1/3 of the usual dose.
6. Muscle rigidity, especially of the muscles of respiration, can result from rapid injection. Should it occur, manage with assisted respiration and neuromuscular blocking agent.
7. Severe and unpredictable potentiation by MAO inhibitors has been reported; avoid use of fentanyl in patients who have received these agents within the previous 14 days.
8. Use with caution in patients who are susceptible to respiratory depression, e.g., comatose patients with head injury or brain tumor. This drug may also obscure clinical signs of these conditions.
9. Safety for use in children less than 2 years of age has not been established.
10. Safety for use in pregnancy and during delivery has not been established.

Precautions
1. The initial dose must be reduced in the elderly, debilitated and other poor-risk patients. Reaction to initial dose should determine subsequent doses.
2. When used as an adjunct to regional or general anesthesia, the respiratory depression associated with this drug and the anesthesia can be potentiated.
3. Hypotension can occur; treat with head-down position if possible, and fluids. Pressor agents can also be used (**except** epinephrine).
4. Use with caution in patients with chronic obstructive pulmonary disease, and those with potentially compromised respiration.
5. Respiratory depression caused by narcotic analgesics can be managed by narcotic antagonists (such as naloxone) and assisted ventilation. See page 237 for information about naloxone.
6. When fentanyl is administered with droperidol (as separate drugs or combined as Innovar) pulmonary arterial pressure may be decreased.
7. This drug has potentiating effects with other CNS depressants (narcotics, barbiturates, tranquilizers, general anesthetics). When used concomitantly

fentanyl citrate
(continued)

with any of these agents, the dosage of each should be reduced.

8. This drug can cause bradycardia. Atropine may be used to reverse this. Use with caution in patients with preexisting bradyarrhythmias.
9. Administer with caution in the presence of liver or kidney impairment.

Adverse Reactions
1. Most common: respiratory depression, apnea, bradycardia, muscle rigidity. If these are untreated, respiratory or cardiac arrest can result.
2. Dizziness, hypotension, blurred vision, nausea, vomiting, laryngospasm, diaphoresis.
3. When fentanyl and droperidol are given in combination: chills, elevated blood pressure, restlessness, postop. hallucinations can occur. Also, extrapyramidal symptoms, which can be controlled with anti-Parkinson agents.

Management of Overdosage
1. Manifestations of overdosage:
   a. Respiratory depression— hypoventilation and apnea
   b. Muscle rigidity
   c. Bradycardia, circulatory depression (hypotension)
2. Treatment:
   a. Assisted ventilation, oxygen, maintenance of patent airway.
   b. If muscle rigidity is present, an intravenous neuromuscular blocking agent may be needed to allow assisted ventilation.
   c. Maintain body warmth and adequate hydration.
   d. A narcotic antagonist such as naloxone (Narcan) should be used for respiratory depression after the above emergency supportive measures have been initiated. The duration of respiratory depression may exceed the duration of effectiveness of the antagonist. Follow individual narcotic antagonist instructions: naloxone, page 237.

□ **Nursing Implications**
1. Patients receiving this drug intravenously should be under constant observation to detect the possible onset of respiratory or circulatory depression. Resuscitative equipment and drugs should be readily available.
2. Monitor heart rate and blood pressure before and every 5–10 minutes after an injection, for 30 minutes. Then monitor these parameters every 15 minutes times 3. The duration of action is 30–60 minutes in patients with normal liver and kidney function and over 60 minutes in the presence of hepatic and renal impairment. Patients with pre-existing arrhythmias should be observed via continuous ECG monitoring during therapy with this drug. Bradycardia (adults: heart rate less than 60/minute) can be treated with atropine 0.5–1.0 mg. Significant hypotension will probably be treated with fluids, vasopressors and/or a narcotic antagonist.
3. For patients not already receiving respiratory assistance, monitor respiratory rate at least every 3–5 minutes following an injection. At the same time, observe for the presence of cyanosis of the oral membranes and nail beds. Monitor for onset of laryngospasm (dyspnea, wheezing, stridor). If the respiratory rate falls, attempt to verbally stimulate the patient to increase the respiratory rate. Frequency of stimulation should be such as to bring the rate to a normal level. If the patient cannot be aroused, begin assisted ventilation with a manual breathing bag (Ambu, Puritan, Hope). Maintain a patent airway with an oral-pharyngeal airway;

administer oxygen if cyanosis develops. Notify physician. Have a narcotic antagonist agent at the bedside. Continue respiratory support until swallow, gag and cough reflexes return, and until the patient's spontaneous respiratory rate is 12–14/minute. Monitor blood gases and remain with the patient for the next several hours. Note that the duration of action of a narcotic antagonist may be less than that of the respiratory depression produced by the fentanyl; additional doses of the antagonist may be needed.

4. Be prepared to manage vomiting to prevent aspiration.

5. If this drug is given to patients who are ambulatory, assist as needed in the event of dizziness, to prevent injury.

fluorouracil ■
(Adrucil, 5-FU, 5-Fluorouracil)

Actions/Indications
Antineoplastic, antimetabolite, cell-cycle specific.

Used for palliative management of carcinoma of colon, rectum, breast, stomach and pancreas when considered incurable by surgery or other means.

Dosage
Adults and Children:
Dosage must be based on weight (use ideal weight if patient is obese or if there has been weight gain due to edema).

12–15 mg/kg/day once a day, for 4 successive days. *Daily dose must not exceed* 800 mg. If no toxicity is observed, 6 mg/kg is given on 6th, 8th, 10th, and 12th days. Discontinue after 12th day dose.

Patients in poor nutritional state (see Contraindications) should receive 6 mg/kg/day for 3 successive days. If no toxicity is seen, 3 mg/kg may be given on 5th, 7th, and 9th days. Daily dose for poor-risk patients should not exceed 400 mg.

If toxicity is not a problem contin-

ue therapy on *either* of the following schedules:

1. Repeat dosage of first course every 30 days after the last day of the previous course, or

2. When toxic signs have subsided, administer a maintenance dose of 10–15 mg/kg/week as a single dose. Do not exceed 1 gm/week.

Dosage reduction in the presence of renal impairment must be based on individual patient response.[1]

Preparation and Storage
Available in 10-ml ampuls containing 500 mg of drug (50 mg/ml).

Slight discoloration does not affect the use of the drug. Protect from light. If a precipitate occurs due to exposure to low temperatures, resolubilize by heating to 140° F (60°C) with vigorous shaking.

Cool to body temperature before administering.

Drug Incompatibilities
Do not mix with any other medication in any manner.

Modes of IV Administration

Injection
Yes
No dilution is required

Intermittent Infusion
Yes
Use D5W or NS 100–200 ml. Infuse over 30–60 min.

Continuous Infusion
No

Contraindications; Warnings; Precautions; Adverse Reactions

Contraindications
1. Poor nutritional state
2. Depressed bone marrow function
3. Presence of serious infection

Warnings
1. Patient must be hospitalized during initial treatment.
2. Use with extreme caution in pa-

fluorouracil
(continued)

tients with a history of high-dose pelvic irradiation, previous use of alkylating agents, those who have bone marrow involvement by metastatic tumors, or who have impaired hepatic or renal function.

3. Safety for use in pregnancy has not been established.
4. There may be mutagenic effects on germinal cells of males and females.
5. Any form of therapy that adds stress, interferes with nutrition, or depresses bone marrow, will increase the toxicity of fluorouracil.

Precautions
1. WBC with differential should be taken prior to each dose.
2. *This drug can cause severe bone marrow depression, GI hemorrhage and even death despite careful adjustment of dosage.*
3. Therapy should be discontinued if any one of the following signs of toxicity appear:
   a. Stomatitis, esophagopharyngitis
   b. Leukopenia, WBC < 3500/cu mm
   c. Vomiting (intractable)
   d. Diarrhea (frequent or watery stools)
   e. GI ulceration or bleeding
   f. Platelet count < 100,000/cu mm
   g. Hemorrhage from any site
4. Avoid extravasation.

Adverse Reactions
1. Gastrointestinal: anorexia, nausea, vomiting, diarrhea, stomatitis, esophagopharyngitis (usually seen on fourth day of a loading dose therapy and subsides 2–3 days after discontinuation (50% of all patients)
2. Blood: bone marrow depression producing leukopenia and thrombocytopenia; leukopenia nadir—(maximum depression) —at 9–21 days, and thrombocytopenia nadir at 7–17 days

3. Skin: hair loss (reversible), loss of finger- and toenails, rashes (maculopapular, usually on extremities), photosensitivity, Addisonian hyperpigmentation
4. Neurologic: reversible cerebellar ataxia (1% incidence, may last several weeks after discontinuation)
5. Other: photophobia, lacrimation, epistaxis, euphoria, myocardial ischemia.

☐ **Nursing Implications**
1. The patient receiving this medication will be experiencing the emotional and physical effects of the malignancy. Knowledge of the patient's feelings about his disease and its implications will assist in helping him tolerate the chemotherapy. The incidence of uncomfortable side effects and adverse reactions is high. It is within the nurse's role to assist the patient in coping with the discomforts of the disease and its treatment, and to help him work through depression and anger toward acceptance of the disease at his own pace. Despite the unpleasantness this drug may bring, it can be a source of hope for the patient.
2. *Management of gastrointestinal effects*:
   a. See Adverse Reactions No. 1.
   b. Be prepared to administer antiemetics around the fourth day of loading dose therapy. These drugs can be given prophylactically prior to the onset of symptoms.
   c. Small frequent meals, timed with periods when the patient feels his best, are advisable. Bland foods are usually tolerated better than others. Carbohydrate and protein content should be high.
   d. If the patient is anorexic, encourage high nutrient liquids and water to maintain nutrition and hydration.
   e. Keep accurate measurements of emesis volume and total

intake and output to guide the physician in ordering parenteral fluids when necessary.

f. Monitor for the onset of diarrhea. Notify the physician and administer antiperistaltic drugs as ordered. Observe for signs and symptoms of hypokalemia, e.g., muscle weakness and cramps. Maintain hydration.

g. Monitor for signs and symptoms of esophagopharyngitis: sore throat, dysphagia, burning pain in the chest. Notify the physician. Administer antacids as ordered. A bland, mechanical soft diet is advisable.

3. *Management of stomatitis*:

a. Administer preventive oral care every 4 hours and/or after meals.

b. For preventive oral care use a very soft toothbrush (child's) and toothpaste; avoid trauma to the tissues.

c. Examine oral membranes at least once daily (instruct patient and/or family) to detect the onset of inflammation or ulceration.

d. If stomatitis occurs, notify the physician and begin therapeutic oral care:[2]
Mild Inflammation: Remove dentures: use a soft toothbrush and a hydrogen peroxide solution (1 part peroxide and 4 parts saline). Do not use toothpaste. Rinse with the peroxide solution and then water. Replace dentures. This procedure should be carried out every 4 hours and/or after meals.
Severe Inflammation: Remove dentures; use soft gauze pads rather than a toothbrush. Use the peroxide solution as described above. Rinse with water using an asepto syringe and gently suction until returns are clear. Do not replace dentures. It may be necessary to

give this care every 2–4 hours.

e. Order soft, bland diet. If the stomatitis is severe, the patient may need a liquid diet, or be NPO.

f. For patients who can tolerate oral intake, administer Xylocaine Viscous or acetaminophen elixir as a mouthwash prior to meals to decrease pain (do not use aspirin rinses), as ordered by the physician.

g. Parenteral analgesia may be required.

4. *Management of hematologic effects*:

a. The greatest degree of bone marrow depression occurs usually on day 7–14; the time of recovery varies.

b. Be aware of the patient's white blood cell and platelet count prior to each injection.

c. If the WBC falls to 2000/cu mm, take measures to protect the patient from infection such as protective (reverse) isolation, avoidance of invasive procedures, maintaining bodily (especially perineal) cleanliness, carrying out strict urinary catheter care when appropriate, etc. Monitor for infection by recording temperature every 4 hours, and examining for rashes, swellings, drainage and pain. Explain these measures to the patients.

d. If the platelet count falls below 100,000/cu mm, monitor for thrombocytopenic bleeding: petechiae, purpura, hematuria, melena, blood in stools, gum bleeding, vaginal bleeding, epistaxis, hematemesis, etc. Avoid trauma. Transfusions may be ordered.

e. Instruct the patient and family on the importance of follow-up blood studies if the drug is being administered on an outpatient basis.

fluorouracil
(continued)

5. *Management of hair loss:*
   a. Use a scalp tourniquet during injection, if ordered, to help prevent hair loss.
   b. Counsel the patient on the possibility of hair loss to enable him to prepare for this disfigurement.
   c. Reassure him of probable regrowth of hair following discontinuation of the drug.
   d. Provide privacy, and time for the patient to discuss his feelings.
6. *Management of skin problems:*
   a. If rashes occur, administer cool compresses as ordered. Turn the patient on bed rest frequently to prevent skin breakdown.
   b. Reassure the patient that finger- and toenails will grow back after discontinuation of the drug. Protect fingers and toes from trauma.
   c. Warn the patient to avoid exposure to the sun to prevent sunburn. If exposure is unavoidable, suggest the use of a sunblock lotion.
   d. Inform the patient of the transient nature of skin pigmentation changes.
7. If the patient develops ataxia, initiate measures to protect him from injury during dangerous activities such as climbing stairs.

References
1. Shinn, Arthur F., et al.: Dosage Modification of Cancer Chemotherapeutic Agents in Renal Failure. *Drug Intelligence and Clinical Pharmacy,* 11:141, March 1977.
2. Bruya, Margaret Auld, and Madeira, Nancy Powell: Stomatitis After Chemotherapy. *American Journal of Nursing,* 75(8):1351, August 1975.

Suggested Readings
Bruya, Margaret Auld, and Madeira, Nancy Powell: Stomatitis After Chemotherapy. *American Journal of Nursing,* 75(8):1349–1352, August 1975.
Giadquinta, Barbara: Helping Families Face the Crisis of Cancer. *American Journal of Nursing,* 77:1583–1588, October 1977.
Gullo, Shirley: Chemotherapy—What To Do About Special Side Effects. *RN,* 40:30–32, April 1977.
Laatsch, Nancy: Nursing the Woman Receiving Adjuvant Chemotherapy for Breast Cancer. *Nursing Clinics of North America,* 13(2):337–349, June 1978.

furosemide ■
(Lasix)

Actions/Indications
Potent diuretic. Inhibits reabsorption of sodium and chloride in proximal and distal tubules and in loop of Henle. Effect begins within 5 min of injection, peaks in 30 min, lasts 2 hrs.

Used in the treatment of edema in congestive heart failure, cirrhosis, and renal disease. Emergency treatment of pulmonary edema.

Dosage
Adults:
Initial—20–40 mg. A second dose can be given 2 hrs later. If no response, increase dose by 20-mg increments, no sooner than 2 hrs after last dose.
   Pulmonary edema—40 mg followed by another 40 mg in 1–1 1/2 hours.*
Children:
1 mg/kg. If no response, increase by 1 mg/kg in 2 hrs. Doses greater than 6 mg/kg are not recommended.
*Very high doses are sometimes used in renal failure, up to 3000 mg.

Preparation and Storage
Available in 2 ml, 4 ml and 10 ml ampuls and 2 ml and 4 ml prefilled syringes each containing 10 mg/ml.

Store at room temperature. Do not use if solution is yellow. Protect prefilled syringes from light.

Use filtering needle (or syringe filter) when removing from ampuls.

Drug Incompatibilities

Do not mix with:
Invert sugar 10% in Electrolyte #2
Fructose 10% in water
Any strongly acidic solutions such as those containing:
Ascorbic acid
Epinephrine
Levarterenol
Tetracycline

Modes of IV Administration

Injection
Yes
Slowly over 1–2 min. Most effective mode to produce diuresis.

Intermittent Infusion
Yes
Use NS, RL, or D5W *only*.
  Administer at 1 mg/min.

Continuous Infusion
Yes
Use NS, RL, or D5W *only*.
  Infuse within 24 hrs.
  Use this mode for large doses to avoid hearing loss, 2000–3000 mg over 8–10 hrs; do not exceed a rate of 4 mg/min.

Contraindications; Warnings; Precautions; Adverse Reactions

Contraindications
1. Hypersensitivity to furosemide or to sulfonamides; (there may be cross-allergenicity).
2. Anuria
3. Hepatic coma or electrolyte imbalance
4. Pregnancy and in women of childbearing potential (may cause fetal abnormalities)

Warnings
1. Excessive diuresis may result in dehydration, reduction of blood volume and circulatory collapse with the possibility of vascular thrombosis and embolism especially in the elderly
2. Excessive loss of potassium may precipitate digitalis toxicity in patients receiving digitalis glycosides

3. Sudden alterations of fluid and electrolyte balance may precipitate hepatic coma in patients with cirrhosis; observe patient closely.
4. Observe for blood dyscrasias, liver damage, and idiosyncratic reactions.
5. If BUN or oliguria increases during therapy, discontinue drug.
6. Furosemide may potentiate effects of other antihypertensives; patients receiving such drugs may need reduced dosage while on furosemide.
7. This drug may exacerbate or activate systemic lupus erythematosis.
8. This drug is found in breast milk; nursing should be discontinued if furosemide is required.
9. Intravenous administration of this drug increases ototoxicity of aminoglycoside antibiotics, especially in patients with renal disease. Avoid use of furosemide in such patients, except in life-threatening situations.
10. Tinnitus and hearing loss (both reversible and irreversible) have been reported. Ototoxicity is most likely after *rapid* injection of excessively high doses in patients with severe renal disease. In such patients, controlled infusion rate (not to exceed 4 mg/min) is recommended.

Precautions
1. This drug depletes sodium, water and potassium. Monitor serum electrolytes, CO_2 and BUN frequently during therapy and observe for electrolyte imbalance (see Nursing Implications No. 3).
2. Hypokalemia is more likely with: brisk diuresis, cirrhosis or concomitant use of ACTH or corticosteroids.
3. Asymptomatic hyperuricemia may occur. Gout may rarely be precipitated.
4. Avoid dehydration, especially in renal patients; reversible elevations of BUN can occur.

furosemide
(continued)

5. Monitor serum calcium levels; hypocalcemia can occur. Tetany has been reported (rare).
6. Alterations in glucose tolerance with hyperglycemia can occur in diabetics and latent diabetics; check urine and blood glucose periodically.
7. Salicylate toxicity may occur in patients on high doses of salicylates in conjunction with furosemide.
8. Furosemide may increase the nephrotoxicity of cephaloridine.
9. This drug may decrease arterial responsiveness to pressor amine drugs, though not enough to diminish their effectiveness.
10. Furosemide antagonizes the skeletal muscle relaxing effect of tubocurarine and potentiates the action of succinylcholine.

Adverse Reactions

1. Dermatitis: urticaria, pruritus, exfoliative dermatitis, photosensitivity
2. Nausea, vomiting, diarrhea, anorexia
3. Postural hypotension
4. Blurred vision, dizziness, headache
5. Hematologic changes
6. Hearing loss, tinnitus (see Warning No. 10)
7. Other: hyperglycemia, hyperuricemia, urinary bladder spasm, thrombophlebitis

☐ **Nursing Implications**

1. Weigh the patient prior to therapy and daily thereafter.
2. Monitor urine output every 8 hours or more frequently as indicated. Observe for oliguria (adults: less than 30 ml/hour for 2 or more consecutive hours). Observe for bladder distention in susceptible patients. Use a urinary collection device in infants and small children.
3. Monitor for electrolyte imbalance, i.e., hyponatremia, hypokalemia. Signs and symptoms:
   Hyponatremia

Headache
Nausea, diarrhea
Abdominal cramps
Confusion and stupor
Hypotension (late)
Hypokalemia
Weakness
Muscle cramps
Lethargy
Irritability
Abdominal distention
Cardiac arrhythmias (late)
Poor feeding in infants.
Administer potassium supplements as ordered.

4. Monitor for dehydration:
   a. Excessive weight loss
   b. Decreased skin turgor (tenting)
   c. Weakness, lethargy
   d. Decreased urine output
   e. Increased specific gravity
5. Monitor blood pressure every 30 minutes after injection and then every 2 hours or as indicated by the patient's condition. Hypovolemia and fall in cardiac output with subsequent hypotension is likely to occur with excessive diuresis. Fluids will be used to re-establish blood volume. Utilize central circulatory monitoring devices if available, such as pulmonary artery pressure and central venous pressure.

Suggested Readings

Kemp, Ginny, and Kemp, Doug: Diuretics. *American Journal of Nursing,* 78:1007–1010, June 1978 (references).
Plumb, Vance J.: Clinical Hazards of Powerful Diuretics, Furosemide and Ethacrynic Acid. *Modern Concepts of Cardiovascular Disease,* 47(7), July 1978.

gentamicin sulfate ■
(Garamycin 40 mg/ml and Garamycin Pediatric 10 mg/ml)

Actions/Indications

Aminoglycoside antibiotic to treat serious infections due to susceptible strains of the following organisms:

- *Pseudomonas aeruginosa*
- *Proteus* species
- *E. coli*
- *Klebsiella-Enterobacter-Serratia* species
- *Citrobacter* species
- *Staphylococcus* species

Effective in bacterial septicemia and neonatal sepsis and serious bacterial infections of the CNS, urinary tract, respiratory tract, GI tract, skin, soft tissues, and bones.

Dosage

Whenever feasible, particularly in patients with impaired renal function or extensive burns, adjust dosage according to serum concentrations of drug. (See Warning 3b).

In The Presence of Normal Renal Function
Adults:
3 mg/kg/day in equally divided doses every 8 hrs. In life-threatening infections, up to 5 mg/kg/day (reduce as soon as clinically indicated).
Children:
6–7.5 mg/kg/day given in equally divided doses every 8 hours.
Premature or Full-Term Neonates:
< *1 week of age*—5 mg/kg/24 hrs, in equally divided doses every 12 hours.
Infants:
1–6 weeks of age—7.5 mg/kg/24 hrs, in equally divided doses every 8 hrs.
> *6 weeks*—5.0–7.5 mg/kg/24 hrs, in equally divided doses every 6 hrs.

In The Presence of Renal Failure in Adults:[1]

1. Select Loading Dose in mg/kg [LEAN WEIGHT] to provide peak serum level desired. Approximate peak levels from commonly used loading doses are indicated below:

LOADING DOSE	EXPECTED PEAK SERUM LEVEL BASED UPON ONE-HALF HOUR IV INFUSION
2.0 mg/kg	6–8 g/ml
1.75 mg/kg*	5–7 g/ml
1.5 mg/kg	4–6 g/ml
1.25 mg/kg	3–5 g/ml
1.0 mg/kg	2–4 g/ml

*(Recommended for most moderate to severe systemic infections.)

2. Select Maintenance Dose (as percentage of chosen loading dose) to continue peak serum levels indicated above according to patient's creatinine clearance and desired dosing interval.

PERCENTAGE OF LOADING DOSE REQUIRED FOR DOSAGE INTERVAL SELECTED:

Cr. Clear.	8 hrs.	12 hrs.	24 hrs.
90	90%	—	—
80	88	—	—
70	84	—	—
60	79	91%	—
50	74	87	—
40	66	80	—
30	57	72	92%
25	51	66	88
20	45	59	83
15	37	50	75
10	29	40	64
7	24	33	55
5	20	28	48
2	14	20	35
0	9	13	25

Hull and Sarubbi do not recommend adjustments of gentamicin dosage in patients with mild to moderate renal impairment who are receiving carbenicillin concomitantly.[2]

Preparation and Storage

Available in two concentrations:

1. 40 mg/ml—supplied in 2 ml vials containing 80 mg, 20 ml vials containing 800 mg, 1.5 ml prefilled syringes containing 60 mg and 2 ml prefilled syringes containing 80 mg.
2. Pediatric form containing 10 mg/ml—2 ml vials containing 20 mg.

Mix in D5W or NS only. Do not use if solution is discolored or contains a precipitate.

Drug Incompatibilities

Do not mix with:
Amphotericin B
Ampicillin
Carbenicillin
Cephalosporins
Chloramphenicol
Dopamine
Heparin

gentamicin sulfate
(continued)
Nafcillin
Oxacillin
Sulfadiazine
Ticarcillin
Vitamin B complex with C

Modes of IV Administration

Injection
No
Nephrotoxicity, ototoxicity increases with rapid injection.

Intermittent Infusion
Yes
Dilute dose in 50–200 ml NS or D5W.
 Use a smaller volume for infants and children.
 Do not exceed a concentration of 1 mg/ml.
 Infuse over 1/2–2 hours.

Continuous Infusion
No
Therapeutically inappropriate.

Contraindications; Warnings; Precautions; Adverse Reactions

Contraindications
Hypersensitivity

Warnings
1. This drug is potentially nephrotoxic; use with caution in patients with pre-existing renal impairment and those receiving high doses or prolonged therapy. Monitor renal function in all patients. Discontinue if BUN or creatinine rises.
2. This drug can be ototoxic (vestibular and auditory damage) particularly to patients with renal disease or those receiving higher doses or prolonged therapy.
3. To reduce risk of nephrotoxicity and ototoxicity (especially in patients with impaired renal function and the elderly):
   a. Monitor renal and eighth cranial nerve function (see Nursing Implications)
   b. Monitor serum concentration when possible. (Keep peak < 12 mcg/ml, valleys < 2 mcg/ml.)
   c. Avoid concurrent or sequential use of such drugs as cisplatin, cephaloridine, kanamycin, amikacin, neomycin, polymyxin B, colistin, paromomycin, streptomycin, tobramicin, vancomycin, viomycin and potent diuretics such as: ethacrynic acid and furosemide.
4. Safety for use in pregnancy has not been established.

Precautions
1. Respiratory paralysis can occur in patients receiving: anesthetics or mass transfusions of citrate-anticoagulated blood. Prolongation of paralysis secondary to neuromuscular blocking agents (succinylcholine, etc.) may be reversed by calcium salts.
2. Use with caution in patients with neuromuscular disorders (myasthenia gravis or parkinsonism); it may aggravate muscle weakness.
3. Is cross-allergenic with other aminoglycosides.
4. Patient should be well-hydrated during therapy.
5. Overgrowth of nonsusceptible organisms can occur.

Adverse Reactions
(Most likely in patients with known renal impairment or those receiving high doses and prolonged therapy.)
1. Nephrotoxicity.
2. Neurotoxicity: (vestibular and auditory)—dizziness, vertigo, tinnitus, hearing loss, numbness, skin tingling, muscle twitching, convulsions.
3. Wide range of other reported reactions including: respiratory depression, hypersensitivity (fever, rash, urticaria, laryngeal edema, anaphylactoid reactions), laboratory abnormalities (elevated serum transaminase, decreased electrolytes, anemia and other blood dyscrasias).

Management of Overdosage

In the event of overdosage or toxic reactions peritoneal dialysis or hemodialysis will remove drug from the blood.

☐ Nursing Implications

1. Take anaphylaxis precautions; see Appendix.
2. Monitor renal function:
   a. BUN and creatinine—be aware of these values, daily.
   b. Urinary output—monitor for oliguria every 8 hours or as condition indicates.
   c. Urine specific gravity—fall in value may indicate impending failure.
   d. Weight—weigh patients before initiating and daily throughout therapy. Notify physician of changes in renal status.
3. Monitor for eighth cranial nerve damage:
   a. *Auditory damage*—high-frequency hearing, loss as determined by audiometric testing, general hearing loss.
   b. *Vestibular damage*—dizziness, vertigo, tinnitus (ringing in the ears), roaring in the ears.
4. Monitor for signs and symptoms of nonsusceptible organism overgrowth infection:
   a. Fever (take rectal temperature at least every 4–6 hours)
   b. Increasing malaise
   c. Signs and symptoms of localized infection: redness, soreness, pain, swelling, drainage (change in volume or character of pre-existing drainage)
   d. Cough (change in volume or character of pre-existing sputum)
   e. Diarrhea
   f. Oral lesions (thrush) or perineal itching and rash (monilia) secondary to *Candida albicans*

References

1. Hull, J. Heyward, and Sarubbi, Felix A.: Gentamicin Serum Concentrations: Pharmacokinetic Predictions. *Annals of Internal Medicine*, 85:188, August 1976. (Used by permission.)
2. Ibid.

Suggested Reading

Vanderveen, Timothy W.: Aminoglycoside Antibiotics. *American Journal of IV Therapy*, July 1977, pp. 5–13.

glucagon hydrochloride ▓

Actions/Indications

Produced in the pancreas (alpha cells of Isles of Langerhans); causes an increase in blood glucose, by converting liver glycogen to glucose. Used to treat hypoglycemic states associated with diabetes and insulin shock therapy. Also diagnostic aid for relaxation of the stomach, duodenum and small bowel in radiologic exams.

Used by some groups to reverse the adverse effects of propranolol and enhance the effect of digitalis when used for congestive heart failure. (Glucagon can increase the force of myocardial contractility and cardiac output.)

Dosage

In hypoglycemia—
Adults:
0.5–1.0 unit. If patient does not respond in 5–20 min. repeat twice and *administer glucose, 50% by intravenous injection.*
Children:
0.025–1.0 mg/kg/dose. Repeat in 20 min. Maximum total dose is 1 mg. Administer 50% dextrose in water concomitantly.
Neonates:
(The symptomatic newborn of a diabetic mother) 0.30 mg/kg/dose, repeated once in 20 min. Give 50% dextrose in addition.
Insulin Shock Therapy—0.5–1 mg, after one hour of coma. If no response in 10–25 minutes, repeat dose.
As a diagnostic aid—0.5 mg by intravenous injection.

glucagon hydrochloride
(continued)
Preparation and Storage
Available as a powder in vials containing 1 unit (1 mg) and in vials containing 10 units (10 mg) each packaged with special diluent.

Use only diluent provided by manufacturer and no other. Use entire diluent vial. Solution produced is 1 mg/ml. Refrigerate and discard after 90 days.

Drug Incompatibilities
Do not mix with any other medication in any manner.

Modes of IV Administration

Injection
Yes
May administer directly into vein or into the injection port of a running IV, over 1 minute.

Intermittent Infusion
No
Pharmacologically inappropriate.

Continuous Infusion
No
Pharmacologically inappropriate.

Contraindications; Warnings; Precautions; Adverse Reactions

Contraindications
Hypersensitivity

Warnings
1. Give with caution to patients with a history of insulinoma (may cause hypoglycemia) or pheochromocytoma (marked increase in blood pressure can result).
2. The patient must be treated at the first signs of hypoglycemia; prolonged reactions may result in cerebral cortical damage.

Precautions
Liver glycogen stores must be available. If not, supplements of glucose must be given to treat the hypoglycemia.

Adverse Reactions
Nausea and vomiting on awakening from hypoglycemic state

☐ **Nursing Implications**
Hypoglycemia:
1. Stay with the patient with hypoglycemia. Monitor time of awakening. Repeat dose in 20 minutes if there is no response.
2. Maintain an open intravenous line.
3. Have 50% dextrose at the bedside.
4. Prevent aspiration by turning patient on his side. Keep tracheal suction equipment at bedside. Use airways, manual breathing bags, etc. and assist breathing as needed.
5. Observe seizure precautions.
6. If patient does not awaken after 20 minutes and full doses of glucagon and glucose, unconscious state may be due to something other than hypoglycemia.
7. Determine what precipitated the hypoglycemia.
8. Instruct patient and family on:
   a. causes and prevention of hypoglycemia
   b. signs and immediate treatment
   c. Use of glucagon at home (if prescribed by physician)
   d. Complete diabetic self-care

glycopyrrolate injection ■
(Robinul Injectable)

Actions/Indications
Anticholinergic (antimuscarinic) agent, inhibits the action of acetylcholine on structures innervated by postganglionic cholinergic nerves and on smooth muscles that react to acetylcholine. Reverses bronchorrhea, bronchospasm, bradycardia, and intestinal hypermotility induced by anti-cholinesterase agents.

Used preoperatively and intraoperatively: to reduce the reaction of the vagal reflex and thereby reduce salivary, tracheobronchial and pharyngeal secretions; to reduce the volume and free acidity of gastric secretions; and to block cardiac vagal inhibitory reflexes during induction of anesthesia and intubation. This drug can be used intraoperatively to reduce vagal traction reflexes and arrhythmias. It protects against the peripheral muscarinic effects (bradycardia and excessive secretions) of cholinergic agents such as neostigmine and pyridostigmine, and may also be used intravenously in the treatment of peptic ulcer because of its ability to reduce gastric secretions and free acidity.

Dosage
Adults:
  Intraoperative—0.1 mg (0.5 ml) repeated as needed at intervals of 2–3 minutes. See Precaution No. 4.
  To reverse the muscarinic effects of neostigmine and pyridostigmine—0.2 mg (1.0 ml) for each 1 mg of neostigmine or 5.0 mg of pyridostigmine. Administer the neostigmine or pyridostigmine and the glycopyrrolate simultaneously, in the same syringe.
  Peptic Ulcer—0.1 mg (0.5 ml) at 4-hour intervals; for a more profound effect, 0.2 mg (1.0 ml). Frequency should be dictated by patient response, up to 4 times a day.
Children:
  Intraoperative—0.002 mg (0.01 ml)/lb, do not exceed 0.1 mg (0.5 ml) repeated as needed at 2–3 minute intervals.
  To reverse the muscarinic effects of neostigmine and pyridostigmine—0.2 mg (1.0 ml) for each 1 mg of neostigmine or of each 5.0 mg of pyridostigmine.

Preparation and Storage
Supplied in 1 and 2 ml single-dose vials and 5 and 20 ml multiple-dose vials, each containing 0.2 mg/ml. Store at room temperature.

Drug Incompatibilities
This agent **can** be mixed with any of the following medications and fluids:
D5W
D10W
D5 Saline

Fentanyl and droperidol
Hydroxyzine
Lactated Ringers
Meperidine
Morphine
Neostigmine
Pyridostigmine
  Do **not** combine in syringe with:
Chloramphenicol
Dexamethasone
Diazepam
Dimenhydrinate
Pentazocine lactate
Secobarbital
Sodium bicarbonate
Sodium methohexital
Sodium pentobarbital
Thiopental

Modes of IV Administration

Injection
Yes
May be administered undiluted.

Intermittent Infusion
No

Continuous Infusion
No

Contraindications; Warnings; Precautions; Adverse Reactions

Contraindications
1. Known hypersensitivity.
2. In treatment of peptic ulcer where therapy may be prolonged, this agent may be contraindicated in patients who also have: glaucoma, obstructive uropathy, gastrointestinal obstruction, paralytic ileus, intestinal atony of the elderly or debilitated, unstable cardiovascular status in acute hemorrhage, severe ulcerative colitis, toxic megacolon in ulcerative colitis, and myasthenia gravis.

Warnings
1. Use with caution if at all in patients with glaucoma or asthma. This drug may cause an exacerbation of these conditions.
2. May produce drowsiness or blurred vision.

glycopyrrolate injection
(continued)
3. Diarrhea may be an early symptom of incomplete intestinal obstruction, especially in patients with an ileostomy or colostomy, and this agent should not be used.

Precautions
1. Investigate any tachycardia before giving this drug, because it may increase heart rate. Therefore, also use with caution in patients with: coronary artery disease, congestive heart failure, cardiac arrhythmias, hypertension, hyperthyroidism.
2. In treating peptic ulcer, use with caution in the elderly and in all patients with autonomic neuropathy, hepatic or renal disease, ulcerative colitis or hiatal hernia.
3. Overdosage may produce a curare-like action; i.e., muscle weakness or paralysis.
4. Intravenous administration of any anticholinergic in the presence of cyclopropane anesthesia can result in ventricular arrhythmias; therefore, use with caution. Administering in small increments of 0.1 mg or less may reduce the likelihood.
5. Safety for use in pregnancy has not been established. It is not known whether or not this agent is excreted in human milk, administer with caution in nursing mothers.
6. Safety for use in children below 12 years of age has not been established for the treatment of peptic ulcer.

Adverse Reactions
1. Extension of anticholinergic actions: dry mouth, urinary hesitancy and retention, blurred vision (due to mydriasis), photophobia, increased ocular tension, tachycardia, palpitation, decreased sweating, headache, nervousness, drowsiness, weakness, nausea, vomiting, impotence, constipation.
2. Anaphylaxis, urticaria, rashes, mental confusion.

Management of Overdosage
To combat the resultant anticholinergic effects produced by this agent, neostigmine may be given in increments of 0.25 mg in adults. This dosage may be repeated every 5 to 10 minutes or until symptoms are reversed. The maximum dose of neostigmine in this instance is 2.5 mg. Smaller doses should be used in children. Monitor for reduced heart rate and return of bowel sounds.

If there are nervous system symptoms (excitement, restlessness, convulsions) physostigmine should be used because it crosses the blood-brain barrier. Dosage is 0.5 to 2.0 mg slowly administered intravenously, repeated as necessary up to 5 mg in adults. Use smaller doses in children. See page 280 on physostigmine and page 239 on neostigmine.

Treat fever symptomatically. Rarely, a curare-like effect occurs and affects respiratory muscles; support ventilation until adequate spontaneous respiration returns.

☐ **Nursing Implications**
1. When this drug is used during anesthesia, monitor for an increased heart rate. If cyclopropane is the anesthetic agent in use, monitor for ventricular irritability; i.e., premature ventricular contractions and ventricular tachycardia. Be prepared to treat with lidocaine.
2. This drug may cause an acute exacerbation of bronchial asthma and glaucoma. Monitor for onset of these problems and notify the physician if they occur. The signs and symptoms of acute glaucoma are: eye pain, scleral redness, rainbow vision, and blurred vision (remember that this drug itself can cause blurred vision).
3. Maintain patient safety if the patient experiences side effect such as mental confusion, blurred vision, and drowsiness. Use side rails at all times. If

these problems occur, do not leave the patient unattended.
4. Monitor for anaphylaxis.
5. Monitor for signs and symptoms of an intestinal obstruction: diarrhea, constipation, abdominal distention. Check for bowel sounds. Notify the physician if there is the possibility of an obstruction.
6. This drug may cause muscle weakness or paralysis. Monitor quality of respiration and respiratory rate in the event that the muscles of breathing are affected. Maintain a patent airway and assist ventilation with a manual breathing device if respirations fall below 8 per minute. Notify the physician immediately.
7. Neostigmine and physostigmine should be available at all times. These drugs can counteract some of glycopyrrolate's side effects just as glycopyrrolate can reverse the undesirable effect of those agents.
8. If this agent is used over a prolonged period of time for the peptic ulcer patient, constipation may occur. Help to prevent this with encouraging an adequate fluid intake, mild activity as tolerated, high-fiber diet, and stool softeners as ordered.

heparin, sodium ■
(Lipo-Hepin, Panheprin, Sodium Heparin from Beef Lung, Sodium Heparin from Porcine Intestinal Mucosa)

Actions/Indications
Anticoagulant, a mucopolysaccharide formed by the mast cells and present in the human body in minute amounts.

Heparin is thought to act by potentiating the action of a circulating heparin co-factor (antithrombin III) to neutralize activated Factor X preventing the conversion of prothrombin to thrombin. When a hypercoagulable state exists, it inactivates thrombin, preventing the conversion of fibrinogen to fibrin; also prevents formation of a stable fibrin clot. Heparin prolongs clotting time but does not affect bleeding time and does not lyse existing clots.

May also block the action of bioactive amines which are responsible in part for local constriction of bronchi and blood vessels in a pulmonary embolus.
• Used for prophylaxis and treatment of:
  1. Venous thrombosis
  2. Pulmonary embolism
  3. Atrial fibrillation with embolus
  4. Peripheral arterial embolism
• Prevention of cerebral thrombosis
• Diagnosis and treatment of disseminated intravascular coagulation defects
• Prevention of intravascular clotting after arterial or cardiac surgery
• Anticoagulation in: hemodialysis, peritoneal dialysis, transfusion, and extracorporeal circulation.
• Adjunct in coronary occlusion with acute M.I.

Dosage
Titrate dosage with clotting time and/or partial thromboplastin time (PTT). Maintain PTT at 1.5–2 times a control value or clotting time at 2.5–3 times control.
Adults:
Therapeutic anticoagulation—Initially, 10,000 units; follow with 5,000–10,000 units every 4–6 hrs by injection or intermittent infusion; or 5000 units initially by injection, then 20,000 to 40,000 units/24 hrs via continuous infusion, 1000 units/hr.

In *total body perfusion*—150 units/kg, guided by appropriate coagulation studies throughout the procedure.

Extracorporeal dialysis—Follow instructions provided by equipment manufacturer.
Children:
Initially, 50 units/kg; maintenance, 100 units/kg every 4 hrs.

See Management of Overdosage for protamine neutralization of heparin.

heparin, sodium
(continued)

Preparation and Storage

Available in beef lung and porcine intestinal mucosa derivations in the following concentrations:

1000 units/ml
5000 units/ml
10,000 units/ml
20,000 units/ml
40,000 units/ml

Supplied in single dose and multiple dose vials and in prefilled syringes.

Also available as a heparin-lock flush solution in disposable syringes containing 100 units/ml. This preparation is not to be used for anticoagulant therapy.

Drug Incompatibilities

Do not mix with:
Barbiturates
Cephalothin
Diphenhydramine
Erythromycin
Gentamicin
Narcotics
Procainamide
Prochlorperazine
Promazine

If an intermittent scalp-vein needle infusion set (heparin lock) is used, flush the system with NS before these drugs are given.

Modes of IV Administration

Injection
Yes
Give undiluted. May be injected into the tubing of a running IV or into an intermittent scalp-vein needle (heparin-lock).[1]

Intermittent Infusion
Yes
Use 50–100 ml of NS

Continuous Infusion
Yes
Preferred mode of administration. Add 24-hr dose to 1000 ml of NS.
Use an infusion pump.

Contraindications; Warnings; Precautions; Adverse Reactions

Contraindications
1. Hypersensitivity
2. Inability to perform suitable blood coagulation tests
3. Uncontrollable bleeding states (such as cerebral hemorrhage or threatened abortion)

Warnings
1. Use with extreme caution in disease states in which there is an increased chance of hemorrhage, such as subacute bacterial endocarditis, arterial sclerosis, increased capillary permeability; during and immediately following spinal tap or spinal anesthesia; major surgery (especially of brain, spinal cord and eye); hemophilia; thrombocytopenia; inaccessible ulcers or tube drainage of any organ.
2. Appropriate coagulation studies (usually partial thromboplastin time), should be done after initial dose and after any change in dosage.
3. Salicylates may induce bleeding because of their effect on platelet aggregation (the main hemostatic defense of heparinized patients), and the ulcerative action they have on gastric mucosa.
4. Use with caution any drug which prolongs prothrombin time or delays coagulation in any way (such as dextran, acetylsalicylic acid, phenylbutazone, ibuprofen, indomethacin, dipyridamole and hydroxychloroquine).
5. Evidence suggests that heparin may antagonize the action of ACTH, insulin, or corticoids and may also modify or inhibit allergic reactions.
6. Use with caution during pregnancy, especially the last trimester and in the immediate postpartum period due to risk of maternal bleeding. It does not cross the placental barrier but there is no adequate infor-

mation as to whether or not it
may affect fertility or cause fetal
abnormalities.
7. Larger than normal doses of
heparin may be necessary in febrile states.
8. The use of digitalis, tetracyclines, nicotine, and
antihistamines may partially
counteract the anticoagulant action of heparin.
9. An increased resistance to heparin is frequently encountered in
cases of thrombosis, thrombophlebitis, infections with throm-
bosing tendency, myocardial infarction, cancer, and in the
postoperative patient. Increased
dosage and careful monitoring
of coagulation studies may be
needed.

Precautions
1. Use with caution in the presence of mild hepatic or renal
disease, hypertension, and during menstruation.
2. Caution should be used when
administering ACD-converted
blood (blood collected in heparin sodium and later converted
to ACD blood), since heparin
anticoagulant activity persists
without decline for up to 22
days following the conversion
when stored under refrigeration. The coagulation mechanism of the recipient may be
altered by such blood, especially
if large amounts are given.
3. Patients receiving this drug generally should be hospitalized.
4. Because this agent is derived
from animal tissue, it should be
used with caution in patients
with a history of allergy. Before
a therapeutic dose is given to
such a patient, a trial dose of
1000 units should be given.
5. As a result of platelet aggregation, heparin can produce
thrombocytopenia and, rarely,
has been associated with thromboembolism which, if untreated,
may lead to arterial obstruction
and organ infarction. Examine

patient periodically for new
thrombosis and monitor platelet
counts.

Adverse Reactions
1. Hemorrhage including gastrointestinal, urinary, adrenal or
ovarian. (see section on
overdosage)
2. Hypersensitivity: chills, fever,
urticaria, asthma, anaphylaxis
3. Acute reversible thrombocytopenia
4. Osteoporosis and suppression
of renal function long-term
high-dose administration
5. Aldosterone suppression, causing an increased loss of sodium
and water in the urine, and an
increased retention of potassium
6. Delayed transient hair loss
(rare)
7. Rebound hyperlipidemia following discontinuation of the drug
8. Priapism (acute, sustained erec-
tion of the penis), rare

Management of Overdosage
1. Overdosage is indicated by
excessively prolonged clotting
or partial thromboplastin times
or the onset of acute bleeding.
2. Protamine sulfate (1% solution)
by slow infusion will neutralize
the heparin. See page 301 for
detailed description of use.
3. Blood or plasma transfusions
may be necessary. These dilute
heparin and add to the hemostatic properties of the blood
but do not neutralize heparin.

☐ **Nursing Implications**
1. Monitor coagulation studies
(partial thromboplastin time)
with the physician. Be certain
that the values are within therapeutic range before administering subsequent doses.
2. Use correct heparin lock
technique[2] for heparin injections. Use an infusion pump for
continuous infusions.
3. Monitor for signs of bleeding:

heparin, sodium
(continued)

a. Hematuria (may be the earliest sign)
b. Melena, red blood in the stools, positive guaiac (examine all stools)
c. Hematemesis
d. Nose bleeding
e. Gum bleeding
f. Prolonged bleeding after venipunctures or IM injections
g. Ecchymosis
h. Swelling of any muscle group associated with pain and tenderness
i. Vaginal bleeding (advise patients to report the onset of menstruation). If bleeding occurs, hold the next dose of heparin and notify the physician. Monitor vital signs.
4. Monitor for signs and symptoms of allergic reaction.
5. Avoid IM injections and trauma-producing procedures such as catheterizations.
6. Keep protamine on hand; see Management of Overdosage.

Reference
1. Sager, Diane P. and Bomar, Suzanne K.: *Intravenous Medications —A Guide to Preparation, Administration and Nursing Management.* Philadelphia: J. B. Lippincott Company, 1980, p. 149–151.
2. Ibid.

Suggested Readings
Caprini, J. A., Zoellne, J. L. and Weisman, M.: Heparin Therapy, Part 1. *Cardiovascular Nursing*, 13:13–16, May–June 1977 (references).
Geske, Cheryl S.: Anticoagulant Therapy in Acute Myocardial Infarction. *Heart and Lung*, 1:639–648, September–October 1972 (references).
Stein, Myron, Stevens, Paul, and Saffer, Alfred: Recognition and Management of Pulmonary Embolism. *Heart and Lung*, 1:650–654, September–October 1972.

hydralazine hydrochloride ∎
(Apresoline Hydrochloride)

Actions/Indications
Antihypertensive. Produces vascular smooth muscle relaxation to decrease peripheral vascular resistance. Increases cardiac output and renal blood flow.

Used to treat severe essential hypertension, but is not predictably effective in hypertensive emergencies.

Dosage
Adults:
20–40 mg, repeat as necessary. Patients with renal impairment will require lower doses. Blood pressure will fall within a few minutes after injection; maximal decrease within 10–80 min. *Maximum daily dose—* 300–400 mg.
Children:
1.7–3.5 mg/kg/day divided into 4–6 equal doses.

Intravenous route should be used only when the oral route is inappropriate.

Preparation and Storage
Available in 1-ml ampuls, 20 mg/ml. Discard unused portions.

Drug Incompatibilities
Do not inject into IV tubing containing:
Aminophylline
Ampicillin
Calcium disodium edetate
Chlorothiazide
Ethacrynate
Hydrocortisone
Mephentermine
Methohexital
Phenobarbital
Sulfadiazine

Modes of IV Administration

Injection
Yes
May be given undiluted through Y injection site. Inject at a rate of 10 mg/min.

Intermittent Infusion
No
Do not mix with fluids.

Continuous Infusion
No
Do not mix with fluids.

Contraindications; Warnings; Precautions; Adverse Reactions

Contraindications
1. Hypersensitivity
2. Coronary artery disease
3. Rheumatic mitral valve disease

Warnings
1. High, prolonged doses may produce a syndrome resembling systemic lupus erythematosus. Drug should be discontinued in this event. Symptoms will regress with some residua.
2. Complete blood count, LE prep., and antinuclear antibody titers should be done before and periodically during prolonged therapy and if fever, arthralgia, chest pain or malaise occur. Positive results require consideration for discontinuing the drug.
3. Use MAO inhibitors with caution in patients receiving this drug.
4. This drug can cause fetal abnormalities in animals. Do not use in pregnancy unless expected benefits outweigh potential risks to the fetus.
5. Profound hypotension may occur when this drug is administered concomitantly with diazoxide.

Precautions
1. Produces reflex myocardial stimulation which increases myocardial oxygen consumption and can precipitate angina and ECG changes of ischemia. Do not use in patients with coronary artery disease.
2. May cause postural hypotension (may reduce pressor responses to epinephrine).

3. Use with caution in patients with acute cerebral vascular accident; reduced blood pressure may cause relative cerebral ischemia.
4. Evidence suggests that this drug increases renal blood flow in patients with normal renal function. However, use with caution in the presence of advanced renal disease; reduced dosage will be required.
5. Blood dyscrasias have been reported; monitor hemoglobin, RBC, WBC during *prolonged* therapy.
6. May have an antipyridoxine effect requiring supplementary pyridoxine if symptoms such as paresthesias, numbness and tingling develop.

Adverse Reactions
1. Reactions are reversible with discontinuation of the drug or reduction of dosage.
2. Common side effects:
   a. Headache
   b. Palpitations, tachycardia, angina pectoris.
   c. Anorexia, nausea, vomiting.
3. Less common:
   a. Lacrimation, conjunctivitis
   b. Flushing of the face
   c. Peripheral neuritis (see Precaution No. 6).
   d. Dizziness
   e. Tremors
   f. Muscle cramps
   g. Psychotic reactions (depression, anxiety, disorientation)
   h. Hypersensitivity (rashes, urticaria, chills, fever, rarely hepatitis)
   i. Constipation, difficulty in voiding
   j. Blood dyscrasias
   k. Lymphadenopathy, splenomegaly
   l. Hypotension

Management of Overdosage
1. Signs: hypotension, tachycardia, headache, myocardial ischemia, chest pain, arrhythmias, shock.

hydralazine hydrochloride
(continued)
2. Treatment: Support blood pressure with volume expanders; avoid use of pressor agents. If vasopressor is used, select one least likely to produce cardiac arrhythmias. Digitalize as needed. Monitor renal function.

☐ **Nursing Implications**
1. Expect the blood pressure to begin to decrease starting 10–80 minutes after each injection. Monitor the blood pressure (indirect measurements will suffice) every 5 to 10 minutes after the injection for 1 hour, then once an hour for 2 hours, and then every 4 hours until the next injection. Repeat cycle for each dose unless the patient has complications.
2. If the patient has had a recent myocardial infarction or cerebrovascular accident, monitor the blood pressure more frequently than stated above. Report to the physician any fall in blood pressure below the established limits. Be prepared to treat hypotension (see Overdosage).
3. If the patient is able to cooperate, instruct him to report chest pain of any type. Anginal pain could indicate the onset of myocardial ischemia; notify the physician at once, and continue to monitor vital signs, including ECG, frequently.
4. Monitor for the consequences of severely elevated blood pressure if the patient is experiencing a hypertensive crisis:
   a. Encephalopathy—confusion, stupor, nausea, vomiting, visual disturbances, reflex asymmetries
   b. Cerebrovascular accident—paralysis or weakness
   c. Myocardial ischemia and/or infarction—chest pain, ECG changes (see Nursing Implication No. 3)
   d. Left ventricular failure—shortness of breath, orthopnea, elevated central venous pressure (or pulmonary artery pressure), tachycardia, rales, onset of a third and/or fourth heart sound.
   e. Renal failure—oliguria, rising BUN and creatinine.[2] Overdosage of this drug can cause an extreme reduction in blood pressure which can also cause these complications.
5. If the patient is receiving this drug for a noncrisis situation, he may ambulate after the injection when the blood pressure has stabilized. Before the patient ambulates alone, determine if postural hypotension is occurring on rising. If it is, report the lying and standing pressures to the physician. Take the necessary safety precautions to prevent patient injury. Instruct the patient to rise from a lying position slowly and to stand only after having been in the sitting position for 3–5 minutes, and then to rise slowly.
6. Monitor for the onset of a lupus-type syndrome seen with this drug: joint pains and swelling, malaise.
7. If the patient is to receive this drug in its oral form on a chronic basis, he must be instructed on hypertensive self-care prior to discharge from the hospital.

References
1. AMA Committee on Hypertension: The Treatment of Malignant Hypertension and Hypertensive Emergencies. *JAMA*, 228(13):1675, June 24, 1974.
2. Romankiewicz, J. A.: Pharmacology and Clinical Use of Drugs in Hypertensive Emergencies. *American Journal of Hospital Pharmacy*, 34(2):185–193, February 1977.

Suggested Readings
American Medical Association Committee on Hypertension: The Treatment of Malignant Hyper-

tension and Hypertensive Emergencies. *JAMA*, 228:1673–1679, June 24, 1974.

Fleischmann, L. E.: Management of Hypertensive Crisis in Children. *Pediatric Annals*, 6(6):410–414, June 1977.

Jones, L. N.: Symposium on Teaching and Rehabilitation of the Cardiac Patient. Hypertension: Medical and Nursing Implications. *Nursing Clinics of North America*, 11:283–295, June 1976.

Keith, Thomas: Hypertensive Crisis. Recognition and Management. *JAMA*, 237(15):1570–1577, April 11, 1977.

Koch-Weser, Jan: Hypertensive Emergencies. *New England Journal of Medicine*, 290:211–214, January 24, 1974.

Long, M. L., et al.: Hypertension: What the Patient Needs to Know. *American Journal of Nursing*, 76:765–770, May 1976.

Romankiewicz, J. A.: Pharmacology and Clinical Use of Drugs in Hypertensive Emergencies. *American Journal of Hospital Pharmacy*, 34(2):185–193, February 1977 (references).

hydrocortisone sodium succinate (Solu-Cortef) and hydrocortisone sodium phosphate ■
(Hydrocortone)

Actions/Indications
Adrenocorticosteroid, with potent anti-inflammatory, metabolic and other numerous effects. Used in:
- Endocrine disorders such as adrenal insufficiency
- Collagen diseases such as systemic lupus
- Allergic states
- Respiratory diseases
- Shock
- Overwhelming infections
- Rheumatic disorders
- Dermatologic disorders
- Ophthalmic diseases (allergic and inflammatory processes)
- Gastrointestinal disorders (ulcerative colitis, regional enteritis)
- Hematologic disorders
- Neoplastic diseases (palliative management of leukemias and lymphomas)
- Nephrotic syndrome without uremia
- Multiple sclerosis (acute exacerbations)

Dosage
Adults:
Severe shock—Dosage schedules are highly variable. Suggested dosages range from 0.5–2 gm every 2–6 hrs to 50 mg/kg every 24 hrs.

Other clinical situations—100–500 mg initially repeated at intervals of 1, 3, 6 and 10 hours as necessary to obtain an appropriate clinical response.

Children:
Governed by severity of condition and response to initial doses. Use no less than 25 mg/day. Doses of 0.16–1.0 mg/kg or 6–30 mg/M^2 once or twice daily have been recommended.

Gram-neg. shock—initially, 50 mg/kg; then: 50–75 mg/kg day (maximum single dose 500 mg).

Status asthmaticus—10 mg/kg/day

Neonates:
2.5 mg/kg/dose

Preparation and Storage
Supplied as powder in vials containing 100-, 250-, 500-, and 1000-mg of drug. 100-mg size can be reconstituted with 2 ml water for injection, bacteriostatic. Do not use diluents containing benzyl alcohol when administering this drug to neonates. For other vials use diluent provided by the manufacturer. Protect reconstituted form from light; discard after 3 days.

Note that hydrocortisone sodium succinate and sodium phosphate are the only two hydrocortisone preparations that can be given intravenously. Read labels carefully.

Drug Incompatibilities
Do not mix with:
Aminophylline
Amobarbital
Ampicillin
Cephalothin

hydrocortisone sodium succinate and phosphate
(continued)
Colistimethate
Dimenhydrinate
Diphenhydramine
Ephedrine
Heparin
Hydralazine
Kanamycin
Metaraminol
Methicillin
Nafcillin
Oxytetracycline
Pentobarbital
Phenobarbital
Prochlorperazine
Promethazine
Secobarbital
Tetracycline
   Insulin is compatible for up to 8 hours in solution.

Modes of IV Administration

Injection
Yes
Preferred for initial emergency use.
   Inject undiluted through Y injection site of a running IV over 30 seconds to several minutes depending on the dose.

Intermittent Infusion
Yes
Add dose to 50 ml D5W or NS. Infuse over 15–20 min.

Continuous Infusion
Yes
Use D5W, NS or D5/NS. Use no less than 1 ml of IV fluid to dilute 1 mg of drug.

Contraindications; Warnings; Precautions; Adverse Reactions

Contraindications
1. Systemic fungal infections
2. In the absence of a life-threatening situation, avoid in:
   a. Peptic ulcer disease
   b. Viral diseases (especially ocular)
   c. Infectious diseases without antibiotic treatment (especially TB)

   d. Myasthenia gravis
   e. Psychosis
3. Hypersensitivity

Warnings
1. Additional stress during therapy (surgery, trauma, infection, etc.) may require larger doses.
2. There may be a decreased resistance and inability to localize infection as well as masking of signs of infection.
3. Use in pregnancy and lactation requires that potential benefits be weighed against hazard to the fetus. Infants born to mothers on corticosteroids should be observed for signs of hypoadrenalism.
4. Large doses elevate BP, cause salt and water retention, and increase excretion of potassium and calcium. Dietary salt restriction and potassium supplements may be needed.
5. Limit use in TB to disseminated and fulminating types, in which antituberculous drugs are being given. If required for patients with latent TB, observe for reactivation.
6. Anaphylaxis has occurred secondary to this drug.

Precautions
1. In prolonged therapy, drug-induced adrenocortical insufficiency can be minimized by tapering of doses to discontinue.
2. There is an enhanced effect of corticosteroids in patients with hypothyroidism and cirrhosis. (Lower dosage is advisable.)
3. Psychosis can result from therapy. Pre-existing psychiatric problems may be exacerbated.
4. Use with caution in:
   a. Nonspecific ulcerative colitis, especially if there is a danger of abscess or perforation
   b. Diverticulitis
   c. Fresh intestinal anastomoses
   d. Peptic ulcer disease
   e. Renal insufficiency
   f. Hypertension
   g. Osteoporosis
   h. Myasthenia gravis

i. Ocular herpes simplex (corneal perforation can occur)

Adverse Reactions Seen In Short-Term Intravenous Therapy
1. Fluid and electrolyte imbalance: sodium and water retention with possible secondary hypertension, hypokalemia, hypocalcemia.
2. Gastrointestinal: peptic ulcer with possible perforation, pancreatitis, ulcerative esophagitis (prophylactic antacids may be used).
3. Dermatologic: impaired wound healing, petechiae, ecchymosis.
4. Neurologic: increased intracranial pressure, seizures (increasing frequency in patients with pre-existing seizure disorder), vertigo, headaches, mental confusion, euphoria, exacerbation of psychosis.
5. Endocrine: decreased glucose tolerance; increased requirements for insulin or oral hypoglycemics in diabetics.
6. Eye: increased intraocular pressure.
7. Metabolic: negative nitrogen balance secondary to rapid muscle catabolism.
8. Anaphylactoid reaction.

□ **Nursing Implications**
1. Take precautions to prevent infections in wounds by using strict aseptic technique in dressing changes, etc. Avoid invasive procedures such as catheterizations. The skin may become more fragile because of the steroid therapy. Patients on bed rest and those with general body weakening secondary to an acute illness should be turned hourly (except during sleep, then every 2–3 hours) to prevent skin breakdown. Initiate the use of supportive measures such as a flotation pad, water mattress, etc. Administer scrupulous skin care to prevent infection.
2. Hypotension can occur. Monitor blood pressure every 2–4 hours, or as the patient's condition dictates. Monitor blood pressure before and immediately after intravenous injection.
3. Weigh the patient daily to detect for water and sodium retention. Dietary restrictions in sodium may be prescribed by the physician. Examine daily for peripheral edema. Monitor for exacerbation of congestive heart failure in susceptible patients (increasing dyspnea, increasing resting heart rate, fatigue, rales, etc.)
4. There may be delayed healing of wounds; take precautions to prevent dehiscence. Sutures may be left in place longer than usual for this reason.
5. Monitor urine glucose in patients on high-dose therapy and with diabetes. Diabetic individuals may require a larger dosage of insulin or oral agent.
6. Administer antacid therapy as ordered to assist in preventing peptic ulcer. Monitor for signs of the development of an ulcer and/or acute intestinal bleeding: melena, positive stool guaiac, hematemesis, epigastric pain and/or distention, anemia or falling hematocrit.
7. Monitor for signs and symptoms of hypokalemia: weakness, irritability, abdominal distention, poor feeding in infants, muscle cramps.[1] Dietary or pharmacologic potassium supplements may be ordered, guided by serum potassium levels.
8. Monitor for signs and symptoms of hypocalcemia: irritability, change in mental status, seizures, nausea, vomiting, diarrhea, muscle cramps, late effects —cardiac arrhythmias, laryngeal spasm and apnea.[2] Dietary or pharmacologic supplements may be ordered guided by serum calcium levels.
9. Patients with a history of seizure activity may have an increasing number of seizures while on steroid therapy. Apply appropriate safety precautions.

hydrocortisone sodium succinate and phosphate
(continued)

10. Monitor for behavioral changes, which may range from simple euphoria to depression and psychosis. Apply appropriate safety precautions. A change in dosage may relieve such symptoms.
11. When tuberculin testing is indicated, it should be carried out prior to initiation of steroid therapy, if possible. The patient's reactivity to the tuberculin is altered by the drug, giving a false result.
12. Ambulate the patient with caution if vertigo occurs, and initiate the use of side rails and other safety measures to prevent patient injury. Report the onset to the physician.
13. Be alert to the signs of increasing intraocular pressure: eye pain, rainbow vision, blurred vision, nausea and vomiting.[3] Notify the physician immediately.

References
1. Beeson, Paul, and McDermott, Walsh (editors): *Cecil-Loeb Textbook of Medicine,* (14th ed.), Philadelphia: W. B. Saunders Company, 1975, p. 1587.
2. Ibid., p. 1815.
3. Newell, Frank W., and Ernest, J. Terry: *Ophthalmology— Principles and Concepts* (3rd ed.), St. Louis: C. V. Mosby Company, 1974, p. 329.

Suggested Readings
Glasser, Ronald J.: How the Body Works Against Itself; Autoimmune Diseases. *Nursing '77,* September 1977, pp. 34–38.
Melick, M. E.: Nursing Intervention for Patients Receiving Corticosteroid Therapy. In *Advanced Concepts in Clinical Nursing* (2nd ed.), K. C. Kintzel, ed., Philadelphia: J. B. Lippincott Company, 1977, pp. 606–617.
Newton, David W., Nichols, Arlene, and Newton, Marion: You can Minimize the Hazards of Corticosteroids. *Nursing '77,* June 1977, pp..26–33.
Reichgott, Michael J., and Melmon, Kenneth L.: The Role of Corticosteroids in Shock. In *Steroid Therapy* Daniel Azarnoff, ed., Philadelphia: W. B. Saunders Company, 1975, pp. 118–133.

hydromorphone hydrochloride ∎
(Dihydromorphinone HCl, Dilaudid)

Actions/Indications
Morphine derivative; narcotic analgesic. Effect begins within 15 minutes and lasts for more than 5 hours.

Used for relief of moderate to severe pain in the following situations:
- Postoperatively
- Acute myocardial infarction
- Any form of cancer
- Trauma (soft tissue and bone)
- Burns
- Biliary colic
- Renal colic

Dosage
Adults:
2 mg usual; 3–4 mg in very severe pain every 4–6 hrs or as the duration of pain relief dictates.
Children:
Dosage not available for use in children. Adolescents can receive adult dosage.

Preparation and Storage
Available in ampuls containing: 1 mg/ml, 2 mg/ml, 3 mg/ml or 4 mg/ml, and in 10 ml and 20 ml multidose vials each containing 2 mg/ml.

Slight yellowish discoloration does not affect use of the drug.

Do not mix with IV fluids.

This is a Schedule II drug under the Controlled Substances Act of 1970. Maintain hospital or institutional regulations guiding its use.

Drug Incompatibilities
Do not inject into an IV line containing sodium bicarbonate or thiopental sodium.

Modes of IV Administration

Injection
Yes
Dilute dosage in 10 ml sterile water for injection or NS, inject slowly over 2–3 min.

Intermittent Infusion
No
Do not mix with IV fluids.

Continuous Infusion
No
Do not mix with IV fluids.

Contraindications; Warnings; Precautions; Adverse Reactions

Contraindications
1. Hypersensitivity to opiate derivatives
2. Intracranial lesions producing increased intracranial pressure (drug can markedly increase CSF pressure)
3. In depressed ventilatory function (such as COPD, cor pulmonale, emphysema, kyphoscoliosis, status asthmaticus)

Warnings
1. This drug produces dose-related respiratory depression which, along with hypotension, is more likely with rapid injection.
2. Narcotics may obscure diagnosis or clinical course of patients with acute abdominal conditions or head injuries.

Precautions
1. Use with caution in elderly or debilitated patients and those with hepatic or renal disease, hypothyroidism, Addison's disease, prostatic hypertrophy or urethral stricture.
2. Use with caution postoperatively and in patients with pulmonary disease; it suppresses the cough reflex.
3. Use of this drug concomitantly with other narcotic analgesics or other CNS depressants can potentiate the CNS depression;

the dosage of one or both drugs should be reduced.
4. This drug can cause fetal abnormalities in animals; complete information is unavailable in humans. Use in pregnancy only if expected benefits outweigh potential risks to the fetus.
5. Use during labor and delivery can produce respiratory depression in the infant.
6. It is not known whether this drug is excreted in breast milk; nursing should be discontinued if the drug must be given.
7. Safety for use in children has not been established.

Adverse Reactions
1. Sedation, drowsiness, anxiety, dizziness
2. Nausea and vomiting
3. Circulatory depression and cardiac arrest have occurred after rapid injection.
4. Postural hypotension and syncope
5. Spasm of ureters and bladder sphincters, urinary retention
6. Respiratory depression

Overdosage
1. Symptoms: respiratory depression (decreased rate, tidal volume, Cheyne–Stokes respiratory pattern, cyanosis), extreme somnolence progressing to stupor or coma, skeletal muscle flaccidity, cold and clammy skin, bradycardia, hypotension; apnea, and cardiac arrest may follow.
2. Treatment: maintain an open airway and assist or control ventilation as required. Administer narcotic antagonist (naloxone 0.005 mg/kg—see page 237). Repeated doses may be needed since duration of action of hydromorphone exceeds that of the antagonist. Give oxygen, IV fluids, vasopressors as indicated.

☐ Nursing Implications
1. Schedule doses to prevent pain from reaching its maximum intensity. Never withhold an anal-

hydromorphone hydrochloride
(continued)

gesic unless ordered by the physician.

2. Evaluate patient's response to the drug. Notify physician if dosage, frequency, or agent is apparently ineffective.

3. Administer one-half hour prior to treatments, ambulation, or other painful procedures such as coughing or chest physical therapy. Administer at bedtime to promote restful sleep.

4. Administer emotional support positioning and other care measures to enhance analgesic affect of the drug.

5. Monitor for respiratory depression:

   a. Count respiratory rate every 2–3 minutes during and for the first 15 minutes after intravenous injection and every 15–30 minutes for the next 2 hours. Repeat cycle with additional doses.

   b. If respiratory rate falls below 8–10/minute, if respirations become very shallow or if Cheyne–Stokes pattern develops attempt to arouse the patient. If successful, coach him to breathe at a rate of 10–12/minute. Notify the physician; have naloxone or other antagonist at the bedside. Do not leave the patient alone.

   c. If the patient cannot be aroused to increase respiratory rate, begin ventilation with manual breathing bag at a rate of 10–12/minute. Monitor pulse. Administer oxygen if cyanosis develops. Notify the physician. Do not leave the patient alone until a spontaneous respiratory rate of 10–12/minute is reached, and other vital signs have stablilized.

   d. Be prepared to manage respiratory depression in the neonate if the mother has received this drug during labor.

Suggested Readings

McCaffery, Margo, and Hart, Linda L.: Undertreatment of Acute Pain with Narcotics. *American Journal of Nursing,* 76(10):1586–1591, October 1976 (references).

Wiley, Francis M., and Rhein, Marilee: Challenges of Pain Management: One Terminally Ill Adolescent. *Pediatric Nursing,* 3:26–27, July–August 1977.

insulin, regular ■
(Actrapid, Iletin, Velosulin)

Actions/Indications
Hypoglycemic hormone. Promotes the movement of glucose from blood to cell for oxidation; lowers blood glucose level; regulates the formation of glucose from noncarbohydrate sources.

Effects begin immediately and last for 20 minutes.

Used to treat hyperglycemia and diabetic ketoacidosis. Also used to induce hypoglycemic shock in psychotherapy and in polarizing solutions for treatment of acute myocardial infarction. When administered with dextrose, potassium will move from the blood into the cell.

Dosage
Adults:
Dosage must be determined and titrated with blood glucose and acetone levels.

Severe diabetic acidosis—100–200 units initially, followed by additional doses of 20–50 units every 30 min, guided by hourly blood glucose (should not fall below 100 mg/100 ml).

Low-dose infusions can also be used at a rate of 5–10 units/hr, following an initial bolus of 100 units. During infusion, titrate drip rate with hourly blood and urine glucose levels.

Preparation and Storage
Available as beef, pork and beef/pork preparations in U-80 and

U-100 concentrations. Use syringes with the appropriate scale.
Do Not Use U-500 Regular Insulin Intravenously.
Store in refrigerator. Discard if solution is cloudy or has a color change. These changes indicate loss of potency.

There can be adsorption of insulin to the surfaces of glass and plastic solution containers. It has been suggested to add small amounts of normal serum albumin (human) to the infusion to prevent this.[2] Regardless of this adsorption, infusion rates must be guided by serum glucose levels.

Drug Incompatibilities
Do not mix in infusion solution with other medications because of titration dosage. Do not mix in an intravenous line with:
Aminophylline
Amobarbital
Barbiturates
Chlorothiazide
Methylprednisolone
Phenytoin
Sodium bicarbonate
Sulfadiazine
Sulfisoxazole
Thiopental

Modes of IV Administration

Injection
Yes
Through Y injection site.

Intermittent Infusion
No

Continuous Infusion
Yes
When blood glucose is excessively high, NS is usually used as infusion fluid.

D5W can be used when blood glucose is near normal.

Infusion rate is titrated with blood glucose values. Add a sufficient amount of insulin to make calculation of drip rate simple; e.g., 25 units in 500 ml (1 unit/20 ml).

Contraindications; Warnings; Precautions; Adverse Reactions

Contraindications
Hypersensitivity to beef or pork

Warnings
Any change in purity, strength, manufacturer or species source (beef, pork, beef/pork) of the insulin given may require a change of dosage to avoid hypoglycemia or hyperglycemia.

Precautions
Do not allow blood glucose to fall below 100 mg/100 ml.

Adverse Reactions
1. Hypoglycemia (hunger, headache, dizziness, diaphoresis, eventual coma if untreated)
2. Hypersensitivity (generalized rash, shortness of breath, rapid pulse, diaphoresis, hypotension)

☐ Nursing Implications
1. Monitor blood and urine glucose and ketone levels, and serum carbon dioxide during administration of insulin. Do not allow blood glucose to fall below 100 mg/100 ml.
2. Monitor for signs and symptoms of hypoglycemia: diaphoresis; pallor in fair-skinned individuals and ashened color in dark-skinned persons; change in mental status, e.g., confusion, agitation, or lethargy; headache; hunger or nausea; tachycardia; tremors; seizure.
3. Administer supportive care to the comatose patient in ketoacidosis, i.e., prevention of aspiration, respiratory care, prevention of skin breakdown, fluid and electrolyte balance, monitoring of vital signs.
4. Use an infusion pump for continuous infusions for precise control of rate. It is advisable for patients receiving such infusion to be cared for in an intensive care unit.
5. Patients with newly-diagnosed diabetes will require thorough

insulin, regular
(continued)

instruction regarding all aspects of diabetic self-care. The same information should be reviewed with previously known diabetics to help avoid hyperglycemia and hypoglycemia in the future.

References
1. Keisberg, Robert A: Diabetic Ketoacidosis: New Concepts and Trends in Pathogenesis and Treatment. *Annals of Internal Medicine,* 88:686, 1978.
2. Petty, Clayton and Cunningham, Nelson L.: Insulin Adsorption by Glass Infusion Bottles, Polyvinyl Chloride Infusion Containers, and Intravenous Tubing. *Anesthesiology,* 40:400–404, April 1974.

Suggested Readings
Heber, David, Molitch, Mark E., and Sperling, Mark A.: Low-Dose Continuous Insulin Therapy for Diabetic Ketoacidosis. *Archives of Internal Medicine,* 137:1377–1380, October 1977.
———: Low-Dose Insulin Therapy in Diabetic Ketoacidosis. *Archives of Internal Medicine,* 137:1361–1362, October 1977.

isoproterenol hydro-
chloride ■
(Isuprel, Iprenol)

Actions/Indications
Sympathomimetic (produces the effects of epinephrine); a beta adrenergic stimulator. Has the following actions:
• Increased contractility of the heart
• Improved myocardial conductivity
• Increased heart rate
• Increased systolic blood pressure and decreased diastolic pressure
• Relaxation of bronchial and intestinal smooth muscle
Used as an adjunct to the treatment of shock, cardiac standstill, carotid sinus hypersensitivity.
Used in the temporary management of complete heart block and si-nus bradycardia and ventricular arrhythmias requiring increased cardiac activity for treatment.
Also used in the management of bronchospasms during anesthesia.

Dosage
Adults:
Cardiac standstill or complete heart block—bolus injection of 20–60 mcg (1–3 ml of the 1:50,000 solution), followed by 10–200 mcg as needed to elicit a response.
OR
Administer as an infusion; initial rate of 5 mcg/min adjusted to patient response.
OR
As an intracardiac injection, 20 mcg (1.0 ml of the 1:50,000 solution). Repeat as necessary.
Bronchospasm—in anesthesia, or when an attack is unresponsive to inhalation drug administration, 10–20 mcg (0.5–1.0 ml of the 1:50,000 solution) as a direct IV injection.
Shock, carotid sinus hypersensitivity, sinus bradycardia—range, 0.5–30.0 mcg/min via an infusion (use the 1:500,000 solution). Volume rate = 0.25–15 ml/min. Dosage must be regulated by patient response.
Children:
Bradyarrhythmias—0.5–4.0 mcg/min (use the 1:500,000 solution). Titrate with heart rate.
Cardiac standstill—1–4 mcg/min (use the 1:500,000 solution). Titrate with patient response.
A bolus injection may also be used, 10–30 mcg (0.5–1.5 ml of a 1:500,000 solution), followed by an infusion of 200 mcg in 300 ml of fluid, titrated with patient response.
Status asthmaticus (investigational)— 0.8–1.7 mcg/kg/min by infusion. Monitor ECG and titrate with patient response.

Preparation and Storage
Available in 1 ml and 5 ml ampuls of a 1:5000 solution (0.2 mg/ml) (200 mcg/ml).
The following solutions are most commonly used:
1:50,000 (20 mcg/ml). Prepare by

adding 1 ml of the 1:5000 solution to 9 ml diluent.

1:500,000 (2.0 mcg/ml). Prepare by adding 1 ml of the 1:5000 solution to 100 ml diluent *or* add 5 ml of drug to 500 ml diluent.

A more concentrated solution can be used for patients requiring large dosage and a minimum of fluid: 2 mg of drug (10 ml of the 1:5000 solution) in 500 ml of diluent.

Use D5W or NS for infusion.

Drug Incompatibilities

Do not mix with:
Alkaline buffered antibiotics
Aminophylline
Any calcium preparation
Barbiturates
Lidocaine or any other drug which raises the pH above 6.0
Sodium bicarbonate

Modes of IV Administration

Injection
Yes
Use a 1:50,000 solution as described under Preparation and Storage.

Inject over 1 min. This mode is recommended only for cardiac standstill or bronchospasm in *adults*.

Intermittent Infusion
No
Administer by titration; see Continuous Infusion below.

Continuous Infusion
Yes
Using a 1:500,000 solution, begin the infusion with the dosages recommended. Titrate with arterial pressure, heart rate, pulmonary artery pressure and urine flow.

Use an infusion pump, preferably the volumetric type, if available.

Contraindications; Warnings; Precautions; Adverse Reactions

Contraindications
1. Pre-existing tachyarrhythmias (except those ventricular arrhythmias treated by increasing cardiac output)

2. Tachyarrhythmias secondary to digitalis intoxication
3. Idiopathic hypertrophic subaortic stenosis (IHSS)[1]

Warnings
This drug increases myocardial oxygen consumption; its use in patients in cardiogenic shock due to acute MI may be detrimental to myocardial functioning.

Precautions
1. Do not administer concurrently with epinephrine; serious arrhythmias may result.
2. Adjust dosage carefully in patients with coronary insufficiency, diabetes, hyperthyroidism or in patients sensitive to sympathomimetics.
3. Correct any hypovolemia with volume expanders before beginning treatment with this drug.
4. Observe patients in shock closely while this drug is being given. Decrease or discontinue the infusion if heart rate exceeds 110/minute.
5. Use in pregnancy only if expected benefits outweigh potential risks to mother and child.
6. Use with caution in patients receiving cyclopropane anesthesia; arrhythmias can occur.

Adverse Reactions
1. Flushing of the face
2. Sweating
3. Mild tremors
4. Nervousness
5. Headache
6. Palpitations—usually transient and do not require discontinuation of the drug
7. Pulmonary edema has been reported in a patient extremely sensitive to sympathomimetic drugs
8. Precipitation of transient complete heart block
9. Post-resuscitation tachycardia
10. Myocardial irritability producing premature ventricular contractions and ventricular tachycardia

isoproterenol hydrochloride
(continued)
☐ **Nursing Implications**

1. Adequate parameters must be available for monitoring to guide titration of this drug. At a minimum, heart rate, ECG, central venous pressure (CVP), blood pressure (BP) and urine output must be utilized. If possible, it is advisable to use direct arterial blood pressure and pulmonary capillary wedge pressure (PCWP) readings. Because of this drug's vasoconstrictive actions, the indirectly obtained blood pressure may be significantly different from the more accurate intra-arterial blood pressure. The values of these parameters to strive for when titrating the drug must be determined by the physician.

2. Heart rate and blood pressure (direct or indirect) must be recorded prior to and every 2–3 minutes during the initial phase of titration. When the blood pressure stabilizes for at least 1 hour near or at the desired, preset value, frequency of monitoring can be reduced to every 15–30 minutes, or as indicated by the patient's general condition.

3. CVP and PCWP should be recorded prior to and every 30 minutes during titration. A continuous oscilloscopic display of arterial pressure and PCWP is ideal in this situation.

4. Urine output should be recorded hourly during the initial phase of therapy with this drug for shock. Urine flow reflects indirectly the perfusion of the kidneys. A fall in urine output may indicate the need for a change in drug therapy, either an increase in isoproterenol drip rate, or its discontinuation and the initiation of another agent. Notify the physician if urine output falls below 30 ml/hour for 2 consecutive hours in an adult patient.

5. Use a volumetric infusion pump if available. If a pump is not available, use microdrop tubing and perform frequent drip counts.

6. Patients receiving therapy with this drug frequently require respiratory support. Monitor respiratory rate, effort and blood gases with other parameters. Be prepared to initiate manual ventilation.

7. Monitor ECG continuously during infusion; premature ventricular contractions are common during administration. If these occur, decrease infusion rate. If isoproterenol dosage cannot be decreased, a lidocaine infusion may be started at 1–4 mg/minute (dosage during the use of isoproterenol may be greater than normal because of drug-induced improved hepatic perfusion). Other causes for myocardial irritability such as hypoxia must be ruled out. If the heart rate exceeds 110 beats/min (adults), decrease infusion rate while monitoring other parameters.

8. Instruct the patient, if he is able to cooperate, to report chest pain.

9. Avoid extravasation. See Appendix.

References

1. Beeson, Paul B. and McDermott, Walsh (editors) *Textbook of Medicine* (14th ed.) Philadelphia: W.B. Saunders Company, 1975, p. 975.

Suggested Readings

Amsterdam, Ezra A., et al.: Evaluation and Management of Cardiogenic Shock. Part I. Approach to the Patient. *Heart and Lung,* 1(3):402–408, May–June 1972 (references).
————: Evaluation and Management of Cardiogenic Shock. Part II. Drug Therapy. *Heart and Lung,* 1(5):663–671, September–October 1972 (references).

Tarazi, Robert C.: Sympathomimetic Agents in the Treatment of Shock. *Annals of Internal Medicine*, 81:364–371, September 1974 (references).

Woods, Susan L.: Monitoring Pulmonary Artery Pressures. *American Journal of Nursing*, 76:1765–1771, November 1976 (references).

levothyroxine sodium ■
(Levoid, Synthroid)

Actions/Indications
A synthetic form of thyroxine, the principle hormone secreted by the thyroid gland.

Used for replacement therapy for decreased to absent thyroid function.

Intravenous administration is used for myxedema coma and for thyroid hormone replacement when oral administration is not possible and a rapid onset of action is needed.

Dosage
Adults and Children:
0.2–0.5 mg

Effects begin in 6–8 hours but full effects will be evident 24 hrs later. A repeat injection of 0.1–0.3 mg can be given on the second day if significant improvement has not been seen.

Myxedema coma—0.2–0.5 mg.

PBI levels should be monitored and used to guide subsequent dosage.

Preparation and Storage
Supplied in 10 ml vials containing 0.5 mg (500 mcg) of drug in powder form. To reconstitute add 5 ml NS (do not use any diluents containing a bacteriostatic agent). Shake vial to insure thorough mixing.

Solution will contain 0.1 mg/ml.

Use immediately and discard unused portion.

Drug Incompatibilities
No data.

Do not mix with any other medication in any manner.

Modes of IV Administration

Injection
Yes
Inject a solution containing 0.1 mg/ml over 1 min.

Intermittent Infusion
No

Continuous Infusion
No

Contraindications; Warnings; Precautions; Adverse Reactions

Contraindications (Relative)
1. Thyrotoxicosis
2. Acute myocardial infarction
3. Adrenal insufficiency

Warnings
1. Use with caution in patients with cardiovascular disease, especially hypertension. Use a low initial dosage. Decrease dosage if chest pain or other sign of cardiac problems occur.
2. Patients with cardiac problems who are receiving catecholamines (epinephrine) concomitantly or are having surgery should be carefully monitored for arrhythmias.
3. May potentiate anticoagulant effects of warfarin or coumarin.
4. Adrenal insufficiency must be corrected with corticosteroids prior to the administration of thyroid hormones.
5. This drug can unmask previously obscured symptoms of endocrine disorders such as diabetes mellitus, hypopituitarism, adrenal insufficiency and diabetes insipidus. An adjustment in the therapy of these concomitant disorders may be required.
6. Use for treatment of obesity is inappropriate and hazardous.

Precautions
1. Dosage must be delivered in small initial doses and gradual increments.
2. In patients with diabetes, insulin

levothyroxine sodium
(continued)
and oral hypoglycemic agent requirements may increase. The opposite is true if thyroid dosage is decreased.

Adverse Reactions
Excessive dosage may cause the symptoms of hyperthyroidism, e.g., weight loss, palpitations, chest pain, leg cramps, nervousness, sweating, tachycardia and other arrhythmias, headache, insomnia, heat intolerance, fever. Dosage should be decreased.

☐ **Nursing Implications**
1. Full effects of this drug will not be seen until the day after administration.
2. Patients with cardiac problems must be observed by continuous ECG monitoring during and following intravenous injection. Anticipate tachyarrhythmias (atrial fibrillation, paroxysmal atrial tachycardia and premature ventricular contractions).
3. When administering catecholamines or sympathomimetics to patients on this drug and with cardiac problems monitor ECG continuously and be prepared to treat ventricular irritability (premature ventricular contractions, ventricular tachycardia). Keep lidocaine 100 mg at the bedside.
4. If the patient is concomitantly on coumarin or warfarin anticoagulants, monitor closely for bleeding. Be aware that the anticoagulant dosage should be decreased. Frequent prothrombin times will be required.
5. Monitor diabetics for hyperglycemia, e.g., with urine fractionals. Be aware of the fasting blood sugar. Insulin or oral hypoglycemic dosage may have to be increased.
6. Monitor for signs of hyperthyroidism (see Adverse Reactons). Instruct the patient to report symptoms, if he is capable.
7. Patients on IV therapy will

eventually be placed on an oral thyroid preparation. Plan to instruct the patient on long-term self-care.
8. Administer supportive care as indicated for the comatose patient, e.g., skin care, safety precautions. Corticosteroids may be ordered if there is evidence of adrenal steroid insufficiency. See page 175 for information on administration of hydrocortisone.

lidocaine hydrochloride ■
(Xylocaine Intravenous for Cardiac Arrhythmias)

Actions/Indications
Antiarrhythmic. Increases the electrical stimulation threshold of the ventricular myocardium during diastole, with no change in contractility.

Indicated in the acute management of serious or life-threatening ventricular arrhythmias (premature ventricular contractions and ventricular tachycardia) particularly those associated with:
• Cardiac manipulation including cardiac surgery
• Acute myocardial infarction
• The use of drugs producing myocardial irritability (vasopressors, dopamine, etc.)

Dosage
Adults:
Initial—50–100 mg bolus. If no change in the arrhythmia in 5 min, repeat dose.

Use *only* the 5-ml, 100-mg ampuls or prefilled syringes for direct IV injection.

Do not administer more than 200–300 mg in 1 hr. (See Precaution No. 1.)

Maintenance—following an initial bolus, begin a continuous infusion if necessary. Dosage range is 1–4 mg/min. (20–50 mcg/kg/min in the average 70-kg person).

Up to 7 mg/min has been used for short periods; do not exceed this dosage, or 200–300 mg in 1 hr.

Titrate with ECG monitoring.

Children:
Initial (using a 0.2% solution)—0.5–
1.0 mg/kg/dose; repeat in 5–10 min
as needed.
   Maintenance—20–50 mcg/kg/min.
Do not exceed 100 mg in 1 hr.
Infants:
Injection—0.5 mg/kg/dose, repeated
every 5–10 min as needed.[1]

Preparation and Storage
This drug is supplied in several parenteral forms. Use *only* solutions labeled for cardiac arrhythmias:
   For direct IV injection—5 ml ampuls
and prefilled syringes containing
100 mg (20 mg/ml)
   For preparation of infusions—1 gm
and 2 gm vials and additive syringes
containing 40 mg/ml
   To prepare solutions:
1. 0.4% solution (4 mg/ml) pro-
    vides convenient flow rate cal-
    culation and is preferable when
    a fluid restriction is required:

Lidocaine	Vol. of Fluid
2 gm	500 ml
1 gm	250 ml
600 mg	150 ml

2. 0.2% solution (2 mg/ml) may
    be used when fluids are not re-
    stricted:

Lidocaine	Vol. of Fluid
2 gm	1000 ml
1 gm	500 ml
500 mg	250 ml

3. 0.1% solution (1 mg/ml) may
    be used for patients who can
    tolerate larger volumes of flu-
    ids:

Lidocaine	Vol. of Fluid
1 gm	1000 ml
500 mg	500 ml

Also available in premixed bottles
for infusion: 0.2% solution, 500 ml;
0.4% solution, 250 and 500 ml; and
0.8% solution, 250 and 500 ml.

Drug Incompatibilities
Do not mix with sodium bicarbonate, amphotericin B, methohexital or
sulfadiazine in any manner.

Modes of IV Administration

Injection
Yes
At a rate of 25–50 mg/min; more
rapid administration has caused seizures.
   May be given undiluted.
   Allow adequate time for the drug
to reach the site of action before repeating dose (5 min.)
   Bolus injection insures rapid rise
in blood level of the drug and
should precede infusions.

Intermittent Infusion
No
Administer by titration; see Continu-
ous Infusion section below.

Continuous Infusion
Yes
Use any IV fluid (D5W preferred).
Titrate with ECG response (i.e., sup-
pression of premature ventricular
contractions).
**USE AN INFUSION PUMP OR
AT LEAST MICRODROP TUB-
ING TO CONTROL FLOW RATE**

Flow Rates: For 0.4%

4 mg/min	=	1 ml/min
	=	60 microdrops/min
	=	60 ml/hr
3 mg/min	=	3/4 ml/min
	=	45 microdrops/min
	=	45 ml/hr
2 mg/min	=	1/2 ml/min
	=	30 microdrops/min
	=	30 ml/hr
1 mg/min	=	1/4 ml/min
	=	15 microdrops/min
	=	15 ml/hr

Contraindications; Warnings; Pre-
cautions; Adverse Reactions

Contraindications
1. Known hypersensitivity to any
    local anesthetic
2. High grade sinoatrial or atrio-
    ventricular block, Wolff-Parkin-
    son-White Syndrome

Warnings
1. Constant ECG monitoring must
    be used when administering this
    drug for titration of drip rate.

lidocaine hydrochloride
(continued)

2. Signs of prolongation of conduction, i.e., increasing P-R interval or widening of the QRS complex, should prompt discontinuation of the drug. This drug can increase the severity of A-V block.
3. Discontinue if arrhythmias appear or seem to be increased by the drug.
4. Emergency resuscitative equipment, including defibrillator must be readily available.
5. Information for proper use in children is limited.
6. This drug may increase the ventricular rate in the presence of atrial fibrillation.
7. Safety for use in pregnancy has not been established. Expected benefits should be weighed against potential risks to the fetus.

Precautions
1. This drug is metabolized by the liver and excreted by the kidneys. Use with caution in patients with severe impairment of these organs, hypovolemic shock, severe congestive heart failure and in the elderly.[2] Toxicity, especially of the central nervous system, is more likely in these individuals, and persists longer after discontinuation of the drug.
2. Administration for PVC's in the presence of sinus bradycardia, without prior acceleration of the sinus rate (by isoproterenol or pacing), may increase the PVC's and lead to ventricular tachycardia.
3. Treat other factors which can produce premature ventricular contractions, e.g., hypoxia, pain, hypotension, digitalis toxicity, other drugs.

Adverse Reactions
1. NONCARDIAC SIGNS OF TOXICITY:
   a. Numbness of the lips, tongue, pharynx and face, paresthesias.
   b. Dysarthria (difficulty in speaking)
   c. Tremors, twitching
   d. Tinnitus, dizziness
   e. Blurred or double vision
   f. Drowsiness, apprehension, euphoria
   g. Advanced toxicity—seizures, respiratory depression and arrest
2. CARDIAC SIGNS OF TOXICITY:
   a. Prolongation of P-R interval or widening of the QRS complex
   b. Bradycardia (sinus arrest may occur in the presence of sick sinus syndrome)
   c. *Increasing* frequency of premature ventricular contractions
   d. Hypotension, cardiovascular collapse
3. ALLERGIC REACTIONS

Management of Toxicity
1. Stop the infusion immediately with the onset of any one sign or symptom. Signs and symptoms will usually subside within 15–20 minutes.
2. Continue to monitor for the arrhythmia being treated.
3. Have the following drugs readily available to treat adverse reactions:
   a. Hypotension—vasopressors such as norepinephrine (Levophed), dopamine (Intropin), use with caution to avoid further ventricular irritability
   b. Bradycardia—atropine 0.5–1.0 mg. (average adult dose)
   c. Seizures—diazepam 2.5–5.0 mg. (average adult dose)
4. Monitor respiratory status: maintain an open airway and oxygenation.

☐ Nursing Implications

1. Use a volumetric infusion pump to control flow rate and therefore dosage. If a pump is not available, use microdrop administration set and monitor the drip rate frequently. Record the total 8-hour dose in milligrams, and the milligram per minute dose required to control the arrhythmia on an hourly basis.
2. Examine the patient frequently for cardiac and noncardiac signs and symptoms of toxicity. See Management of Toxicity. Be prepared to manage seizures; keep the side rails up at all times. Instruct the patient to report any symptoms when they occur, if he is able. Notify the physician of the onset of toxicity.
3. Monitor blood pressure every 10–15 minutes until the infusion rate has stabilized with the control of the arrhythmia, then every hour. If hypotension occurs, slow the infusion and begin more frequent monitoring of the blood pressure. Notify the physician.
4. When titrating to control the arrhythmia, always use the least amount of drug necessary for control.

References

1. Standards for Cardiopulmonary Resuscitation (CPR) and Emergency Cardiac Care (ECC). *JAMA*, 227(7, Suppl.):859, February 18, 1974.
2. Lie, K. I., et al.: Lidocaine in the Prevention of Primary Ventricular Fibrillation. *New England Journal of Medicine*, December 1974, p. 1235.

Suggested Readings

Andreoli, Kathleen G., et al.: *Comprehensive Cardiac Care* (3rd ed.), St. Louis: C. V. Mosby Company, 1975, pp. 169–177 on premature ventricular contractions and ventricular tachycardia; and pp. 312–313 on administration of lidocaine.

Collinsworth, Ken A., Kalman, Sumner M., Harrison, Donald C.: The Clinical Pharmacology of Lidocaine as an Antiarrhythmic Drug. *Circulation*, 50:1217–1230, December 1974 (references). This article is for advanced readers.

Intravenous Infusion of Vasopressors—Programmed Instruction. *American Journal of Nursing*, 65(11):129–152, November 1965. (Useful information on the theories behind titration that can be applied to all drugs.)

Levitt, Barrie, Borer, Jeffrey S. and Saropa, Arleen: The Clinical Pharmacology of Antiarrhythmic Drugs, Part I: Lidocaine and Procainamide. *Cardiovascular Nursing*, 10(5), September–October 1974.

Mattea, Judith and Mattea, Edward: Lidocaine and Procainamide Toxicity During Treatment of Arrhythmias. *American Journal of Nursing*, 76(9):1429–1431, September 1976.

lorazepam ■
(Ativan)

Actions/Indications

Sedative, tranquilizer. Used as a preanesthetic sedative, producing reduced anxiety and some amnesia to the events related to surgery or procedure.

Central nervous system and respiratory depression does occur but is minimal with recommended doses. Accumulation of the drug in the body is also minimal.

Onset of action after intravenous injection is 8–15 minutes with a peak at 15–30 minutes. Duration of action is 4 hours.

This agent is excreted through the kidneys after metabolism in the liver.

Dosage
Adults:

2 mg or 0.02 mg/lb. (0.05 mg/kg), whichever is smaller. Do not exceed this dose in patients over 50 years of age. Do not exceed 4 mg in any patient. Larger doses as high as 0.05

lorazepam
(continued)
mg/kg up to a total of 4 mg can be used with caution if absolutely necessary.

Administer 15–20 minutes prior to the procedure.
Children:
Not recommended.

Preparation and Storage
Supplied in Tubex cartridges and multidose vials, containing 2 mg/ml and 4 mg/ml.

Immediately prior to intravenous injection dilute with an equal volume of sterile water for injection, sodium chloride injection or D5W.

Drug Incompatibilities
Do not mix with any other medication in any manner.

Modes of IV Administration

Injection
Yes
Dilute in equal volume of sterile water for injection, D5W, or NS. Do not exceed an injection rate of 2 mg/minute.

Intermittent Infusion
No

Continuous Infusion
No

Contraindications; Warnings; Precautions; Adverse Reactions

Contraindications
1. Known hypersensitivity to benzodiazepines, polyethylene glycol, propylene glycol, or benzyl alcohol.
2. Acute narrow-angle glaucoma.
3. Intra-arterial injections are contraindicated (see Warnings No. 1).

Warnings
1. **TAKE ALL PRECAUTIONS TO AVOID INTRA-ARTERIAL INJECTION AND PERIVASCULAR EXTRAVASATION.** Intra-arterial injection can produce arteriospasm resulting in gangrene which may require limb amputation.
2. The level of sedation produced may lead to airway obstruction when a greater than recommended dose has been given, or with the recommended dose in conjunction with other sedating drugs. Be prepared to maintain an open airway and to assist ventilation.
3. Use of this drug in patients in coma, shock or acute alcohol intoxication is not recommended.
4. While this drug may be used with caution in a reduced dosage in patients with mild renal or hepatic impairment, it is not recommended in the presence of renal or hepatic failure.
5. Patients over 50 years of age may have a more profound and prolonged sedation with this drug; use lowest recommended dose.
6. Combinations of this drug and scopolamine may produce increased sedation, hallucinations, and irrational behavior.
7. This agent may cause fetal damage when given to pregnant women and should not be used during pregnancy or delivery.
8. It is not recommended that this drug be used for outpatient procedures. Inpatient use requires recovery room observation of the patient.
9. Pharyngeal reflexes are not affected when this agent is used for peroral endoscopic procedures; therefore, topical or regional anesthesia is recommended to reduce reflex activity.

Precautions
1. Additive central nervous system depression will occur with concomitant use of phenothiazines, narcotic analgesics, barbiturates, scopolamine and monoamine oxidase inhibitors.
2. Administer with *extreme* caution to patients who are elderly, very ill, and to those with limited pulmonary reserve. This drug

may cause hypoventilation, hypoxia, and ultimately resulting cardiac arrest. See Warning No. 2.
3. Alcohol, other sedatives and tranquilizers should be avoided for 24–48 hours after the use of this drug.
4. This drug should not be administered to nursing mothers.

Adverse Reactions
1. Extension of central nervous system depression, more likely in patients over 50: restlessness, confusion, depression, delirium, visual hallucinations, dizziness, diplopia, blurred vision, and mild hearing loss.
2. Hypo- and hypertension.
3. Respiratory depression.
4. Skin rash, nausea, and vomiting.
5. Abuse of this drug may lead to a limited dependence.

Management of Overdosage
Symptoms are oversedation from drowsiness to coma. Ataxia, hypotonia, and hypotension have occurred. Treatment is supportive until the drug is eliminated from the body; e.g., monitoring vital signs, maintaining fluid and electrolyte balance, adequate airway and assisted ventilation. Forced diuresis with fluids may accelerate elimination from the body if renal function is normal. Osmotic diuretics such as mannitol may help. In critical situations renal dialysis and blood exchange may be indicated. Published reports indicate that intravenous infusion of 0.5 to 4.0 mg of physostigmine at the rate of 1 mg/min may reverse signs and symptoms of central anticholinergic overdosage. However, the use of physostigmine is not without hazard, see page 280 on this drug.

☐ Nursing Implications
1. Take all precautions to avoid intra-arterial or perivascular injection (see Warning No. 1). Normally some burning can be expected during injection; this should disappear after flushing of the vein. If it is suspected that such an accident has occurred, monitor the limb and affected area for blanching, loss of pulses, pain, and coldness. Notify the physician. Protect the area and continue to monitor for arterial insufficiency. Gangrene can occur. See Appendix.
2. Monitor respiratory rate and depth after injection. Be prepared to use mechanical means to maintain a patent airway, and assist ventilation. Oxygen, airways, manual breathing bags and suction should be readily available. The patient should not be left unattended following an injection.
3. Monitor for prolonged sedation, confusion, visual hallucinations, restlessness, blurred vision, reduced hearing. See "Overdosage" above. These effects may occur more frequently in the elderly or debilitated. Protect the patient from injury; use side rails, etc. Reassure him of the temporary nature of these effects. Provide supportive treatment as ordered.
4. Monitor blood pressure and heart rate frequently following injection.
5. Be prepared to manage vomiting to prevent aspiration.
6. This drug may cause an acute exacerbation of glaucoma; observe for the onset. Signs and symptoms may be: scleral redness, eye pain, blurred vision, and rainbow vision. Notify the physician.
7. Warn patients that they may experience amnesia and prolonged sedation. Alcohol or other central nervous system depressant drugs should not be used for 24–48 hours following the use of this agent. Hazardous tasks should also be avoided during this post-injection time period. This drug is usually not used for outpatient procedures because of the long duration of action.

magnesium sulfate ■

Actions/Indications
Central nervous system depressant.
Also depresses smooth cardiac and
skeletal muscle. Is an antagonist of
calcium to the CNS. Used to treat:
- Seizures in toxemia (eclampsia) of
  pregnancy
- Hypomagnesemia
- Uterine tetany secondary to large
  doses of oxytocin
- Cerebral edema (as an osmotic
  agent)
- Barium poisoning
- Hypertension or encephalopathy
  in children with acute nephritis

Raises serum magnesium levels
immediately and the effects last 30
min.

Dosage
Adults:
Anticonvulsant—1 gm repeated as
needed.
  Eclampsia—10–14 gm total dose.
Usually given by infusion, titrated
with frequency of seizures: use a solution of 4–5 gm in 250 ml D5/NS
(2% solution), repeating as necessary. Do not exceed a 24-hr dose of
30–40 gm. (May also be given IM.)
  Magnesium deficiency—1–2 gm. Repeat until relief of symptoms is seen
or the serum level of magnesium has
returned to normal.
  Uterine tetany—1–2 gm by infusion
titrated with uterine tone. (Use infusion described under eclampsia
above.)
  Cerebral edema—2.5 gm. Repeat as
needed.
  Barium poisoning—1–2 gm by infusion titrated with presence or absence of muscle spasms.
  When giving this drug for the
above indications in repeated doses
or infusions, the patient's knee jerk
reflex should be tested before each
additional dose, or periodically during an infusion. If the reflex is absent, the administration of the drug
should be stopped until the reflex
returns.
  Administration of the drug beyond the point where the knee jerk
disappears may lead to apnea.
  Total parenteral nutrition—1 gm
(8.1 mEq)/day, depending on serum
magnesium level.
Children:
Total parenteral nutrition—0.5 gm (4
mEq)/day, depending on serum
magnesium level.
  Magnesium deficiency—25 mg/kg
every 6 hrs for 3–4 doses,
depending on serum magnesium
level. (Usually given IM.)
  In acute nephritis—100 mg/kg *IM*
(0.2 ml of a 50% solution) as needed; 100–200 mg/kg in a 1%–3% solution IV, if convulsions are life-
threatening.
  Dosage for other indications not
available.

Preparation and Storage
Supplied in the following concentrations and containers:
100 mg/ml (10% solution), 10 ml
  and 20 ml ampuls
250 mg/ml (25% solution), 10 ml
  ampuls
500 mg/ml (50% solution), 2 ml, 10
  ml and 20 ml ampuls, and in 30
  ml multidose vials (Also in disposable syringes of 10% and 50%
  concentrations.)
  Use a 5% solution for infusion
made by adding 5 gm of drug to
100 ml D5/NS. The concentration
of any infusion should never exceed
20%.

Drug Incompatibilities
Do not mix with:
Aminophylline
Sodium bicarbonate
Any calcium preparation
Novobiocin
Vitamin B complex
Clindamycin
Tobramycin
Polymyxin
Chlorpromazine

Modes of IV Administration

Injection
Yes
Do not exceed a rate of 1.5 ml/min
of a 10% solution (150 mg/min).

Infusion is preferred mode.

Intermittent Infusion
Yes
At a rate not to exceed 3 ml of a
5% solution/min (150 mg/min) until effects are obtained. Do not exceed 150 mg/min of a 10% solution.

Continuous Infusion
Yes
At a rate not to exceed 3 ml of a
5% solution/min (150 mg/min) until effects are obtained. Do not exceed 150 mg/min of a 10%
solution.

**Contraindications; Warnings; Pre-
cautions; Adverse Reactions**

Contraindications
1. Any degree of heart block
2. Myocardial damage (acute myocardial infarction,
   myocardopathy, etc.)

Precautions
1. Administer with caution in the
   presence of renal disease; no
   more than 2 gm should be giv-
   en within a 48-hour period.
   Monitor serum magnesium levels. High plasma magnesium
   levels will produce flushing,
   sweating, hypotension, shock,
   depressed cardiac and CNS
   function, weakness. Overdosage
   will cause respiratory
   depression and eventually paralysis and apnea.
2. This drug decreases serum calcium.
3. Decrease dosage of barbiturates,
   narcotics, or other CNS depressants while administering magnesium to prevent overdepression.
4. Administer with extreme caution if the patient has received
   digitalis. Treating magnesium
   toxicity with calcium in the digitalized patient is hazardous. Serious alterations in A-V
   conduction including complete
   heart block can occur.

5. Calcium gluconate or calcium
   gluceptate should be readily
   available for IV administration
   as an antidote in the event that
   high serum magnesium levels
   develop. (See Nursing Implication No. 5.) In adults, 10 to 20
   ml of calcium gluconate 10%
   solution will usually reverse respiratory depression or heart
   block due to hypermagnesemia.
6. Magnesium should not be administered to the patient in preeclampsia or eclampsia within
   24 hours of delivery. Infants of
   mothers who have received
   magnesium may have neuromuscular and/or respiratory
   depression at birth.

Adverse Reactions
Magnesium intoxication (serum level
greater than 4 mEq/liter); see Nursing Implications No 6.

☐ **Nursing Implications**
1. Normal serum magnesium is 1.5
   –2.0 mEq/liter.
2. Low serum magnesium will produce: CNS irritability (seizures,
   spasticity), personality changes,
   tremor, cardiac tachyarrhythmias.
3. Do not leave the patient alone
   during infusion.
4. Monitor for effectiveness of the
   magnesium infusion:
   a. Anticonvulsant effect
   b. Relaxation of spastic muscles
      and tremors
   c. Resolution of arrhythmias
      Infusion is usually stopped
      when these signs appear.
5. Monitor urine output. Slow or
   stop infusion if urinary output is
   less than 100 ml in 4 hours. Notify the physician.
6. Monitor for symptoms of high
   serum magnesium (usually begin at serum levels of 4
   mEq/liter):
   a. Loss of knee-jerk reflex
      (check every 5 minutes or
      prior to each dose)
   b. Decreased respiratory rate
      and depth (count every 5

magnesium sulfate
(continued)

   minutes); respiratory paralysis may occur.
   c. Flushing of the skin (especially the face)
   d. Diaphoresis
   e. Flaccidity
   f. Hypotension (monitor blood pressure every 5–10 minutes during infusion)
   If one or more of these signs appear, slow or stop the infusion and notify physician.
7. Be prepared to manage respiratory failure. Keep the following equipment readily available: airways, suction, oxygen, endotracheal tubes and laryngoscope, manual breathing bag and mask.
8. Calcium gluconate or calcium gluceptate infusion can be a specific antidote to combat high magnesium levels and resultant respiratory failure. (See page 42 on calcium infusions.) When using calcium infusions, place the patient on continuous ECG monitoring. Be prepared to manage arrhythmias, especially if the patient is on a digitalis preparation.
9. Be prepared to administer respiratory assistance to the infant of a mother who received this drug within 24 hours of delivery.

Suggested Readings

Butts, Priscilla: Magnesium Sulfate in the Treatment of Toxemia. *American Journal of Nursing,* 77:1294–1298, August 1977 (reference).

Elbaum, Nancy: Detecting and Correcting Magnesium Imbalance. *Nursing '77,* August 1977, pp. 34–35.

mannitol ■

Actions/Indications

Osmotic diuretic; a sugar-alcohol that increases the osmolarity of the blood to draw fluid from the intracellular and extracellular spaces. Prevents the reabsorption of water in the renal tubules. The result is obligatory diuresis. Uses:
• To evaluate glomerular filtration rate
• To prevent or treat oliguria secondary to renal insufficiency
• To reduce intraocular pressure, therapeutically or prior to surgery
• To reduce intracranial pressure and to treat cerebral edema by reducing brain mass
• To promote the urinary excretion of toxic substances
• Along with other diuretics for management of nephrotic, cirrhotic or cardiac edema.

Dosage

Adults:
To prevent or treat oliguria
   Test dose—200 mg/kg (or 12.5 gm) given over 3–5 min. If there is an increase in urine output after 5 min, the full dose can be given by infusion.
   Infusion—50–200 gm, in 24 hrs. Rate is adjusted to maintain a urine flow of 30–50 ml/hr. Use 5, 10 or 15% solution.
   Treatment of increased intracranial or intraocular pressure—1.5–2.0 gm/kg over 30–60 min. Use a 15 or 20% solution.
   To promote excretion of toxic substances—up to 200 gm over 30–60 min, repeated until blood levels of the substance show clearance. Use a 5 or 10% solution.
   To evaluate glomerular filtration—100 ml of a 20% solution added to 180 ml NS, infused over 30 min (normal urinary output response is 125 ml/min in males and 116 ml/min in females).
   For diuresis—100 gm administered as a 10 to 20% solution over 2 to 6 hours.
Children:
(all indications):
   Test dose—200 mg/kg or 6 gm/M^2 over 3–5 min.
   Infusion—2 gm/kg or 60 gm/M^2 titrated with urine output or desired effect. See Warning No. 8.

Preparation and Storage

Supplied in the following concentrations:

Percent solution	Grams/ 100 ml	mg/ml
5%	5	50
10%	10	100
15%	15	150
20%	20	200
25%	25	250

If crystals are present in the vial, place it in warm water (50°C) until the crystals are dissolved. Cool to body temperature or room temperature before administration. *Always* use an in-line IV filter, regardless of the mode of administration.

Drug Incompatibilities

Do not mix in any manner with:
Potassium chloride
Blood
Cephalosporins

Modes of IV Administration

Injection
Yes
Slowly, over 3–5 min. Use an in-line filter. See table under Preparation section to convert gm/ml to mg/ml.

Intermittent Infusion
Yes
Time of infusion is usually 30–60 min. Use an in-line filter. Titrate with desired result. 5, 10, 15 or 20% solutions are usually used. See table under Preparation section to convert gm/ml to mg/ml.

Continuous Infusion
Yes
Titrate with desired result. Use an in-line filter. 5, 10, 15 or 20% solutions are usually used. See table under Preparation section to convert gm/ml to mg/ml.

Contraindications; Warnings; Precautions; Adverse Reactions

Contraindications
1. Well established anuria due to renal disease

2. Renal failure that fails to respond to a test dose within 3–5 min
3. Severe dehydration
4. Active intracranial bleeding except during craniotomy
5. Congestive heart failure and pulmonary edema (and pulmonary edema secondary to abnormal capillary permeability); or the appearance of failure during administration

Warnings
1. Administer with caution to patients with compromised renal reserve.
2. Infusion should be stopped if oliguria or azotemia develops.
3. Large doses may produce circulatory overload and cardiac decompensation.
4. Water intoxication may occur if large doses are given to patients unable to excrete the drug rapidly enough.
5. There may be serious electrolyte and fluid imbalances secondary to this drug. Monitor serum sodium and potassium levels.
6. Reduction of intracranial pressure may increase intracranial bleeding if occult active bleeding exists.
7. Safety for use in pregnancy has not been established.
8. Dosage requirements for patients under 12 years of age have not been established.

Precautions
1. Monitor renal function (BUN and creatinine levels) and hydration (central venous pressure, blood pressure, urine specific gravity and skin turgor).
2. Reduction of urine output (less than 100 ml/hr) should prompt discontinuation of the drug unless oliguria is secondary to a nonrenal condition. Correct nonrenal causes.
3. Do not administer concomitantly with whole blood. If unavoidable, add at least 20 mEq NaCl to the mannitol.

mannitol
(continued)
4. Avoid extravasation.
5. Monitor cardiac status, i.e., heart rate, blood pressure, signs of congestive heart failure.
6. Can increase the chances of eighth cranial nerve damage when given with kanamycin.
7. The urinary excretion of lithium will be increased, therefore the dosage may need to be increased.

Adverse Reactions
1. Rapid infusion leads to circulatory overload, pulmonary edema, water intoxication.
2. Sodium and chloride loss in the urine may be excessive
3. Renal adverse reactions—osmotic nephrosis
4. Convulsions, dizziness
5. Headache, chest pain, arm pain
6. Nausea, vomiting, thirst
7. Hypo- and hypertension
8. Allergic reactions of all forms

☐ Nursing Implications
1. Monitor renal function, i.e., responsiveness to the drug:
   a. Hourly or half-hourly urinary output. Drug infusion rate is usually titrated against urine output. Infusion is usually stopped if after a routine dose the output falls below 100 ml/hour. (The kidneys must be able to excrete the fluids drawn into the vascular compartment by the drug.)
   b. Specific gravity—use collection device in children if appropriate.
   c. Hydration via CVP, skin turgor.
   d. Be aware of the patient's BUN and creatinine levels, elevation of either value not due to other causes should prompt discontinuation of the mannitol.
   e. Monitor ability to urinate; check for bladder distention *hourly*. Use a pediatric collection device in children under 2 years or as indicated.
2. Monitor cardiac status:
   a. Blood pressure and pulse every hour, or as patient's condition dictates.
   b. Observe for increased respiratory rate, orthopnea, dyspnea, rales.
   c. If there is known cardiac disease, CVP, arterial pressure or pulmonary artery (wedge) pressure should be monitored to indicate the onset of compromise in left ventricular function. Deviations should prompt discontinuation of the infusion and notification of the physician.
   d. Be prepared to treat cardiac decompensation—oxygen, rotating tourniquets, thiazide diuretics, digitalis.
3. Be aware of the patient's serum sodium and potassium. Monitor for signs of hyponatremia and hypokalemia:
   a. Hyponatremia—headache, nausea, abdominal cramps, disorientation, diarrhea, hypotension (late).
   b. Hypokalemia—weakness, lethargy, muscle cramps, irritability, abdominal distention, cardiac arrhythmias (late).
4. In the presence of head injury when mannitol is administered to reduce intracranial pressure, monitor change in neurologic signs that could indicate intracranial bleeding:
   a. Pupillary reaction to light
   b. Hand grip
   c. Orientation
   d. Movement of extremities
   These signs may also be monitored to evaluate reduction in intracranial pressure secondary to the administration of mannitol.
5. Take extravasation precautions; see Appendix.
6. When this drug is being used to decrease intraocular pressure,

monitor for effectiveness by patient symptoms, e.g., decreased ocular pain and blurred vision, resolution of rainbow vision. Scleral redness should also resolve.

mechlorethamine hydrochloride ■
(Mustargen, Nitrogen Mustard)

Actions/Indications
Alkylating agent; has a cytotoxic action that inhibits the growth of rapidly proliferating cells. Used for the palliative treatment of Hodgkin's disease (Stages III and IV), lymphosarcoma, chronic myelocytic or lymphocytic leukemia, polycythemia vera, mucosis fungoides and bronchogenic carcinoma.

Dosage
Dosage must be based on ideal dry body weight. In the presence of edema or ascites the actual weight must be estimated.
Adults and Children:
0.4 mg/kg given as a single dose or over 4 succesive days a dose of 0.1 mg/kg day. This can be repeated in 3 to 6 weeks when the patient has recovered hematologically from the previous treatment.

Preparation and Storage
This drug is a powerful vesicant, use extreme caution in preparing it for use. Avoid inhalation of its dust or vapors, and contact with skin, mucous membranes or eyes. Use rubber gloves. See Precaution No. 1.
Prepare solution *immediately* before administration.
Each vial contains 10 mg of drug. Inject 10 ml of sterile water for injection or sodium chloride injection into the vial. With the needle in place in the rubber stopper, shake the vial to promote dissolution, withdraw desired amount. Resulting solution will contain 1 mg/ml. Do not use the solution if it is discolored.
Discard unused portion. Discard syringe and needle carefully to avoid human contact with the solution.

Drug Incompatibilities
Do not mix with any other medication in any manner.

Modes of IV Administration

Injection
Yes
Inject into the "Y" injection site of a running IV to reduce vein irritation. Inject over 3–5 min. Flush vein with 10 ml NS after injection.

Intermittent Infusion
No

Continuous Infusion
No

Contraindications; Warnings; Precautions; Adverse Reactions

Contraindications
1. Use in patients with widely disseminated, inoperable neoplasms should probably be avoided.
2. Use in patients with leukopenia, thrombocytopenia and anemia due to tumor invasion of the bone marrow carries greater than usual risk. The drug may promote improvement in bone marrow function by reducing tumor activity, but hematopoiesis may be further compromised leading to a fatal outcome.
3. Infectious diseases.
4. Tumors of the bone marrow and nerve tissue respond poorly to this drug.

Warnings
1. Extravasation of this drug into subcutaneous tissues results in a painful inflammation, induration and tissue sloughing. If infiltration occurs, prompt injection of sterile isotonic sodium thiosulfate (1/6 molar) solution into the infusion appliance and with a 25 ga. needle into the affected area should be carried out. Ice

mechlorethamine hydrochloride
(continued)
compresses should then be applied for the next 6 to 12 hours.

2. The hematologic status of the patient should be determined before therapy is started.

3. This drug may contribute to extensive and rapid development of amyloidosis, and should be used only if foci of acute and chronic suppurative inflammation are absent.

4. Nitrogen mustards can produce fetal abnormalities, especially if they are used in early pregnancy. Use in the first two trimesters should be avoided if possible. The patient should be informed of the risks involved. Breast-feeding should be stopped prior to treatment.

Precautions
1. **This drug is highly toxic in the powder and solution forms.** Handle with care, avoid contact with skin, mucous membrane or eyes. If contact with eyes occurs, immediately irrigate with copious amounts of normal saline or balanced salt ophthalmic irrigating solution. Skin contact also requires irrigation with water for at least 15 minutes followed by 2% sodium thiosulfate solution.

2. Administer with *extreme caution* before or after x-ray therapy or therapy with other cytotoxic agents that affect bone marrow function. Marrow recovery must be seen before any form of therapy is initiated or reinitiated.

3. Use of this agent may be associated with an increased incidence of a second malignant tumor, especially when other antineoplastic agents or radiation therapy are also used.

4. Hyperuricemia may develop. Urate precipitation should be anticipated, especially in the treatment of lymphomas. Therapy for this should be instituted including adequate fluid intake.

5. Drug toxicity, especially sensitivity to bone marrow failure, is more common in patients with chronic lymphatic leukemia. Use with extra caution if at all in this condition.

Adverse Reactions
1. The clinical use of this drug is usually accompanied by toxic reactions.

2. Local toxicity: thrombosis and thrombophlebitis at injection site, especially if venous pressure is elevated.

3. Gastrointestinal: nausea and vomiting usually occur 1 to 3 hours after injection and can last for 24 hours. Diarrhea may be severe enough to be dose-limiting. Stomatitis is also seen.

4. Hematologic toxicity: hemolytic anemia may occur in patients with lymphomas and chronic lymphocytic leukemia. Lymphocytopenia usually occurs within 24 hours after the first injection; granulocytopenia occurs within 6 to 8 days and lasts 10 to 21 days. Agranulocytosis appears infrequently. Recovery from leukopenia is complete within 2 weeks of the maximum reduction. Thrombocytopenia usually parallels granulocytopenia in onset and duration. Bleeding may occur because of the low platelet count. Severe hematopoietic depression can occur with normal clinical doses. Persistent pancytopenia has been reported. Erythrocyte and hemoglobin levels may fall during the first 2 weeks after administration of the drug, rarely to significant levels. Depression of the blood-producing system may last up to 50 days after the initial dose. Dosage over that recommended can lead to severe bone marrow depression and even death.

5. There may be immunosuppressive activity, predisposing the patient to bacterial, fungal or viral infection. This is more likely to occur when steroids are also

used. Treatment should be discontinued if a herpes zoster infection occurs.
6. Rashes, erythema multiforme.
7. Treatment may be followed by delayed catamenia, oligomenorrhea or temporary or permanent amenorrhea. Impaired spermatogenesis, azoospermia, and total germinal aplasia have been reported. Spermatogenesis may return in patients in remission.
8. Hepatotoxicity can occur and will be evidenced by jaundice.
9. Alopecia is common. Hair growth usually returns after cessation of treatment.
10. Neurotoxicity can cause eighth cranial nerve damage. Auditory changes include tinnitus and diminished hearing. Vestibular damage will be evidenced by vertigo.

☐ **Nursing Implications**
1. The patient receiving this medication will be experiencing the emotional and physical effect of the malignancy or other condition being treated. Knowledge of the patient's feelings about his disease and its implications will assist in helping him tolerate the chemotherapy. The incidence of uncomfortable side effects and adverse reactions is high. It is within the nurse's role to assist the patient in coping with the discomforts of the disease and its treatment, and to help him work through depression and anger toward acceptance of the disease at his own pace. Despite the unpleasantness this drug may bring, it can be a source of hope for the patient.
2. Management of nausea and vomiting:
   a. Many patients experience fewer injection side effects (e.g., nausea and vomiting) when they are placed in a prone or reclining position during the administration of this drug.
   b. Usually occurs 1–3 hours after injection. Vomiting may subside after 8 hours, but nausea can persist for 24 hours.
   c. Administer at night if possible to correlate with normal sleep patterns, accompanied by sedation and an antiemetic. To be effective, antiemetics should be administered 1 hour prior to the injection of the drug.
   d. Small frequent meals, timed with a period when the patient feels his best, are advisable. Bland foods usually are tolerated. Carbohydrate and protein content should be high.
   e. If the patient is anorexic, encourage high nutrient liquids and water to maintain hydration (hydration helps to avoid complications of hyperuricemia).
   f. Keep accurate measurements of emesis volume and total intake and output to guide the physician in ordering parenteral fluids when necessary.
3. Management of stomatitis:
   a. Administer preventive oral care every 4 hours, and/or after meals or vomiting.
   b. Use a soft toothbrush and toothpaste, avoid trauma to oral membranes.
   c. Examine mouth and gum tissue daily to detect the onset of inflammation or ulceration. Instruct the patient and family on how to do this.
   d. If stomatitis occurs, notify the physician and administer therapeutic oral care as ordered.
   e. Order a bland, mechanical soft diet if inflammation is mild. If it is severe, the patient may need to be NPO.
   f. For patients who tolerate oral intake, administer Xylocaine Viscous or acetaminophen elixir as a mouthwash

mechlorethamine hydrochloride
(continued)

prior to meals to decrease pain. Do not use aspirin rinses.

g. Patients with severe inflammation and ulceration may require parenteral analgesia.

4. Take all precautions to prevent extravasation. If extravasation occurs or is suspected notify the physician immediately, follow directions under Warning No. 1. Keep sodium thiosulfate on hand. See Appendix.

5. Thrombophlebitis can occur at the injection site. Notify the physician at onset; apply warm compresses as ordered, elevate the extremity. Protect the area from trauma.

6. Management of hematologic effects:

a. Be aware of the patient's white blood cell and platelet counts prior to each injection.

b. If the WBC falls to 2000/cu mm, take measures to protect the patient from infection, such as protective (reverse) isolation, avoidance of invasive procedures, maintenance of bodily (especially perineal) cleanliness, carrying out strict urinary catheter care when appropriate, etc. Monitor for infection by recording temperatures every 4 hours, examining for rashes, swellings, drainage and pain. Explain these measures to the patient.

c. If the platelet count falls below 100,000/cu mm, monitor for thrombocytopenic bleeding: petechiae, purpura, hematuria, melena, blood in stools, gum bleeding, vaginal bleeding, epistaxis, hematemesis, etc. Avoid trauma. Transfusions may be ordered.

d. Instruct the patient and family on the importance of follow-up blood studies, and the reporting of the signs and symptoms listed in "b" and "c" above if the drug is being administered on an outpatient basis.

7. Management of hair loss:

a. Use scalp tourniquet or ice packs during and for 5–10 minutes after injection, if ordered.

b. Counsel the patient on the possibility of hair loss to enable him to prepare for this disfigurement.

c. Reassure him of the possibility of regrowth of hair following discontinuation of the drug.

d. Provide privacy and time for the patient to discuss his feelings.

8. If rashes occur, report them to the physician and administer cool compresses as ordered. Turn the patient frequently to prevent skin breakdown.

9. Monitor for jaundice; notify physician at onset.

10. Monitor for hearing loss, tinnitus, and vertigo which indicate the onset of auditory and vestibular nerve damage. Notify the physician.

11. The positive expected outcomes from therapy are: regression of tumor size, decreased pain, increased appetite and exercise tolerance.

meperidine hydrochloride ■
(Demerol Injection)

Actions/Indications
Narcotic analgesic, synthetic opiate. Actions similar to morphine. For relief of moderate to severe pain, as a preoperative medication, for support of anesthesia, for obstetrical analgesia.

Dosage
Adults:
For pain—10–100 mg every 2–4 hrs.
  Preoperative—10–50 mg.

Anesthesia support—injection or infusion, titrate to patient need and effects obtained.
See Preparation Section For Solution.
Children:
IV administration not recommended.

Preparation and Storage
Must be diluted prior to injection.
Solution for infusion is prepared by adding enough meperidine to a desired volume of fluid to produce a concentration of 1 mg/ml. Use D5W or NS.
This is a Schedule II drug under the Controlled Substances Act of 1970. Maintain hospital or institutional regulations guiding its use.

Drug Incompatibilities
Do not mix with any other drug in IV bottle; and do not inject into an IV line containing:
Aminophylline
Barbiturates
Heparin
Methicillin
Morphine
Phenytoin
Sodium bicarbonate
Sodium iodide

Modes of IV Administration

Injection
Yes
Very slowly, diluted in an equal amount of NS.
See Warning No. 4.

Intermittent Infusion
Yes
Only by anesthesiologist. Titrate to obtain desired effect without producing adverse reactions.
Use a 1 mg/ml solution.

Continuous Infusion
Yes
Only by anesthesiologist. Titrate to obtain desired effect without producing adverse reactions.
Use a 1 mg/ml solution.

Contraindications; Warnings; Precautions; Adverse Reactions

Contraindications
1. Hypersensitivity
2. Patients who are receiving or have received MAO inhibitors (Marplan, etc.) in the past 2 weeks

Warnings
1. Physical and psychic dependence occurs. Tolerance may also occur after repeated doses.
2. Use with caution and in reduced dosage in patients who are concurrently on other narcotic analgesics, general anesthetics, phenothiazines, other tranquilizers, sedative-hypnotics, and any other CNS depressants, including alcohol. Respiratory depression, hypotension and coma can result.
3. In the presence of a head injury, intracranial lesion, or in any case of increased intracranial pressure, this drug may further increase cerebrospinal fluid pressure and can depress respirations. Use caution in these situations.
4. Rapid IV injection can lead to severe respiratory depression, apnea, shock, and cardiac arrest. A narcotic antagonist, naloxone, and respiratory support equipment must be at the bedside. The patient must be lying down during administration.
5. Use with *extreme* caution in patients with an acute asthmatic attack, chronic obstructive lung disease, cor pulmonale, decreased respiratory reserve (chest trauma, surgery, cancerous lesions, malformations), or pre-existing respiratory depression, hypoxia or hypercapnia (increased blood pCO_2). Apnea can result.
6. Administer with extreme caution to patients with hypovolemia, acute blood loss, or who have received phenothiazines. Severe hypotension can result.

meperidine hydrochloride
(continued)

7. May produce orthostatic hypotension; keep patient at rest.
8. Do not use in pregnant patients prior to the labor period, unless benefits outweigh risks to the fetus. Can produce respiratory depression in the infant when given during labor. Resuscitation of the infant may be required.
9. This drug is secreted in breast milk.
10. See Nursing Implications for treatment of overdosage and adverse reactions.

Precautions
1. Use with caution in patients with atrial flutter and other supraventricular arrhythmias; increased ventricular rate may result.
2. May aggravate pre-existing seizure disorders.
3. May obscure symptoms used to diagnose patients with acute abdominal symptoms.
4. Reduce dosage and use with caution in the elderly or debilitated, in patients with severe hepatic or renal impairment, hypothyroidism, Addison's disease, prostatic hypertrophy or urethral stricture. These patients are more likely to have adverse reactions.

Adverse Reactions
1. Respiratory depression and apnea
2. Circulatory depression, i.e., fall in blood pressure, cardiac arrest
3. Light-headedness, dizziness, sedation
4. Nausea, vomiting
5. Diaphoresis
6. Transient hallucinations, disorientation, euphoria, weakness
7. Constipation, biliary tract spasm
8. Tachycardia, bradycardia, palpitations
9. Urinary retention
10. Hypersensitivity reactions ranging from rashes to anaphylaxis
11. Visual disturbances
12. Dry mouth

☐ **Nursing Implications**
1. Monitor closely for respiratory depression and extreme somnolence during the first hour after an injection. If the respiratory rate falls below 8 per minute, attempt to stimulate the patient to increase his respiratory rate. Firmly instruct him to breathe, repeating instructions to make him breathe at least 10–12 times a minute.[1] If the patient does not respond to this, begin to support respirations manually using mouth-to-mouth breathing or a manual breathing bag and mask. Call for the physician to administer a narcotic antagonist such as naloxone (Narcan). Prepare 0.1–0.4 mg for an initial dose. (See page 237 for full information on naloxone.) Fluids and vasopressors may be required for the patient who becomes hypotensive.

   Monitor the newborn for respiratory depression when the mother has received meperidine. Be prepared to assist ventilation. Naloxone administration may be necessary.
2. If the patient receiving meperidine has a pre-existing respiratory problem which makes him more vulnerable to breathing difficulties or depression (e.g., hypoxia, pulmonary infection, chest trauma, chest surgery, any patient immediately postanesthesia, chest malformations, those who have received neuromuscular blocking agents, other respiratory depressing agent or who are in shock), keep the following equipment at the bedside:
   a. Oxygen if not already in use
   b. Oral-pharyngeal airways
   c. Suction equipment
   d. Endotracheal tubes and a laryngoscope (if not already in use)
   e. Manual, self-inflating breathing bag.

Follow resuscitation guidelines as listed in No. 1 above. Such patients should not be left alone during the first hour after injection. Meperidine causes the same amount of respiratory depression as does morphine (contrary to popular belief). Peak depression will occur within 1 hour of injection (usually 15 minutes after an IV injection). Normal respirations return within 2 hours.[2]

3. Monitor for further rise in intracranial pressure in patients with a pre-existing problem. Neurologic signs, blood pressure and heart rate should be evaluated at least every 30 minutes.
4. When used in patients with atrial tachyarrhythmias, monitor ECG continuously for increased ventricular response and possible subsequent cardiac decompensation (fall in blood pressure, signs of pulmonary edema).
5. Take seizure precautions for patients with pre-existing seizure disorders.
6. Monitor for urinary retention in patients with prostatic hypertrophy or urethral stricture. Palpate bladder size every 4 hours. Measure urine output every 8 hours or as patient's condition warrants.
7. Be prepared to manage nausea and vomiting. Take aspiration precautions in patients with weakened gag reflex. Keep suction at the bedside.
8. Take safety precautions in the elderly in the event of disorientation to prevent patient injury; use side rails and soft restraints as necessary.
9. Take precautions to prevent constipation in patients on prolonged therapy with this drug (hydration, stool softeners, enemas as necessary).
10. Administer successive doses when pain is just beginning to return. Do not wait until it re-

turns to full intensity. Dosage intervals must be determined by patient response rather than time intervals. Notify physician if pain is returning before the time interval he has prescribed is reached.

References
1. McCaffery, Margo, and Hart, Linda L.: Undertreatment of Acute Pain with Narcotics. *American Journal of Nursing*, 76:1589, October 1976.
2. Ibid.

Suggested Readings
McCaffery, Margo, and Hart, Linda L.: Undertreatment of Acute Pain with Narcotics. *American Journal of Nursing*, 76:1586–1591, October 1976 (references).
McCaffery, Margo: When Your Patient's Still In Pain Don't Just Do Something: Sit There. *Nursing '81*, 11:58–61, June 1981 (references).
Smith, Dorothy W., and Germain, Carol P. Hanley: *Care of the Adult Patient* (4th ed.), Philadelphia: J. B. Lippincott Company, 1975, pp. 134–146 (references).

methicillin sodium ■
(Staphcillin, Celbenin)

Actions/Indications
Antibiotic, penicillinase-resistant. Synthetic penicillin. Used to treat infections due to penicillinase-producing staphylococci. Susceptibility tests must be performed.

Also effective in treating infection due to susceptible *Strep. pneumoniae,* group A beta-hemolytic streptococci and penicillin G-resistant and penicillin G-sensitive staphylococci.

Dosage
Adults:
1 gm every 6 hrs. Higher doses are used in severe infections.
Older Children:
100–400 mg/kg/24 hrs in divided doses every 4–6 hrs.

methicillin sodium
(continued)
Neonates:[1]
0–14 days of age, 2,000 gm or less in weight—50 mg/kg/24 hrs in equally divided doses every 12 hrs.

0–14 days of age, over 2,000 gm in weight—75 mg/kg/24 hrs in equally divided doses every 8 hrs.

15–30 days of age, 2,000 gm or less in weight—75 mg/kg/24 hrs in equally divided doses every 8 hrs.

15–30 days of age, over 2,000 gm in weight—100 mg/kg/24 hrs in equally divided doses every 6 hrs.

Therapy should be continued for at least 48 hrs after the patient has become afibrile and asymptomatic and cultures are negative.

Preparation and Storage

Reconstitute powder with sterile water for injection or sodium chloride injection:
1-gm vial—add 1.5 ml
4-gm vial—add 5.7 ml
6-gm vial—add 8.6 ml

The concentration of each preparation is 500 mg/ml.

Shake vial vigorously. Discard unused solution after 24 hours if stored at room temperature, or 4 days if stored in refrigerator.

Use the following fluids for infusion of methicillin:
NS
D5W
D5/NS
10% D-Fructose in Water
10% D-Fructose in NS
M/6 Sodium r-Lactate
Lactated Ringer's
Lactated Potassic Saline
5% Plasma Hydrolysate in Water
10% Invert Sugar in Water
10% Invert Sugar plus 0.3% Potassium Chloride in Water
Travert 10% electrolyte #1, #2, #3

Solutions of 2 mg/ml, 10 mg/ml and 20 mg/ml of this drug in the above fluids are stable for 8 hours. Drug concentration and rate and volume of the solution used should be adjusted so that the total dose is administered before the drug loses its stability.

Drug Incompatibilities

Do not mix with any other medication in any manner.

Modes of IV Administration

Injection
Yes
Further dilute each 1 ml of reconstituted form with 25 ml NS, inject at a rate of 10 ml/min.

Intermittent Infusion
Yes
Further dilute the reconstituted form with the following amounts of sterile water or compatible IV fluid (see Preparation section)
Infuse over 30–60 min.

Continuous Infusion
Yes
Add a 6-hour dose to 500–1,000 ml of the fluids listed in Preparation section.

Infuse over the appropriate amount of time.

Contraindications; Warnings; Precautions; Adverse Reactions

Contraindications
Hypersensitivity to any penicillin

Warnings
1. There may be cross-allergenicity with cephalosporins.
2. Anaphylaxis can occur.

Precautions
1. Use with caution in patients with allergies.
2. Monitor renal, hepatic, and hematopoietic systems during therapy. This drug rarely precipitates renal impairment in infants and adults.[2] The incidence is only slightly higher in children.[3]
3. There is a possibility of overgrowth of non-susceptible organisms.
4. Safety for use during pregnancy has not been established.
5. Lower dosage and close blood level monitoring is necessary in premature or immature infants and patients with renal failure.

Adverse Reactions

1. Hypersensitivity: rash, urticaria, anaphylaxis, serum sickness
2. Oral lesions: glossitis and stomatitis (rare)
3. Blood dyscrasias: hemolytic anemia, thrombocytopenia, leukopenia, agranulocytosis (usually only seen in high-dose, prolonged therapy)
4. Signs of renal impairment: hematuria, casts, azotemia, oliguria, pyuria. These disappear with discontinuation of the drug.
5. Overgrowth infection secondary to organisms not susceptible to methicillin

☐ **Nursing Implications**

1. Take anaphylaxis precautions; see Appendix.
2. Monitor for signs and symptoms of overgrowth infections:
   a. Fever (take rectal temperature at least every 4–6 hours in all patients)
   b. Increasing malaise
   c. Newly appearing localized signs and symptoms; redness, soreness, pain, swelling, drainage (increased volume or change in character of pre-existing drainage)
   d. Monilial rash in perineal area (reddened areas with itching)
   e. Cough (change in pre-existing cough or sputum production)
   f. Diarrhea
3. Complete blood counts should be performed during therapy. Patients on prolonged high-dose therapy may experience decreasing white cell and platelet counts. If this occurs, usually the drug is discontinued. Infections secondary to low white-cell counts usually occur only after the count reaches 2,000/cu mm or less. If this occurs, place the patient in protective (reverse) isolation, avoid invasive procedures, and monitor for signs and symptoms of infec-

tion. Bleeding secondary to a low platelet count usually begins only after the count falls below 100,000/cu mm. If the count reaches this level, monitor for unusual bleeding and avoid traumatic procedures.

4. Monitor for signs of renal impairment (occurrence is rare):
   a. Be aware of the patient's BUN and serum creatinine.
   b. Send urine for analysis at least weekly while the patient is on intensive intravenous therapy (see Adverse Reaction No. 4).
   c. Notify the physician of the onset of hematuria.
   d. Monitor for oliguria, urine output less than 240 ml per 8-hour period in adults.
5. Monitor for stomatitis, examine oral membranes for inflammation or ulceration at least daily.
   a. If stomatitis occurs, notify the physician and begin therapeutic oral care as ordered.
   b. Order a bland, mechanical, soft diet for patients with mild inflammation. If stomatitis is severe, the patient may be placed on NPO status by the physician.
   c. For patients who can tolerate oral intake, administer Xylocaine Viscous or acetaminophen elixir as a mouthwash prior to meals to decrease pain (do not use aspirin rinses) as ordered by the physician.
   d. Patients with severe stomatitis may require parenteral analgesia.

References

1. McCracken, George H.: *Antimicrobial Therapy for Newborns*, New York: Grune and Stratton, 1977, p. 23.
2. Appel, Gerald, and Neu, Harold C.: The Nephrotoxicity of Antimicrobial Agents. *New England Journal of Medicine*, 296(12):644, March 24, 1977.
3. McCracken, p. 23.

methotrexate sodium ■
(Mexate, Amethopterin)

Actions/Indications
Antimetabolite, used for antineo-
plastic chemotherapy in the follow-
ing malignancies:
- Acute lymphoblastic leukemia
- Acute lymphocytic and meningeal
  leukemia
- Severe, disabling psoriasis
- Choriocarcinoma
- Chorioadenoma destruens
- Hydatidiform mole
- Lymphosarcoma
- Mycosis fungoides
- Breast malignancies
- Epidermoid cancer of the head
  and neck
- Osteogenic sarcoma
- Lung malignancies, especially
  squamous cell and small cell types

Dosage
The intravenous route is
recommended *only* for the following
indications at the following dosages:
Acute Leukemias in Children:
3.3 mg/M^2 daily by injection or
short-term infusion, usually for 4 to
6 weeks to induce remission. Usually
given with prednisone. To maintain
remission, 2.5 mg/kg once every 14
days with prednisone.
   If relapse occurs, repeat entire
regimen.
   Meningeal forms of the disease
are treated with intrathecal injections of preservative-free methotrexate.
   Psoriasis—10–25 mg once a week
by injection or short-term infusion,
until adequate response is seen. Do
not exceed a dose of 50 mg per
week. Oral dose regimens have also
been used. Adjust dosage and
schedule to obtain desired results.
Once an optimal clinical response
has been achieved, reduce the dosage to the lowest possible level with
the longest rest period between dosages. Topical therapy should be
restarted as soon as possible.
   Other indications—Dosage regimens
for the following indications utilize
oral or *intramuscular* administration of
the drug (consult manufacturer's

package insert or institutional proto-
col for dosages):
- Choriocarcinoma
- Chorioadenoma destruens
- Hydatidiform mole
- Lymphosarcoma
- Mycosis fungoides

Dosage regimens for the following
indications vary greatly from institution to institution; many are considered experimental; consult
institutional protocol:
- Lung malignancies
- Breast malignancies
- Epidermoid malignancies

High-dose therapy for osteogenic
sarcoma is considered to be experimental at this time; consult the literature.

Preparation and Storage
Supplied by Lederle Laboratories
and Bristol Laboratories in the following forms:
   Lederle—5 and 50 mg vials of a
2.5 mg/ml and 25 mg/ml solution
respectively; and 20, 50, and 100 mg
vials of drug powder.
   Bristol—20, 50, and 100 mg vials
of drug powder.
   Reconstitute powder with 2 to 10
ml of a preservative-free diluent
such as sterile water for injection.
Use immediately. Discard unused
portions. Protect unopened vials
from light. Investigational forms of
this drug are also available, see
package insert for preparation information.
   Intrathecal administration of this
drug requires special dilution and
preparation, see the manufacturer's
literature. A preservative-free preparation is available.
   Avoid contact of drug with the
skin. If contact occurs, flush area
with running water for 10 minutes.

Drug Incompatibilities
Do not mix with any other medication in any manner.

Modes of IV Administration

Injection
Yes
Check vein patency; further dilute

the reconstituted solution with 2 ml sterile water for injection for each 5 mg of drug. Inject into the "Y" injection site of a running intravenous line at the rate of 10 mg/minute. Flush vein and tubing with 15–20 ml NS following injection.

Intermittent Infusion
Yes
Add dose to 50–100 ml D5W or NS and infuse over 30–60 minutes.

Continuous Infusion
No
Used only in *experimental* high-dose therapy.

Contraindications; Warnings; Precautions; Adverse Reactions

Contraindications
1. Pregnancy
2. Psoriatic patients with severe renal, hepatic, or bone marrow disorders.

Warnings
1. This drug has many toxic side effects; patients who are on intravenous regimens should be hospitalized.
2. Patients and/or significant others must be informed of the severe and potentially hazardous toxic reactions that can result from therapy.
3. Use in psoriasis must be limited to severe, disabling cases, refractory to other therapies. Deaths have been reported with the use of this drug for psoriasis.
4. This drug may produce marked depression of the bone marrow causing anemia, leukopenia, and thrombocytopenia. Concomitant use of the agents that can potentially depress the marrow should be avoided.
5. Monitor renal, hepatic, pulmonary, and hematologic systems before and frequently during therapy. Liver atrophy, necrosis and cirrhosis have occurred.
6. Administer with extreme caution in the presence of hepatic

dysfunction. Concomitant use of other drugs that cause liver damage, including alcohol, must be avoided.
7. Fetal deaths and congenital anomalies have occurred when the mother has received this drug during pregnancy. Women should be advised to avoid conception during and for a time following therapy.
8. Diarrhea and ulcerative stomatitis are frequent toxic side effects and require interruption of therapy; to continue therapy could lead to hemorrhagic enteritis and death.
9. Rapid intravenous injection can cause syncope.

Precautions
1. Use with caution in the presence of infections and previously existing bone marrow depression.
2. Discontinue at the first signs of oral erythema, ulceration, bleeding from any body area, chills and fever, or hematologic depression.
3. Do not administer the following drugs concomitantly with methotrexate: sulfonamides of any kind or salicylates; they may increase the toxicity of this drug. Vitamin preparations containing folic acid may alter the body's response to methotrexate.
4. Use with extreme caution in the presence of peptic ulcer, ulcerative colitis, debility or extremes of age.
5. This drug is excreted primarily by the kidneys. In the presence of renal insufficiency there may be an accumulation of the drug and further renal damage. In this event the dosage should be reduced or discontinued until pretreatment function returns.

Adverse Reactions
1. Hematologic: bone marrow depression resulting in leukopenia, thrombocytopenia and anemia.
2. Gastrointestinal: nausea,

methotrexate sodium
(continued)
vomiting, diarrhea, enteritis, intestinal ulceration, stomatitis, hepatic damage.
3. Dermatologic: rashes, alopecia, depigmentation, pruritus.
4. General: malaise, fatigue, chills, fever.
5. Genitourinary: renal impairment, cystitis, impaired spermatogenesis, and oogenesis, menstrual irregularities, spontaneous abortion, fetal defects.
6. Central nervous system: headaches, dizziness, seizures, neurologic deficits such as paresis.
7. Pneumonitis
8. Osteoporotic effects.

Overdosage
Leucovorin (folinic acid) can neutralize the immediate toxic effects of this drug on the hematopoietic system. When large doses of methotrexate have been given, administer leucovorin up to 75 mg by intravenous infusion within 12 hours of the methotrexate. Follow the infusion with 12 mg of leucovorin IM every 6 hours for 4 doses. When average doses of methotrexate have adverse effects, give 6 to 12 mg of leucovorin IM every 6 hours for 4 doses. When an overdosage is suspected, the dose of leucovorin should be equal to or higher than the doses of methotrexate and should also be administered within one hour of the overdosage.

☐ **Nursing Implications**
1. The patient receiving this medication will be experiencing the emotional and physical effects of the malignancy or the psoriasis. Knowledge of the patient's feelings about his disease and its implications will assist in helping him tolerate the chemotherapy. The incidence of uncomfortable side effects and adverse reactions is high. It is within the nurse's role to assist the patient in coping with the discomforts of the disease and its treatment, and to help him work through depression and anger toward acceptance of the disease at his own pace. Despite the unpleasantness this drug may bring, it can be a source of hope for the patient.
2. Notify the physician if jaundice develops.
3. Administer supportive care for generalized discomforts such as fatigue, malaise, fever and chills. These reactions will be depressing and frustrating for the patient.
4. Monitor urine output during intensive therapy. Oliguria can be an indication of renal impairment. Notify the physician if the urine output falls below 240 ml (in adults) for an 8-hour period. Be aware of the patient's BUN.
5. Keep the patient hydrated and encourage frequent fluid intake (at least every 2 hours) to prevent cystitis secondary to drug metabolites in the urine. Encourage voiding every 2–3 hours to remove the drug-containing urine from the bladder. Signs and symptoms of chemical cystitis include: frequency, urgency, dysuria, hematuria (micro- and macroscopic). Report these to the physician.
6. Report any signs or symptoms of pneumonitis to the physician: cough, shortness of breath, rales, changes on x-ray, chest pain.
7. Management of gastrointestinal disturbances:
   a. Nausea and vomiting are usually mild and of short duration.
   b. Administer an antiemetic, if needed, to correspond to the time when the most uncomfortable symptoms occur.
   c. Small frequent meals, timed with periods when the patient feels his best, are advisable. Bland foods are usually tolerated most easily. Carbohydrate and protein content should be high.
   d. If the patient is anorexic, en-

courage high nutrient liquids and water. Maintain hydration.

e. Keep an accurate measurement of emesis and stool volumes and total intake and output to guide the physician in ordering parenteral fluids when necessary.

f. Administer constipating agents as needed for diarrhea. Monitor for signs of hypokalemia (weakness, muscle cramps).

g. Monitor for the onset of obstructive ileus (abdominal pain, distention, obstipation).

h. Monitor stools for visible and occult blood.

i. Administer laxatives and stool softeners as ordered if constipation occurs.

8. Management of hematologic effects:

a. Be aware of the patient's white blood cell and platelet count prior to each injection.

b. If WBC falls to 2000/cu mm, take measures to protect the patient from infection, such as protective (reverse) isolation, avoidance of invasive procedures, maintenance of bodily (especially perineal) cleanliness, carrying out strict urinary catheter care when appropriate, etc. Monitor for infection: temperature every 4 hours, examination for rashes, swellings, drainage and pain. Explain measures to the patient.

c. If platelet count falls below 100,000/cu mm, monitor for thrombocytopenic bleeding: petechiae, purpura, hematuria, melena, blood in stools, gum bleeding, vaginal bleeding, epistaxis, hematemesis, etc. Avoid trauma. Transfusions may be ordered.

d. Instruct the patient and/or family on the importance of follow-up blood work and

reporting of the signs and symptoms listed in "b" and "c" if the drug is being administered on an outpatient basis.

9. Management of neurologic side effects:

a. Instruct the patient and/or family to report numbness, paresthesias, pain, headaches. Inform the physician at the onset.

b. If the patient is on high-dose therapy, monitor for seizures.

c. Monitor for signs and symptoms of mental depression that are related to drug administration. Inform the physician and administer supportive care. Knowing the etiology can relieve the patient of some anxiety.

10. Management of stomatitis:

a. Onset of stomatitis may indicate the presence of more serious intestinal ulceration.

b. Administer preventive oral care every 4 hours and/or after meals.

c. For preventive care use a very soft toothbrush (child's) and toothpaste; avoid trauma to tissues.

d. Examine oral membranes at least daily (instruct patient and/or family) to detect the onset of inflammation and erythema.

e. If stomatitis occurs, notify the physician and begin therapeutic oral care as ordered.

f. Order a soft, bland diet for patients with inflammation. If stomatitis is severe, the patient may be placed on NPO status by the physician.

g. For patients who can tolerate oral intake, administer Xylocaine Viscous or acetaminophen elixir as a mouthwash prior to meals to decrease pain (do not use aspirin rinses), as ordered by the physician.

h. Patients with severe stomati-

methotrexate sodium
(continued)

tis may require parenteral analgesia.

11. If rashes occur, administer cool compresses and topical agents as ordered. Keep the patient's environment cool. Turn frequently to prevent skin breakdown.

12. Management of hair loss:
   a. Counsel the patient on the possibility of hair loss to enable him to prepare for this disfigurement.
   b. Reassure him of regrowth of hair following discontinuation of the drug.
   c. Provide privacy, and time for the patient to discuss his feelings.

Suggested Readings

Asperheim, Mary K. and Eisenhaur, Laurel: *The Pharmacology Basis of Patient Care* (3rd ed.), Philadelphia: W. B. Saunders Company, 1977, p. 476.

Bender, John F., Grove, William R, and Fortner, Clarence L: High-Dose Methotrexate with Folinic Acid Rescue, *American Journal of Hospital Pharmacy*, 34:961–965, September 1977.

Bruya, Margaret Auld and Madeira, Nancy Powell: Stomatitis After Chemotherapy, *American Journal of Nursing*, 75(8):1349–1352, August 1975.

Giadquinta, Barbara: Helping Families Face the Crisis of Cancer, *American Journal of Nursing*, 77:1583–1588, October 1977.

Gullo, Shirley: Chemotherapy—What To Do About Special Effects. *RN*, 40:30–32, April 1977.

Laatsch, Nancy: Nursing the Woman Receiving Adjuvant Chemotherapy for Breast Cancer, *Nursing Clinics of North America*, 13(2):337–349, June 1978.

Morrow, Mary: Nursing Management of the Adolescent: The Effect of Cancer Chemotherapy on Psychosocial Development. *Nursing Clinics of North America*, 13(2):319–335, June 1978.

Nirenberg, Anita: High-Dose Methotrexate for the Patient with Osteogenic Sarcoma, *American Journal of Nursing*, 76:1776–1780, November 1976.

Sovik, Corinne: The Nursing Care of Lung Cancer Patients, Emphasizing Chemotherapy, *Nursing Clinics of North America*, 13(2):301–317, June 1978

Vietti, Teresa J., and Valeriote, Frederick: Conceptual Basis for the Use of Chemotherapeutic Agents and Their Pharmacology, *Pediatric Clinics of North America*, 23:67–92, February 1976.

methyldopate hydrochloride ■
(Aldomet Ester HCl Injection)

Actions/Indications

Antihypertensive. Reduces both supine and standing blood pressure. The mechanism of action is probably due to its metabolism to alpha-methylnorepinephrine, which then lowers arterial pressure by stimulation of central inhibitory alpha-adrenergic receptors, false neurotransmission, and/or reduction of plasma renin activity. Used to manage hypertensive crisis or any hypertensive situation where parenteral administration is needed, but where *rapid* reduction of blood pressure is not essential.[1]

Lowering of the blood pressure begins in 4–6 hours and lasts 10–16 hours.

Dosage

Adults:
Range—100–1000 mg.
   Usual adult dose—250–500 mg at 6 hour intervals.
   Maximum recommended dose—1000 mg every 6 hours.
Children:
IV route is reserved for hypertensive crises—20–40 mg/kg/day or 600–1200 mg/M^2/day in divided doses every 6 hrs. (maximum total dose 65 mg/kg/day).

Dosage may need to be reduced in the presence of renal insufficiency.

Preparation and Storage
Supplied in 5-ml vials, 50 mg/ml.
Add only to D5W for infusion.

Drug Incompatibilities
Do not combine with any other drug
in IV bottle; do not add to an IV
line containing antibiotics.

Modes of IV Administration

Injection
No
Not recommended.

Intermittent Infusion
Yes
Add dose to 100 ml D5W. Infuse
over 30–60 min.

Continuous Infusion
No
Maximum effects cannot be achieved
via this route.

Contraindications; Warnings; Precautions; Adverse Reactions

Contraindications
1. Active hepatic disease
2. If previous therapy with methyldopa or methyldopate has been associated with liver impairment
3. Hypersensitivity
4. Eclampsia

Warnings
1. *Positive Coombs' test, hemolytic anemia, and liver impairment may occur and have been fatal. These reactions are usually seen after several months of therapy.*
2. If positive Coombs occurs, it should be determined if hemolytic anemia exists.
3. CBC should be carried out before and during therapy to monitor for anemia.
4. Discontinue the drug if Coombs-positive hemolytic anemia occurs, and do not use again.
5. If patient needs a transfusion during therapy, obtain direct and indirect Coombs. If there is a positive *direct* test, there will be no problem typing and cross-matching. A *positive* indi-

rect test will cause problems in correct matching.
6. Monitor hepatic function. If fever, abnormal liver function tests, or jaundice appears, discontinue the drug. Findings will revert to normal. This represents a hypersensitivity reaction. Do not use this drug in these patients again.
7. There may be reduction in WBC; that is reversible.
8. In pregnancy, the potential benefits for the mother must be weighed against possible risks to the fetus. This drug crosses the placental barrier, appears in cord blood and in breast milk.

Precautions
1. Use with caution in the presence of liver disease.
2. May interfere with the following lab studies:
   a. Uric acid (by phosphotungstate method)
   b. Creatinine (by alkaline picrate method)
   c. SGOT (by colorimetric method)
   d. Urine catecholamine; will be falsely high (could interfere with the diagnosis of pheochromocytoma)
3. Paradoxical hypertensive response has been reported.
4. Do not use to manage hypertension in pheochromocytoma.
5. Urine may darken on exposure to air.
6. Chorealike movements have been reported in patients with known severe bilateral cerebrovascular disease. If it occurs, discontinue the drug.
7. Patients on this drug will require lower dosage of anesthetics. Hypotension may occur during surgery and can be controlled with vasopressors.
8. Blood levels are reduced with hemodialysis.
9. Edema may occur; if it progresses or is associated with congestive heart failure, discontinue therapy.
10. Blood pressure may return to

methyldopate hydrochloride
(continued)
pretreatment levels within 48 hours after discontinuation. Oral therapy should be initiated during this time.

Adverse Reactions
1. Sedation during initial period, may decrease with time. Headache and weakness may also be seen.
2. Central nervous system: in addition to No. 1, dizziness, paresthesias, parkinsonism, Bell's palsy, mild psychosis, nightmares, depression.
3. Cardiovascular: bradycardia, aggravation of angina pectoris, orthostatic hypotension, edema
4. Gastrointestinal: nausea, vomiting, constipation, diarrhea, sore tongue, dryness of mouth
5. Hepatic: see Warning No. 6
6. Hypersensitivity: rash, drug fever, anaphylaxis
7. Breast enlargement, gynecomastia
8. Rashes.

☐ **Nursing Implications**
1. If the patient is in hypertensive crisis, be prepared to monitor arterial blood pressure preferably by direct arterial cannulation. Indirect measurements by sphygmomanometer can be used if direct measurement is not available, or if the patient is not in crisis.
2. If the patient is in a hypertensive crisis (this drug is used less often than more rapid-acting agents in these situations), monitor blood pressure every 15 minutes until stabilized, and then every 2–4 hours as the patient's condition dictates. Repeat the cycle with each dose. This drug's action is delayed for 3–5 hours after the infusion.
3. For noncrisis situations, check the blood pressure before the infusion and every 4–6 hours after. Be aware that the cumulative effects of this drug can produce severe hypotension after

several doses. The physician should order blood pressure limits to govern administration.
4. Patients with coronary artery disease (history of myocardial infarction or angina) or history of arrhythmias should have continuous ECG monitoring during infusions.
5. Observe for jaundice, notify the physician.
6. Administer this drug after hemodialysis treatments (manufacturer's suggestion).
7. Report any unusual chorealike movements to the physician (See Precaution No. 6).
8. Weigh the patient daily; report unusual gains, or observable peripheral edema to the physician.
9. If the patient's blood pressure is severely elevated, monitor for the consequences:
   a. Encephalopathy—confusion, stupor (the sedation produced by this drug may interfere with evaluation for this complication), reflex asymmetries, nausea, vomiting, visual disturbances
   b. Cerebrovascular accident
   c. Myocardial ischemia or infarction—chest pain, ECG changes, arrhythmias
   d. Left ventricular failure— shortness of breath, orthopnea, elevated central venous or pulmonary artery pressure, tachycardia, rales, third and/or fourth heart sound
   e. Renal failure—oliguria, rising BUN and creatinine[2] Excessive *reduction* in blood pressure can also precipitate these complications. Check the patient's blood pressure prior to each dose. The physician should set pressure limits for therapy.
10. Patients who are not in crisis can be ambulated after intermittent infusions; do so *with caution.* Measure lying and then standing pressures to detect postural hypotension. Instruct the patient to arise slowly from sitting and lying positions to prevent

postural hypotension-induced dizziness and syncope. If sedation is pronounced, keep the patient on bed rest until the problem resolves.
11. Patients who will be receiving this drug in its oral form on a chronic basis must be instructed on hypertensive self-care.

References
1. American Medical Association Committee on Hypertension: The Treatment of Malignant Hypertension and Hypertensive Emergencies. *JAMA* 228(13):1675, June 24, 1974.
2. Ibid., p. 1675.

methylprednisolone sodium succinate ■
(Solu-Medrol)

Actions/Indications
Corticosteroid, anti-inflammatory agent. Indicated as effective in:
* Endocrine disorders
* Rheumatic disorders
* Collagen diseases
* Dermatologic disease
* Allergic states
* Ophthalmic diseases
* Gastrointestinal diseases
* Acute exacerbations of multiple sclerosis
* Respiratory diseases
* Hematologic disorders
* Neoplastic disease
* Edematous states
May be effective in:
* Generalized neurodermatitis
* Acute rheumatic fever
* Septic shock
* Other forms of shock
* Croup
* Esophageal burns

Dosage
Adults:
Range—10–500 mg every 6 hrs. Larger doses (30 mg/kg) have been given in extreme cases of septic shock with other supportive care. Do not give massive doses for over 72 hrs.
Usual dose—10–40 mg repeated as needed, usually every 4 to 6 hours.

Children:
Dosage must be according to condition of the patient and his response; no dosage less than 0.5 mg/kg/day.

Preparation and Storage
Use only Mix-o-Vial diluent or diluent accompanying the drug for reconstitution. Use within 48 hours.
This is the only methylprednisolone preparation for intravenous use.

Drug Incompatibilities
Do not combine in syringe with any other medication. Do not mix in solution or IV tubing with:
Chlorpromazine (Thorazine)
Digitoxin
Diphenhydramine (Benadryl)
Metaraminol (Aramine)
Promethazine (Phenergan)
Tetracycline
Thiamylal (Surital)
Sodium thiopental
Tolazoline (Priscoline)
Vitamins

Modes of IV Administration

Injection
Yes
To initiate therapy in emergencies, at a rate no greater than 0.5 gm over 10 min. (see Warning No. 10.)

Intermittent Infusion
Yes
Add prepared solution to D5W, NS or D5/NS in any volume. Infuse over 30–60 min.

Continuous Infusion
Yes
Add prepared solution to D5W, NS or D5/NS. The concentration of the infusion fluid must be no greater than 0.25 mg/ml for the solution to remain stable up to 24 hours. More concentrated solutions are stable for only 6 hours and should be infused within that amount of time.

Contraindications; Warnings; Precautions; Adverse Reactions

Contraindications
1. Systemic fungal infections

methylprednisolone sodium succinate
(continued)

2. Considered by some groups to also be relatively contraindicated (in long-term and short-term therapy) in peptic ulcer disease, chickenpox, congestive heart failure, diabetes mellitus, diverticulitis, new intestinal anastomoses, hypertension, myasthenia gravis, osteoporosis, pregnancy, thromboembolism.

Warnings

1. Dosage should be increased before and during unusual stress such as surgery.
2. May mask signs of infection. There may also be decreased ability to localize infection.
3. Prolonged use may produce cataracts, glaucoma, optic nerve damage, and enhance the establishment of viral or fungal infections.
4. Use in pregnancy should be after benefits are weighed against risks. Infants born of mothers who have received this drug during pregnancy should be observed for hypoadrenalism.
5. May cause elevation of blood pressure even in normal doses. Use with caution in patients with a history of, or currently treated, hypertension.
6. Will cause sodium and water retention, and potassium and calcium excretion. Use with caution in patients with renal insufficiency.
7. Do not vaccinate against smallpox or other diseases during therapy.
8. Use in TB should only be for fulminating or disseminated forms and when other supportive therapy is used.
9. Hypersensitivity has occurred, including anaphylaxis.
10. Circulatory collapse has occurred following rapidly administered large doses (greater than 0.5 gm in 10 min).

Precautions

1. Drug-induced secondary adrenocortical insufficiency will be reduced by gradual reduction of dosage rather than abrupt cessation. This is probably not necessary following short-term therapy where adrenocortical suppression is minimal.
2. There is an enhanced response to steroids in hypothyroidism and cirrhosis.
3. Use lowest possible dosage.
4. Psychic disturbances of all forms occur. Pre-existing psychiatric problems, especially psychoses, may be aggravated.
5. Use aspirin with caution, especially if there is hypoprothombinemia.
6. Use with caution if at all, in the following gastrointestinal conditions: impending gastrointestinal perforation, abscess or other infection, diverticulitis, new intestinal anastomoses, peptic ulcer disease. See Contraindications.
7. Use with caution in the presence of myasthenia gravis, osteoporosis.
8. Monitor major organ systems during therapy, e.g. renal, hepatic, endocrine, etc.
9. Use with caution in patients with ocular herpes simplex because of possible corneal perforation.

Adverse Reactions Seen In Short-Term Intravenous Therapy

1. Fluid and electrolyte imbalance: sodium and water retention with possible secondary hypertension, hypokalemia, hypocalcemia
2. Gastrointestinal: peptic ulcer with possible perforation, pancreatitis, ulcerative esophagitis
3. Dermatologic: impaired wound healing.
4. Neurologic: increased intracranial pressure, seizures (increasing frequency in patients with pre-existing seizure disorder), vertigo, headaches, mental con-

fusion, euphoria, exacerbation of psychosis
5. Endocrine: decreased glucose tolerance, increased requirements for insulin or oral hypoglycemic agents in diabetics.
6. Eye: increased intraocular pressure.
7. Metabolic: negative nitrogen balance secondary to rapid muscle catabolism.

□ **Nursing Implications**
1. Take precautions to prevent infections in wounds by using strict aseptic technique in dressing changes, etc. Avoid traumatic procedures such as catheterizations. The skin may become more fragile because of the steroid therapy. Patients on bed rest and those with general body weakening secondary to an acute illness should be turned hourly (except during sleep, then every 2–3 hours) to prevent skin breakdown. Initiate the use of supportive measures such as flotation pads, water mattress, etc. Administer scrupulous skin care to prevent infection.
2. Monitor blood pressure every 2–4 hours, or as the patient's condition dictates. Monitor blood pressure before, during and immediately after intravenous administration; hypotension can occur.
3. Weigh the patient daily to detect for water and sodium retention. Dietary restriction in sodium may be prescribed by the physician. Examine daily for peripheral edema. Monitor for exacerbation of the congestive heart failure in susceptible patients (increasing dyspnea, increasing resting heart rate, fatigue, rales, etc.)
4. There may be delayed healing of wounds; take precautions to prevent dehiscence. Sutures may be left in longer than usual for this reason.
5. Monitor urine glucose in pa-

tients on high-dose therapy and with diabetes. Diabetic individuals may require a larger dosage of insulin or oral agent.
6. Administer antiulcer therapy as ordered to assist in preventing peptic ulcer. Monitor for signs of the development of an ulcer and/or acute intestinal bleeding; melena, positive stool guaiac, hematemesis, epigastric pain and/or distention, anemia or falling hematocrit.
7. Monitor for signs and symptoms of hypokalemia:[1] weakness, irritability, abdominal distention, poor feeding in infants, muscle cramps. Dietary or pharmacologic potassium supplements may be ordered, guided by serum potassium levels.
8. Monitor for signs and symptoms of hypocalcemia:[2] irritability, change in mental status, seizures, nausea, vomiting, diarrhea, muscle cramps; late effects: cardiac arrhythmias, laryngeal spasm and apnea. Dietary or pharmacologic supplements may be ordered, guided by serum calcium levels.
9. Patients with a history of seizure activity may have an increasing number of seizures while on steroid therapy. Apply appropriate safety precautions.
10. Monitor for behavioral changes, which may range from simple euphoria to depression and psychosis. Apply appropriate safety precautions. A change in dosage may relieve such symptoms.
11. Tuberculin testing should be carried out prior to initiation of steroid therapy if possible. The patient's reactivity to the tuberculin is altered by the drug, giving a false result.
12. Ambulate the patient with caution if vertigo occurs, and initiate the use of side rails to prevent patient injury. Report the onset to the physician.
13. Be alert to the signs of increasing intraocular pressure; eye pain, rainbow vision, blurred vi-

methylprednisolone sodium succinate
(continued)

sion, nausea and vomiting.[3] Notify the physician immediately.

References

1. Beeson, Paul, and McDermott, Walsh (editors): *Cecil-Loeb Textbook of Medicine* (14th ed.), Philadelphia: W. B. Saunders Company, 1975, p. 1587.
2. Ibid., p. 1815.
3. Newell, Frank W., and Ernest, J. Terry: *Ophthalmology—Principles and Concepts* (3rd ed.), St. Louis: C. V. Mosby Company, 1974, p. 329.

Suggested Readings

Glasser, Ronald J.: How the Body Works Against Itself: Autoimmune Disease. *Nursing '77*, September 1977, pp. 34–38.
Melick, M. E.: Nursing Intervention for Patients Receiving Corticosteroid Therapy. In *Advanced Concepts in Clinical Nursing* (2nd ed.), K. C. Kintzel, ed., Philadelphia, J. B. Lippincott Company, 1974, pp. 606–617.
Newton, David., Nichols, Arlene, and Newton, Marion: You Can Minimize the Hazards of Corticosteroids. *Nursing '77*, June 1977, pp. 26–33.
Reichgott, Michael J., and Melmon, Kenneth L.: The Role of Corticosteroids in Shock. In *Steroid Therapy*, Daniel Azarnoff, ed., Philadelphia, W. B. Saunders Company, 1975 pp. 118–133.

metoclopramide hydrochloride ■
(Reglan)

Actions/Indications

Stimulates motility of the upper gastrointestinal tract without stimulating gastric, biliary or pancreatic secretions, by inhibiting dopaminergic mechanisms. Used to facilitate small bowel intubation in adults and children in whom the tube does not pass the pylorus with conventional maneuvers. May also be used in radiological examinations of the stomach and small intestine to promote emptying of barium.

Onset of action is 1 to 3 minutes; effects persist for 1 to 2 hours; excretion is through the kidneys.

Dosage
Adults:
10 mg
Children:
6–14 yrs.—2.5–5.0 mg
    Under 6 yrs.—0.1 mg/kg

Preparation and Storage

Supplied in 2 ml ampuls containing 10 mg (5 mg/ml). Store at room temperature. Protect prepared solutions for infusion from light (use ultraviolet light screening bag over bottle).

Drug Incompatibilities
Do not mix with any other medication in any manner.

Modes of IV Administration

Injection
Yes
Slowly over 1 to 2 min.

Intermittent Infusion
Yes
Use D5W, NS, D5/0.45%, NaCl or RL, 25–100 ml. Infuse over 15–30 minutes. Protect solution from light.

Continuous Infusion
No

Contraindications; Warnings; Precautions; Adverse Reactions

Contraindications
1. When stimulation of gastrointestinal motility may be hazardous; e.g., in hemorrhage, obstruction, perforation.
2. In pheochromocytoma, drug may precipitate a hypertensive crisis.
3. Known hypersensitivity or intolerance to this drug.
4. In patients with seizures or who are taking other drugs which

are likely to cause extrapyramidal reactions; the frequency and severity of these seizures or reactions may be increased.

Warning
Extrapyramidal symptoms may occur and are more frequently seen in children and young adults. Symptoms are: restlessness, involuntary movements of limbs, facial grimacing; rarely torticollis, oculogyric crisis, rhythmic protrusion of tongue, bulbar type of speech.

Precautions
1. Rapid injection can cause a transient intense feeling of anxiety and restlessness followed by drowsiness.
2. The gastrointestinal effects of this drug are antagonized by anticholinergics and narcotic analgesics.
3. Additional sedative effects can occur when this drug is given with alcohol, sedatives, or any central nervous system depressant.
4. Absorption of other drugs from the stomach may be decreased (e.g., digoxin) and absorption from the small intestine may be increased (e.g., acetaminophen, tetracycline).
5. Safety for use in pregnancy has not been established. Nursing mothers should not receive this agent.

Adverse Reactions
1. Restlessness, drowsiness, fatigue, and lassitude.
2. Less frequently, insomnia, headache, dizziness, nausea, or bowel disturbances.

Overdosage
Symptoms: drowsiness, disorientation, and extrapyramidal reactions. These may be controlled with anticholinergic, narcotic, analgesic, or antiparkinson drugs. Symptoms are usually self-limiting, lasting less than 24 hours.

□ **Nursing Implications**
1. Monitor for extrapyramidal and other central nervous system effects: restlessness, facial grimacing, confusion, changes in speech or eye movements. Do not leave the patient unattended; protect him from injury; e.g., side rails, and attempt to allay his fears. These effects are usually self-limited, but may last for up to 24 hours.
2. Monitor blood pressure every five minutes during the first 30 to 60 minutes after injection. Patients with pheochromocytoma may experience a hypertensive crisis; other patients may develop hypotension. Notify physician of deviations from prior values.
3. Take seizure precautions in susceptible patients; this agent may precipitate seizures in some patients.
4. Anticipate extension of sedative effects of central nervous system depressants administered with this drug. The patient should be under protective care until full recovery has been made. Ambulate with caution when the patient appears ready. Outpatients should be accompanied home by an adult and should not drive a car for 12 to 24 hours following the injection or infusion.

metronidazole hydrochloride ▓
(Flagyl IV; Flagyl IV RTU [Ready-to-use])

Actions/Indications
Antibacterial, synthetic. Exerts a bactericidal action against many gram-positive and gram-negative anaerobic bacteria.
    Indicated in the treatment of the following serious infections caused by susceptible anaerobic bacteria:
• Intra-abdominal: *Bacteroides* species, *Clostridium* species, *Eubacterium* species, *Peptococcus* species, and *Peptostreptococcus* species.
• Skin and soft tissue: *Bacteroides*

metronidazole hydrochloride
(continued)

species, *Clostridium* species, *Peptococcus* species, *Peptostreptococcus* species, *Fusobacterium* species.
- Gynecological: *Bacteroides* species, *Clostridium* species, *Peptococcus* species, *Peptostreptococcus* species.
- Septicemia: *Bacteroides* species, *Clostridium* species.
- Bone and joint: *Bacteroides* species
- CNS: *Bacteroides* species
- Lower respiratory tract: *Bacteroides* species.
- Endocarditis: *Bacteroides* species

Dosage
Adults:
Loading Dose—15 mg/kg given over 1 hr.
Maintenance Dose—7.5 mg/kg given 6 hrs after the loading dose; then every 6 hrs.
Do not exceed 4.0 gm maximum dose during a 24 hr. period.
Children:
Not recommended.

Preparation and Storage
Available in single dose vials containing 500 mg of drug and in 100 ml-sized RTU (ready-to-use) vials containing 500 mg solution.
To reconstitute vials, add 4.4 ml sterile water for injection, bacteriostatic water for injection, NS or bacteriostatic NS. MIX THOROUGHLY. Concentration is 100 mg/ml. Solution should be clear, pale yellow to yellow green in color.
Reconstituted solutions may be stored at room temperature. Discard after 96 hours.
DILUTION AND NEUTRALIZATION OF VIALS IS REQUIRED PRIOR TO ADMINISTRATION (see Intermittent Infusion section below). (RTU [ready-to-use] vials DO NOT require dilution or buffering.)
DO NOT USE SYRINGES WITH ALUMINUM NEEDLES OR HUBS.

Drug Incompatibilities
Do not mix with any other drug in any manner.

Modes of IV Administration

Injection
No
The reconstituted drug has a very low pH (0.5 to 2.0).

Intermittent Infusion
Yes
DUE TO THE LOW PH, BOTH DILUTION AND NEUTRALIZATION ARE REQUIRED BEFORE ADMINISTRATION.
Dilution: Add reconstituted dose to one of the following fluids: NS, D5W, RL; use a volume to provide a final concentration of no more than 8 mg/ml (e.g., use at least 75 ml for 500 mg dose); mix thoroughly.
Neutralization: Add 5 mEq of sodium bicarbonate injection for each 500 mg of drug. MIX THOROUGHLY. Use within 24 hours. DO NOT REFRIGERATE NEUTRALIZED SOLUTION.
RTU (ready-to-use) form does not require further dilution or neutralization.
Infuse final solution over one hour.

Continuous Infusion
No

Contraindications; Warnings; Precautions; Adverse Reactions

Contraindications
Hypersensitivity to metronidazole or other nitroimidazole derivatives.

Warnings
1. Seizures and peripheral neuropathy have been reported; appearance of neurological reactions requires evaluating expected benefits against risks of continuing therapy.
2. Metronidazole has been shown to be carcinogenic in animals and mutagenic (cause mutations) in bacteria; the risk in humans has not been resolved.
3. This drug crosses the placental barrier. Animal studies have revealed no fetal damage, but

data regarding safety in human pregnancy are incomplete. Use in pregnancy only when clearly needed.
4. This drug is secreted in breast milk. Breast-feeding should be discontinued if this drug is required.
5. Safety and efficacy for use in children has not been established.

Precautions
1. Patients with severe hepatic disease require reduced dosage due to slower metabolism of the drug.
2. Each ready-to-use (RTU) vial contains 14 mEq (322 mg) of sodium. Use with caution in patients predisposed to edema or CHF and in those receiving corticosteroids.
3. Known or latent candida infections may present increased symptoms in patients receiving metronidazole. Treatment with a candicidal agent may be required.
4. Use with care in patients with a history of blood dyscrasias; mild leukopenia has been reported. Leukocyte counts should be done before and after therapy.
5. This drug can potentiate the anticoagulant effect of warfarin and other coumarin anticoagulants and thus prolong the prothrombin time.
6. False-decrease in SGOT values has been observed in patients on metronidazole.

Adverse Reactions
1. Neurologic: seizures, peripheral neuropathy with numbness and paresthesia (see Warning No. 1), headache, dizziness, syncope.
2. Gastrointestinal: nausea, vomiting, diarrhea, abdominal discomfort.
3. Skin: erythematous rash and pruritus.
4. Local: thrombophlebitis
5. Other: fever, darkened urine.

☐ **Nursing Implications**
1. Monitor neurological signs and observe for any seizure activity, especially in patients with a previous history of seizures. Initiate seizure precautions. Observe for symptoms of peripheral neuropathy (numbness, paresthesia) and report to physician.
2. Monitor patients with history of CHF, renal disease, and other susceptible patients for cardiac failure (increasing dyspnea, increasing heart rate, fatigue, rales) or edema secondary to sodium retention. Dietary restriction of sodium may be required.
3. Monitor patients for appearance or worsening of candidal infections: oral lesions (thrush) or perineal itching and rash (monilia). Promote good oral and perineal hygiene.
4. Patients on oral anticoagulant therapy must be monitored closely due to potentiating effect of metronidazole. Prothrombin time should be done frequently. Observe for bleeding from any site.

miconazole ▓
(Monistat I.V.)

Actions/Indications
Synthetic antifungal agent used in the treatment of the following severe systemic fungal infections: coccidioidomycosis, candidiasis, cryptococcosis, paracoccidioidomycosis, chronic mucocutaneous candidiasis. Culture studies must be performed. This drug is metabolized in the liver and excreted in the urine.

Dosage
Adults:
May vary with diagnosis and causative agent, from 200 to 1200 mg/infusion. See table on page 220.
Children:
20–40 mg/kg/day. Do not exceed 15 mg/kg per infusion; follow guide-

miconazole
(continued)
lines for duration suggestions in the table below.
   Repeated courses may be necessitated by relapse or reinfection. Intrathecal administration or bladder instillation may be needed if the infection is meningeal or in the bladder respectively.

Preparation and Storage
Available in 20 ml ampuls (10 mg/ml).
   Dilute in at least 200 ml of diluent, and use immediately. Use 0.9% sodium chloride or D5W for infusion. This solution may darken over time; this is a sign of deterioration. Do not expose to heat.

Drug Incompatibilities
Do not mix with any other medication in any manner.

Modes of IV Administration

Injection
No

Intermittent Infusion
Yes
Infuse over 30 to 60 minutes in 200 ml of NS or D5W only.

Continuous Infusion
No

Contraindications; Warnings; Precautions; Adverse Reactions

Contraindications
1. Known hypersensitivity to this agent.
2. Trivial fungal infections.

Warning
Rapid infusion of undiluted drug may produce transient tachycardia or other arrhythmias.

Precautions
1. Hypersensitivity tests should be performed prior to administration. An initial dose of 200 mg. should be given with a physician in attendance.
2. Monitor hemoglobin, hematocrit, electrolytes, triglycerides and cholesterol during therapy.
3. Safety for use in pregnancy and lactation has not been established.
4. There may be enhancement of the anticoagulant effect of warfarin and other anticoagulant drugs. Carefully titrate anticoagulant dosage with blood tests.
5. Administer with caution to patients with hepatic or renal impairment who may not be able to metabolize and/or excrete this drug adequately.

Adverse Reactions
1. Phlebitis at infusion site.
2. Pruritus, rash, flushes of the skin.
3. Nausea and vomiting, diarrhea, anorexia. (Nausea and vomiting may be avoided by adherence to infusion rate recommendations.)
4. Drowsiness.
5. Transient lowering of hematocrit; thrombocytopenia, hyperlipidemia.
6. Electrophoretic abnormalities of the lipoprotein (usually does not require cessation of treatment).

Dosage and Duration of Therapy for Miconazole

Fungal Infection	Dosage Range*	Duration of Successful Therapy (Weeks)
Coccidioidomycosis	1800–3600 mg/day	3 to over 20
Cryptococcosis	1200–2400 mg/day	3 to over 12
Candidiasis	600–1800 mg/day	1 to over 20
Paracoccidioidomycosis	200–1200 mg/day	2 to over 16

*Divide over 3 equally sized, equally spaced doses by infusion.

☐ Nursing Implications
1. Prevent nausea and vomiting with correct infusion rate. Avoid administering the drug at mealtimes. If nausea does occur, slow the infusion rate. Dosage may need to be reduced by the physician; if it cannot be reduced, administer an antihistamine or antiemetic as ordered to lessen side effects.
2. Monitor for anaphylaxis during the administration of the first dose. A physician should be in attendance. Be prepared with emergency drugs and resuscitation equipment. See Appendix.
3. Be aware of the patient's prothrombin time prior to each dose of an anticoagulant (warfarin-type).
4. Monitor infusion site for phlebitis, change site if it occurs, and administer local care to the area of inflammation.
5. Notify the physician if a rash develops. Keep the patient as comfortable as possible, a cool room temperature, soapless baths, and medications as ordered for symptomatic relief.

minocycline hydrochloride ■
(Minocin, Vectrin)

Actions/Indications
Antibiotic, long-acting derivative of tetracycline.
Indicated in infections caused by:
- Rickettsiae
- *Mycoplasma pneumoniae*
- Agents of psittacosis and ornithosis
- Agents of lymphogranuloma venereum and granuloma inguinale
- Agent of relapsing fever
The following gram-negative organisms:
- *Hemophilus ducreyi*
- *Pasteurella pestis* and *tularensis*
- *Bartonella bacilliformis*
- *Bacteroides* species
- Brucella
- Others as indicated in sensitivity tests.

The following gram-positive organisms:
- Certain Streptococcus species, e.g., *Streptococcus pneumoniae*
- *Staph. aureus* (for skin and soft tissues only)
When penicillin is contraindicated, this drug can be used as an alternative in infections due to:
- *Neisseria gonorrhoeae*
- *Treponema pallidum* and *T. pertenue*
- *Listeria monocytogenes*
- *Clostridium* species
- *Bacillus anthracis*
- *Fusobacterium fusiformis*
- *Actinomyces* species

Dosage
Usual Adult Dose:
200 mg initially followed by 100 mg every 12 hrs. Do not exceed 400 mg in 24 hrs.
Children (Over 8 Years of Age):
4 mg/kg initially followed by 2–4 mg/kg every 12 hrs. (See Warnings No. 7 and 8.)

Preparation and Storage
Supplied in vials of 100 mg.
Reconstitute dry powder with any volume of D5W, NS, D5/NS or RL. Solutions can be stored at room temperature for 24 hours only, then discard.
Further dilute reconstituted solutions as instructed in Continuous Infusion and Intermittent Infusion sections. Use no other infusion fluids than those listed. Do not use a drug-fluid solution if a precipitate has formed.

Drug Incompatibilities
Do not mix with any magnesium- or calcium-containing solutions.

Modes of IV Administration
Injection
No

Intermittent Infusion
Yes
Add dose to 100 ml D5W, NS, D5/NS or RL for each 10 mg of drug. Infuse over 60 minutes.

minocycline hydrochloride
(continued)
Continuous Infusion
Yes
In 12-hour infusions of 500–1000 ml of NS, D5W, D5/NS, or RL.

Contraindications; Warnings; Precautions; Adverse Reactions

Contraindications
Hypersensitivity to any tetracycline

Warnings
1. There may be a rise in BUN during therapy. This is not significant in normal renal function.
2. The drug should be avoided in patients with renal insufficiency. It may directly exacerbate renal dysfunction, indirectly causing an antianabolic state with acidosis and increasing azotemia.[1] Excessive systemic accumulation of the drug may also be seen, which can lead to liver toxicity.
3. May cause liver impairment secondary to fatty infiltration without necrosis, usually seen in intravenous doses over 2 gm/day or in normal doses in patients with renal failure.
4. Use in pregnant patients with renal dysfunction has been associated with maternal death due to acute hepatic failure.
5. This drug is not readily hemodialyzable.[2]
6. When need for this drug outweighs the risks involved with its use during pregnancy or in the presence of renal or hepatic impairment, perform renal and liver function studies before and during therapy. Follow serum tetracycline levels. In renal impairment, excessive levels may occur and dosage should be reduced accordingly. The blood level should not exceed 15 mcg/ml. Other potentially hepatotoxic agents should not be used concomitantly.
7. The use of tetracycline during tooth development may cause permanent discoloration of the child's teeth. There may also be enamel hypoplasia.
8. This drug can affect bone growth in children (also see Warning No. 7).
9. Abnormalities in fetal development have been reported.
10. This drug is secreted in breast milk.

Precautions
1. There may be overgrowth of nonsusceptible organisms including fungi. If a superinfection occurs, the drug should be discontinued and appropriate therapy instituted.
2. Patients who are on anticoagulant therapy may require lower dosage of that anticoagulant while on minocycline.
3. All infections secondary to group A beta-hemolytic streptococcus should be treated for at least 10 days.
4. Avoid using tetracyclines and penicillins together. The actions of penicillin can be reduced by this drug.

Adverse Reactions
1. Gastrointestinal: anorexia, nausea, vomiting, diarrhea, glossitis, dysphagia, enterocolitis, monilial infections of the anogenital region
2. Skin: maculopapular and erythematous rashes, photosensitivity
3. Renal: rise in BUN (dose-related); see Warnings No. 1, 2, 3, 4
4. Hypersensitivity: urticaria, angioneurotic edema, anaphylaxis, exacerbation of lupus erythematosus
5. Blood: hemolytic anemia, thrombocytopenia, neutropenia, eosinophilia
6. Phlebitis at injection site
7. Vertigo
8. In infants: Bulging fontanels, papilledema (pseudotumor cerebri); usually disappears on discontinuation of the drug.

☐ Nursing Implications

1. Take anaphylaxis precautions; see Appendix.
2. If gastrointestinal disturbances occur, notify the physician. If disturbances such as nausea, vomiting and diarrhea are pronounced, the drug will probably be discontinued. Antiemetics, antacids, and constipating agents can be ordered to control symptoms. Monitor intake and output to assist the physician in planning for parenteral fluid replacement. Maintain hydration orally when possible.
3. If the patient will be taking the oral form of this drug as an outpatient, instruct him on the possibility of photosensitivity and the advisability of avoiding exposure to the sun (sun-block lotions may be of help if exposure cannot be avoided).
4. Women of childbearing age and potential and mothers of children who may receive this drug should be informed of Warnings No. 4, 7, 8, 9, and 10 by the physician. Assist in the interpretation of these warnings to the patient.
5. Even though blood dyscrasias are infrequently caused by this agent, be aware of the patient's complete blood cell count during therapy. If the platelet count begins to fall, the drug will probably be discontinued. Bleeding secondary to a low platelet count usually begins only after the count falls below 50,000/cu mm.
6. Monitor for signs and symptoms of overgrowth infections:
   a. Fever (take rectal temperature at least every 4–6 hours in all patients)
   b. Increasing malaise
   c. Newly appearing localized signs and symptoms: redness, soreness, pain, swelling, drainage (increased volume or change in character of pre-existing drainage)
   d. Monilial rash in perineal area (reddened areas with itching)
   e. Cough (change in pre-existing cough or sputum production)
   f. Diarrhea
7. Report the onset of any rash to the physician. Keep the patient's environment comfortably cool and the skin clean. Diphenhydramine (Benadryl) may be ordered to relieve itching.
8. Report the onset of jaundice to the physician.
9. Report the onset of bulging fontanels, and other signs of increasing intracranial pressure, to the physician.
10. Be aware of this drug's relationship with renal function. Most tetracyclines are usually not given to patients with renal impairment because:
    a. The drug accumulates in the body because of decreased excretion.
    b. The presence of the drug may cause further deterioration in renal function.
    c. It may cause a catabolic state with metabolic acidosis, increasing BUN, and possibly death due to uremia.[3]

    Know what the patient's pretreatment BUN and creatinine levels are. Monitor for changes in these values with initiation of treatment.

    Monitor urine output in renal patients receiving the drug. Report increasing oliguria to the physician. Send urine for analysis at least every other day.

References

1. Barza, Michael, and Schiefe, Richard T.: Antimicrobial Spectrum, Pharmacology and Therapeutic Use of Antibiotics. Part I: Tetracyclines. *American Journal of Hospital Pharmacy*, 34:51, January 1977.
2. Ibid.
3. Ibid.

mithramycin ■
(Mithracin)

Actions/Indications
Antineoplastic agent, cell-cycle specific. Used in the treatment of malignant tumors of the testes when
surgery or radiation are impossible.
Not recommended for any other
neoplasm. Tumor regression is usually evident in 3–4 weeks. Also used
to treat symptomatic patients with
hypercalcemia and hypercalciuria in
other advanced neoplasms.

Dosage
Testicular Tumors:
25–30 mcg/kg/day (use actual body
weight or *ideal* weight in the presence of edema). Continue for 8–10
days unless significant toxic effects
are seen. Do not exceed 10 daily
doses. Do not exceed 30 mcg/kg per
dose. Courses of therapy can be repeated at monthly intervals.
Hypercalcemia and Hypercalciuria:
25 mcg/kg for 3–4 days. May use
single weekly dose to control condition. Use *only* in hypercalcemia and
hypercalciuria unresponsive to other
therapy. Patients with renal impairment will require a 25–40% reduction in dosage based on dosage
suggested above.[1]
If desired effects are not seen with
initial course, it can be repeated at
intervals of 1 week.

Preparation and Storage
Supplied in vials of 2500 mcg of
drug powder. To reconstitute add
4.9 ml sterile water for injection and
shake to dissolve.
Each ml = 500 mcg (0.5 mg).
Discard unused portion. Prepare
fresh on the day of use.

Drug Incompatibilities
Do not mix with any other medication.

Modes of IV Administration

Injection
No
Use of this mode has been associated with a higher incidence and
greater severity of side effects.[2]

Intermittent Infusion
Yes
Daily dose in 500–1000 ml D5W
over 4–6 hours.

Continuous Infusion
No

Contraindications; Warnings; Pre-cautions; Adverse Reactions

Contraindications
1. Thrombocytopenia, thrombocy-
   topathy, coagulation disorders,
   or increased susceptibility to
   bleeding due to other causes
2. Impaired bone marrow function
3. The unhospitalized patient

Warnings
1. **Severe thrombocytopenia, a
   hemorrhagic tendency and
   death may occur** (this complication is usually seen following
   doses of 30 mcg/kg or duration
   longer than 10 days).
2. The possibility of achieving
   therapeutic benefit must be
   weighed against the risk of
   hazardous toxicity *before* administering this drug, especially in
   advanced malignancies.

Precautions
1. The following studies should be
   carried out before, during and
   after therapy: platelet count,
   prothrombin time, bleeding
   time. Thrombocytopenia or
   prolongation of prothrombin or
   bleeding time must prompt
   discontinuation of the drug.
   Onset may be rapid and occur
   at anytime during therapy.
2. Prior to treatment, electrolyte
   imbalance, such as hypocalcemia, hypokalemia, and hypo-
   phosphatemia, must be
   corrected.
3. Use with extreme caution in the
   presence of renal or hepatic
   dysfunction. Abnormal liver
   function tests may occur, even
   in normal subjects. These

changes are reversible on discontinuation of the drug.
4. Facial flushing is an indication to discontinue therapy.[3]
5. Patients receiving this drug must be hospitalized.

Adverse Reactions
1. Hematopoietic:
    a. Bleeding syndrome due to thrombocytopenia, elevation in prothrombin, clotting and bleeding times; seen in 5–12% of patients treated, usually heralded by an episode of epistaxis, may advance to widespread GI bleeding
    b. Leukopenia (seen in approximately 6% of patients treated)
    c. Decreased hemoglobin
2. Gastrointestinal: anorexia, nausea, vomiting, diarrhea, stomatitis
3. Skin: facial erythema (see Precaution No. 4), edema, increased pigmentation; rashes
4. Fever (common)
5. Hepatic: elevation of SGOT, SGPT, LDH, alkaline phosphatase, serum bilirubin.
6. Renal: elevation in BUN and serum creatinine, proteinuria (secondary to drug-induced renal insufficiency)
7. Electrolyte balance: decreased serum calcium, phosphorus, and potassium
8. Miscellaneous: drowsiness, weakness, lethargy, mental depression

☐ **Nursing Implications**
1. The patient receiving this medication will be experiencing the emotional and physical effects of malignancy. Knowledge of the patient's feelings about his disease and its implications will assist in helping him tolerate the chemotherapy. The incidence of uncomfortable side effects and adverse reactions is high. It is within the nurse's role to assist the patient in coping with the discomforts of the

disease and its treatment, and to help him work through depression and anger toward acceptance of the disease at his own pace. Despite the unpleasantness this drug may bring, it can be a source of hope for the patient.
2. Management of hematologic effects:
    a. See Adverse Reaction No. 1., Warning No. 1., and Precaution No. 1.
    b. Be aware of the patient's platelet count, the prothrombin, clotting and bleeding times prior to each injection of this drug.
    c. Monitor for bleeding if the platelet count falls below 100,000/cu mm, if the prothrombin time begins to exceed control by 2–3 times, if clotting (coagulation) time exceeds 6–17 minutes (Lee-White method using glass tubes), or if bleeding time exceeds 4 minutes (Ivy method). The bleeding syndrome this drug can precipitate is secondary to depression of hepatic synthesis of several coagulation factors.
       Signs of bleeding: petechiae, purpura, hematuria, melena, blood in the stools, gum bleeding, vaginal bleeding, epistaxis, hematemesis, shock, etc. Avoid traumatic procedures and patient injury. Transfusions of fresh whole blood or platelets may be ordered.
    d. Leukopenia occurs rarely. Be aware of the patient's white blood cell count prior to each injection of this drug. If the WBC falls below 2000/cu mm, take measures to protect the patient from infection such as protective (reverse) isolation, avoidance of invasive procedures, maintaining bodily (especially perineal) cleanliness, carrying out strict urinary catheter care when appropri-

mithramycin
(continued)
ate, etc. Monitor for infection by recording temperatures every 4 hours, examining for rashes, swellings, drainage and pain. Explain these measures to the patient.
3. Management of gastrointestinal symptoms:
   a. Administer antiemetics when they appear to be most effective, e.g., prior to the injection and/or 1 hour prior to meals, etc.
   b. Small frequent meals, timed with periods when the patient feels his best, are advisable. Bland foods are usually tolerated better than others. Carbohydrate and protein content should be high. If the patient is anorexic, encourage high nutrient liquids and water to maintain hydration.
   c. Keep accurate measurements of emesis volume and total intake and output to guide the physician in ordering parenteral fluids when necessary.
   d. Monitor for the onset of diarrhea and notify the physician. Administer antiperistaltics as ordered. Maintain hydration. Monitor for hypokalemia, e.g., muscle cramps and weakness.
4. Management of stomatitis:
   a. Administer preventive oral care every 4 hours and/or after meals.
   b. For preventive care, use a very soft toothbrush (child's) and toothpaste; avoid trauma to tissues.
   c. Examine oral membranes at least daily (instruct patient and/or family) to detect the onset of inflammation or ulceration.
   d. If stomatitis occurs, notify the physician and begin therapeutic oral care.
   e. Order a bland, mechanical soft diet for patients with inflammation. If stomatitis is severe, the patient may be placed on NPO status by the physician.
   f. For the patients who can tolerate oral intake, administer Xylocaine Viscous or acetaminophen elixir as a mouthwash prior to meals to decrease pain (do not use aspirin rinses), as ordered by the physician.
   g. Patients with severe stomatitis may require parenteral analgesia.
5. Monitor for facial flushing. Notify the physician; this is an indication to discontinue the drug.
6. If rashes occur, administer cool compresses as ordered. If the patient is on bed rest, turn him frequently to prevent skin breakdown. Keep room temperature cool.
7. Monitor for fever (differentiation will have to be made between drug fever and temperature elevation secondary to infection).
8. Be aware of the patient's BUN and serum creatinine. If these values rise above normal, begin monitoring urine output every 8 hours. Report oliguria (urine output less than 240 ml in 8 hours) to the physician.
9. Monitor for signs and symptoms of hypocalcemia:[4] muscle cramps and aches, paresthesias, nausea and vomiting, diarrhea.
10. Monitor for hypokalemia (secondary to increased renal excretion of potassium):[5] muscle cramps, weakness, irritability, abdominal distinction.
11. Observe for signs of mental depression. The patient should be informed that the drug is likely to cause such feelings. Give the patient time to express feelings and concerns. Elicit assistance from the family and/or significant others.
12. Avoid extravasation; see Appen-

dix. Moderate heat should be applied to the area as soon as possible.

References

1. Shinn, Arthur F., et al.: Dosage Modifications of Cancer Chemotherapeutic Agents in Renal Failure. *Drug Intelligence and Clinical Pharmacy*, 11:141, March 1977.
2. Trissel, Lawrence A.: *Handbook on Injectable Drugs*, Washington, DC: American Society of Hospital Pharmacists, 1977, p. 235.
3. Silver, Richard T., Lauper, R. David, and Jarowski, Charles I.: *A Synopsis of Cancer Chemotherapy*, The York Medical Group, New York: Dun-Donnelley Publishing Company, 1977, p. 98.
4. Beeson, Paul, and McDermott, Walsh (editors): *Cecil-Loeb Textbook of Medicine* (14th ed.), Philadelphia: W. B. Saunders Company, 1975, p. 1815.
5. Ibid., p. 1587.

Suggested Readings

Bruya, Margaret Auld, and Madeira, Nancy Powell: Stomatitis After Chemotherapy. *American Journal of Nursing*, 75(8):1349–1352, August 1975.

Giadquinta, Barbara: Helping Families Face the Crisis of Cancer. *American Journal of Nursing*, 77:1583–1588, October 1977.

Gullo, Shirley: Chemotherapy—What to Do About Special Side Effects. *RN*, 40:30–32, April 1977.

mitomycin ■
(Mutamycin)

Actions/Indications

Antineoplastic antibiotic that is cell-cycle nonspecific. Used in combination with other agents in disseminated adenocarcinoma of the stomach, breast or pancreas, carcinoma of the head or neck, and chronic myelogenous leukemia.

Dosage

Adults:

Single dose—10–20 mg/M^2 every 6–8 weeks. Repeat doses are adjusted based on the hematologic response to previous doses. See Table below.

Multiple doses—2 mg/M^2/day for 5 days; 2 days no dose; then 2 mg/M^2/day for 5 days. If after two courses there is no improvement, discontinue.

No repeat dosage should be given until the leukocyte count has returned to 3000 and the platelet count to 75,000.

When used in combination with other agents, dosage must be individualized.

Manufacturer's Suggested Dosage Guide

Leukocytes	Lowest cell count after prior dose Platelets	Percentage of prior dose to be given
>4000	>100,000	100%
3000–3999	75,000–99,999	100%
2000–2999	25,000–74,999	70%
<2000	<25,000	50%

Preparation and Storage

Supplied in vials of 5 mg and 20 mg of powder. Reconstitute by adding 10 ml or 40 ml of sterile water for injection, respectively. Shake to dissolve. If dissolution is not immediately seen, allow the vial to stand at room temperature for several minutes, shake again. The resulting solution contains 0.5 mg/ml.

The reconstituted solution is stable if refrigerated for 14 days; discard after that time (7 days if unrefrigerated).

If the drug is added to large volumes of solution, it will be stable for the following times at room temperature:

D5W—3 hours
NS—12 hours
Sod. Lactate—24 hours

Drug Incompatibilities

Do not mix with any other medication except heparin.

mitomycin
(continued)
Modes of IV Administration

Injection
Yes
Into the "Y" site of a running IV.
No need to further dilute reconstituted solution. Flush vein with NS after injection.

Intermittent Infusion
Yes
Use D5W or NS, 100–200 ml, infused immediately after mixing, over 30–60 minutes.

Continuous Infusion
No

Contraindications; Warnings; Precautions; Adverse Reactions

Contraindications
1. Hypersensitivity
2. Thrombocytopenia or other coagulation disorders and increased bleeding tendency due to other causes

Warnings
1. **There is a high incidence of sometimes irreversible bone marrow suppression—thrombocytopenia and leukopenia.** Perform appropriate studies before, during and for at least 7 weeks after therapy.
2. Discontinue if platelet count falls below 150,000/cu mm or if WBC is below 4000/cu mm. Death has resulted secondary to septicemia with low white count.
3. Monitor for renal toxicity. Discontinue if serum creatinine exceeds 1.7 mg/100 ml.
4. Safety for use in pregnancy has not been established. Fetal malformations have been seen in test animals.
5. Avoid extravasation.

Adverse Reactions
1. Bone marrow toxicity: usually reversible thrombocytopenia and leukopenia; suppression is cumulative. After a single dose, the peak suppression occurs in 3–4 weeks. Thrombocytopenia persists for 2–3 weeks and leukopenia for 1–2 weeks. Recovery after cessation of therapy is usually complete in 8 weeks.[1] Twenty-five percent do not recover.
2. Skin and mucous membranes: stomatitis and hair loss, cellulitis at injection or extravasation site.
3. Gastrointestinal: anorexia, nausea and vomiting (14% of patients).
4. Renal: rise in creatinine and BUN (toxicity is in the form of glomerular sclerosis) occurs several months after therapy (2% of patients)
5. Fever (rare)
6. Headache, blurred vision, fatigue, edema of the extremities, syncope (all rare)

☐ **Nursing Implications**
1. The patient receiving this medication will be experiencing the emotional and physical effects of the malignancy. Knowledge of the patient's feelings about his disease and its implications will assist in helping him tolerate the chemotherapy. The incidence of uncomfortable side effects and adverse reactions is high. It is within the nurse's role to assist the patient in coping with the discomforts of the disease and its treatment, and to help him work through depression and anger toward acceptance of the disease at his own pace. Despite the unpleasantness this drug may bring, it can be a source of hope for the patient.
2. Management of hematologic effects:
   a. See Adverse Reaction No. 1, and Warnings Nos. 1 and 2.
   b. Be aware of the patient's white blood cell and platelet counts prior to each dose and daily if the patient is on multiple doses of this drug.
   c. If WBC falls to 2000/cu mm, take measures to pro-

tect the patient from infection such as: protective (reverse) isolation, avoidance of invasive procedures, maintain bodily (especially perineal) cleanliness, carry out strict urinary catheter care when appropriate. Monitor for infection by recording temperatures every 4 hours; examine for rashes, swellings, drainage and pain. Explain these measures to the patient.

d. If the platelet count falls below 100,000/cu mm, monitor for thrombocytopenic bleeding: petechiae, purpura, hematuria, melena, blood in stools, gum bleeding, oozing from an incision, vaginal bleeding, epistaxis, hematuria, etc. Avoid trauma. Transfusions may be ordered.

e. Instruct the patient and family on the importance of follow-up blood work if the drug is being administered on an outpatient basis.

3. Take all precautions to avoid extravasation; see Appendix. If it occurs, notify the physician immediately. Observe the affected area for tissue ulceration, necrosis or sloughing. Protect tissues from further damage. Treat as a burn.

4. Management of nausea and vomiting:
   a. Usually occurs during the first 12–24 hours after an injection.
   b. Administer antiemetic 1 hour prior to injection and/or prior to meals, whichever schedule relieves the symptoms most efficiently.
   c. Small frequent meals, timed with periods when the patient feels his best, are advisable. Bland foods are usually tolerated more readily by a patient who is anorexic or nauseated. Carbohydrate and protein content should be high.

d. If the patient is anorexic, encourage high nutrient liquids and water to maintain nutrition and hydration.

e. Keep accurate measurements of emesis volume and total intake and output to guide the physician in ordering parenteral fluids when necessary.

5. Management of Hair Loss:
   a. Counsel the patient on the possibility of hair loss to enable him to prepare for this disfigurement.
   b. Reassure him of the possibility of regrowth of hair following discontinuation of the drug.
   c. Provide privacy and time for the patient to discuss his feelings.
   d. The scalp tourniquet technique or cooling may be ineffective in preventing hair loss because of this drug's prolonged presence in the blood.

6. Management of Stomatitis:
   a. Administer preventive oral care every 4 hours and/or after meals.
   b. For preventive care, use a very soft toothbrush (child's) and toothpaste; avoid trauma to the tissues.
   c. Examine oral membranes at least once daily (instruct patient and/or family) to detect onset of inflammation and erythema.
   d. If stomatitis occurs, notify the physician and begin therapeutic oral care.
   e. Order a bland, mechanical soft diet for patients with inflammation. If severe stomatitis with ulceration is present, the patient may be placed on NPO status by the physician.
   f. For patients who can tolerate oral intake, administer Xylocaine Viscous or acetaminophen elixir as a mouthwash prior to meals to decrease pain (do not use

mitomycin
(continued)

aspirin rinses), as ordered by the physician.

g. Patients with severe stomatitis may require parenteral analgesia.

7. Patients should be monitored for change in renal status for several months after discontinuation of therapy to detect the onset of renal insufficiency. Stress the importance of follow-up blood studies.

References

1. Silver, Richard T., Lauper, R. David and Jarowski, Charles I.: *A Synopsis of Cancer Chemotherapy*, The York Medical Group, New York: Dun-Donnelly Publishing Company, 1977, p. 88.

Suggested Readings

Bruya, Margaret Auld, and Madeira, Nancy Powell: Stomatitis After Chemotherapy, *American Journal of Nursing*, 75(8):1349–1352, August 1975.

Giadquinta, Barbara: Helping Families Face the Crisis of Cancer. *American Journal of Nursing*, 77:1583–1588, October 1977.

Gullo, Shirley: Chemotherapy— What To Do About Special Side Effects. *RN*, 40:30–32, April 1977.

morphine sulfate ■

Actions/Indications

Narcotic analgesic.

Affects psychic function, making the patient more tolerant of pain, and interferes centrally in the brain to decrease pain conduction. Depresses the respiratory center and cough reflex. For relief of severe pain and accompanying apprehension.

In the treatment of pulmonary edema, this drug produces vasodilation (reduces venous return to the heart) and decreases anxiety.

Maximum analgesic effect occurs in 20 minutes after IV injection, and lasts 4–7 hours.

Dosage

Adults:
Range—5–20 mg.
Usual—10 mg. May be repeated in 2–4 hrs. (Lower doses are required in patients concomitantly receiving other sedative or anesthetic drugs.)
Children:
IV administration not recommended

Preparation and Storage

Supplied in ampuls of 8, 10, and 15 mg/ml, and disposable, prefilled syringes of the same concentrations.

This is a Schedule II drug under the Controlled Substances Act of 1970. Maintain hospital or institutional regulations guiding its use.

Drug Incompatibilities

Do not mix with any other medication. Do not inject into IV tubing containing:
Aminophylline
Heparin
Methicillin
Novobiocin
Phenobarbital
Sodium bicarbonate
Sodium iodide
Thiopental

Modes of IV Administration

Injection
Yes
Add dose to 10 ml sterile water for injection or NS. Administer through Y injection site or 3-way stopcock. Inject over 2–4 min.

Intermittent Infusion
No
Do not add to IV fluid.

Continuous Infusion
No
Do not add to IV fluid.

Contraindications; Warnings; Precautions; Adverse Reactions

Contraindications
1. Bronchial asthma
2. Respiratory depression
3. Hypersensitivity

Warnings
1. May be habit-forming, resulting in psychic and physical dependence.
2. Tolerance may develop after repeated doses.
3. **Fatalities have occurred** when this drug has been administered to patients with increased intracranial pressure, acute asthmatic attack, chronic obstructive lung disease, cor pulmonale, preexisting respiratory depression, hypoxia, or hypercapnia.
4. Severe hypotension may result in the presence of shock secondary to depleted blood volume or with concomitant use of phenothiazines or certain anesthetics.
5. Syncope and orthostatic hypotension can occur in ambulatory patients.
6. Rapid IV injection or large doses will cause sudden respiratory depression.
7. Use in pregnancy requires that expected benefits outweigh the risks to mother and fetus.

Precautions
1. As an analgesic, this drug can mask important symptoms in head injuries (increasing intracranial pressure) and abdominal conditions (acute intestinal obstruction).
2. Caution is advised when administering the initial dose to: elderly or debilitated patients, those with hepatic or renal dysfunction, history of asthma, hypothyroidism, toxic psychoses, Addison's disease, prostatic hypertrophy, or urethral stricture. These patients are more likely to exhibit severe adverse reactions.
3. In supraventricular tachyarrhythmias (atrial flutter, fibrillation or tachycardia), the ventricular rate may be increased by morphine.
4. There may be aggravation of convulsive disorders.
5. Reduce dosage when the patient is concomitantly receiving other narcotic analgesics, general anesthetics, phenothiazines, other tranquilizers, sedative-hypnotics, antidepressants, or any CNS depressant.
6. Naloxone, a narcotic antagonist, should be readily available to combat respiratory depression, see page 237 for further information.

Adverse Reactions
1. Respiratory depression including respiratory arrest; bronchospasm
2. Circulatory depression (vasodilatation producing hypotension)
3. Minor effects: nausea, vomiting, light-headedness, sedation, diaphoresis (may be alleviated with a supine position)
4. Psychic changes: euphoria, agitation, hallucinations, confusion, visual changes
5. Constipation
6. Urinary retention, especially in the presence of prostatic hypertrophy or urethral stricture
7. Hypersensitivity: rash, urticaria, anaphylaxis

☐ **Nursing Implications**
1. Patient should be on bed rest with side rails up during, and for the first hour after, injection. Then ambulate when appropriate with caution.
2. Respiratory support equipment must be readily available in the event of respiratory depression —narcotic antagonist agent: naloxone (see page 237); airways, endotracheal tube and laryngoscope, suction, oxygen, manual breathing bag (Ambu, Hope, Puritan).
3. Monitor for respiratory depression: Count respiratory rate every 3–5 minutes during and after the injection for the first 15 minutes, then every 5–10 minutes for the next hour, then every 30 minutes for the next 2 hours. Repeat cycle for additional doses. If respiratory rate falls below 10/minute, notify physician and be prepared to

morphine sulfate
(continued)

assist ventilation. Observe for cyanosis (central: lips and tongue; peripheral: nailbeds), shallow respirations, change in mental status, and cardiac irregularities. Do not leave the patient unattended for the first 30 minutes. See Warning No. 3.

Take measures to prevent aspiration in the event of vomiting. Begin manual breathing assistance and use of airway if the patient cannot be aroused to increase his own respiratory rate and if the respiratory rate falls below 6 per minute or if cyanosis develops.

4. Monitor blood pressure and apical pulse before injection and every 3–5 minutes for the first 15 minutes, then every 5–10 minutes for the next hour, then every 30 minutes for the next 2 hours. The physician must determine acceptable blood pressure limits. Be prepared to treat hypotension with vasopressors.
5. Any patient with a supraventricular arrhythmia should be monitored with extreme care for an inordinate increase in ventricular rate. Notify physician if rate exceeds 110/minute. Such patients could develop or have an exacerbation of congestive heart failure secondary to rapid heart rate.
6. Seizure precaution in patients with a history of seizures.
7. Be prepared to manage hallucinations and disorientation.
8. Monitor for urinary retention in susceptible patients (see Adverse Reaction No. 6). Palpate bladder size every 4 hours; measure urinary output every 8 hours.
9. Patients on prolonged therapy may require laxatives or stool softeners to prevent constipation. Maintain hydration and high-fiber diet.
10. When scheduling doses, do not make the patient wait for total

return of the pain before repeating a dose; to do so will reduce the effectiveness of the analgesic. Never withhold the drug when it is needed unless a contraindication arises, and then notify the physician for assistance.

Suggested Readings

Smith, Dorothy W., and Germain, Carol P. Hanley: *Care of the Adult Patient* (4th ed.), Philadelphia, J. B. Lippincott Company, 1975, Chapter 10, The Patient in Pain.

Mark, Lester C.: When to Use Narcotics Intravenously. *Drug Therapy* (Hospital Edition), June 1978, pp. 16–20.

McCaffery, Margo, and Hart, Linda: Undertreatment of Acute Pain with Narcotics. *American Journal of Nursing*, 76(10):1586–1591, October 1976.

Grad, Rae Krohn, and Woodside, Jack: Obstetrical Analgesics and Anesthesia: Methods of Relief for the Patient in Labor. *American Journal of Nursing*, 77(2):242–245, February 1977.

Vismara, Louis A., Mason, Dean T., and Amsterdam, Ezra A.: Cardiocirculatory Effects of Morphine Sulfate: Mechanisms of Action and Therapeutic Application. *Heart and Lung*, 3(3):495–499, May–June, 1974 (references).

nafcillin, sodium ■
(Nafcil, Unipen)

Actions/Indications
Semisynthetic penicillin.
    Antibiotic, penicillinase-resistant.
    Wide gram-positive spectrum.
Used for infections due to:
• *Staphylococcus aureus*—penicillin G resistant and susceptible
• Pneumococci
• Group A beta hemolytic streptococcus
    Susceptibility tests must be performed. (Usually used only in infections secondary to penicillinase-producing *Staph. aureus*.)

Dosage

Adults:
Dosage varies with severity of infection. 500–1000 mg every 4 hrs. (No need to adjust dosage in the presence of renal failure.)
Infants and Children:
60 mg/kg/24 hrs
or
1.8 g/M^2/24 hrs divided into 6 doses. For severe infections, double the above doses.[1]

Preparation and Storage

To reconstitute powder, use sterile water for injection, bacteriostatic water for injection (do not use bacteriostatic diluent if drug is being administered to a neonate); or 0.9% sodium chloride in the following volumes: 500 mg, add 1.8 ml; 1 gm, add 3.4 ml; 2 gm, add 6.6 ml. These solutions will contain 250 mg/ml.

Solutions are stable for 3 days at room temperature or 7 days when refrigerated. May be frozen for up to 3 months.

Available also in piggyback bottles for infusion. Dilute as follows:

1-gm bottle—add 49 ml sterile water for injection or NS (concentration will be 20 mg/ml), or add 99 ml diluent to make a concentration of 10 mg/ml.

2-gm bottle—add 49 ml sterile water for injection or NS (concentration will be 20 mg/ml), or add 99 ml diluent to make a concentration of 10 mg/ml.

4-gm bottle—add 97 ml diluent to make a concentration of 40 mg/ml.

Drug Incompatibilities

Do not mix in any manner with:
Aminophylline
Sodium bicarbonate
Metaraminol
Vitamins
Gentamicin and other
   aminoglycosides
Hydrocortisone

Modes of IV Administration

Injection
Yes
Dilute dose in 15–30 ml Sterile Water for Injection or NS. Administer over 5–10 min, into injection site of a running IV.

Intermittent Infusion
Yes
Use NS, D5W, D5/½ NS, RL, M/6 sodium lactate, in any appropriate amount, usually 100–200 ml.
   Infuse dose over 30–60 min.

Continuous Infusion
Yes
Infusion must be completed in 24 hours.
   Use NS, D5W, D5/½ NS, RL, or M/6 sodium lactate, in an amount to make a concentration between 2–30 mg/ml.

Contraindications; Warnings; Precautions; Adverse Reactions

Contraindications
Hypersensitivity to any penicillin

Warnings
1. Anaphylaxis has been reported.
2. There may be cross-allergenicity with cephalosporins.

Precautions
1. Monitor renal, hepatic, and hematopoietic function before and during therapy, especially if therapy is prolonged.
2. Bacterial and fungal overgrowth of nonsusceptible organisms can occur.
3. Safety for use in pregnancy has not been established.
4. May cause thrombophlebitis at injection site.
5. Oral route should not be relied upon in patients with decreased gastrointestinal absorption, or who have gastrointestinal disturbances.

Adverse Reactions
1. Hypersensitivity reactions: anaphylaxis, interstitial nephritis, neutropenia, rashes, serum sickness, cross-allergenicity with penicillin and cephalosporins[2]
2. Positive Coomb's test
3. Diarrhea

nafcillin, sodium
(continued)
4. Glossitis and stomatitis (rare)
5. Overgrowth infections (1% of recipients)[3]
6. Thrombophlebitis at injection site, especially in the elderly.

☐ **Nursing Implications**
1. Take anaphylaxis precautions; see Appendix.
2. Examine oral membranes daily for signs of inflammation. Administer careful oral care at least twice daily. If inflammation occurs, notify the physician and administer therapeutic care as ordered. Order a bland, mechanical soft diet. The patient with severe inflammation and ulceration may be placed on NPO status.
   For patients who can tolerate oral intake, administer Xylocaine Viscous or acetaminophen elixir as a mouthwash prior to meals to decrease pain (do not use aspirin rinses) as ordered by the physician.
   Maintain hydration with bland liquids (avoid fruit juices) and parenteral fluids if needed. Severe inflammation and ulceration may require parenteral analgesia.
3. Monitor for signs and symptoms of overgrowth infections:
   a. Fever (take rectal temperature at least every 4–6 hours in all patients)
   b. Increasing malaise
   c. Newly appearing localized signs and symptoms: redness, soreness, pain, swelling, drainage (increased volume or change in character of preexisting drainage)
   d. Monilial rash in perineal area (reddened areas with itching)
   e. Cough (change in preexisting cough or sputum production)
   f. Diarrhea
4. Change infusion site at first sign of phlebitis.

References
1. Shirkey, Harry C.: *Pediatric Drug Handbook*, Philadelphia: W. B. Saunders Company, 1977, p. 46.
2. Barza, Michael: Antimicrobial Spectrum, Pharmacology and Therapeutic Use of Antibiotics. Part 2: Penicillins. *American Journal of Pharmacy*, January 1977.
3. Ibid, p. 62.

nalbuphine hydrochloride ■
(Nubain)

Actions/Indications
Potent synthetic narcotic analgesic with narcotic agonist/antagonist properties. Potency is comparable to morphine on a milligram basis. Onset of action is 2 to 3 minutes after intravenous administration. Clinical analgesic activity is 3 to 6 hours.

Used for relief of moderate to severe pain, postoperatively, as an adjunct to anesthesia, and during labor.

The drug is metabolized in the liver and excreted in the form of metabolites and in an unchanged form in the feces as a result of biliary secretion, and through the kidneys.

Dosage
Adults:
10 mg for a 70 kg person (approximately 0.14 mg/kg), may be repeated every 3 to 6 hours. Maximum recommended dose is 20 mg or 160 mg in 24 hours. See Warnings for situations requiring dosage adjustments.
Children:
Not recommended.

Preparation and Storage
Supplied in ampuls of 1 and 2 ml, each containing 10 mg/ml. Store at room temperature. Even though this drug is a narcotic, it is not under the Controlled Substances Act regulations.

Drug Incompatibilities
Do not mix with any other medication in any manner.

Modes of IV Administration

Injection
Yes
Dilution not required; inject slowly.

Intermittent Infusion
No

Continuous Infusion
No

Contraindications; Warnings; Precautions; Adverse Reactions

Contraindication
Hypersensitivity

Warnings
1. This drug has a low abuse potential. However, psychological and physical dependence and tolerance may follow abuse or misuse. Use with caution in patients with a history of abuse. Abrupt discontinuation after prolonged use has been followed by abdominal cramps, nausea, vomiting, rhinorrhea, lacrimation, restlessness, anxiety, elevated temperature, and piloerection.
2. There may be impairment in the ability to perform hazardous tasks such as driving a car. Use with caution in ambulatory patients.
3. Use in children is not recommended.
4. Safety for use in pregnancy has not been established except for use during labor. This drug can produce respiratory depression in the neonate, and should be used with caution in women delivering premature infants.
5. The respiratory depressant effects and the potential to elevate the cerebrospinal fluid pressure may be exaggerated in the presence of head injuries, intracranial lesions, or a preexisting increase in intracranial pressure. This drug, like other analgesics, can obscure the clinical manifestations of brain injuries or lesions (e.g.,

change in mental status). Use with extreme caution under these circumstances.
6. This drug has an additive effect when administered with other narcotics, anesthetics, phenothiazines, tranquilizers, sedatives, hypnotics, or any CNS depressant. Dosages must be modified accordingly.

Precautions
1. Some respiratory depression occurs with the normal dose of 10 mg. This depression though similar to that seen with morphine, is not increased greatly with increasing dosages. The depression produced can be reversed with naloxone hydrochloride (see page 237). There should be a reduction in dosage in patients with preexisting respiratory depression regardless of cause.
2. A reduction in dosage may be necessary in patients with impaired renal function.
3. Use with caution in patients with myocardial infarction who have nausea and vomiting; this drug may increase the severity of these problems.
4. Administer with caution to patients about to undergo surgery of the biliary tract since it may cause spasm of the sphincter of Oddi.
5. Narcotic-dependent persons may experience withdrawal symptoms with the use of nalbuphine. If symptoms are serious they may be controlled with small intravenous doses of morphine. In patients who may have withdrawal problems, small doses of nalbuphine can be given (1/4 normal). Progressively larger doses can be given if symptoms do not occur until a desirable level of analgesia is obtained.

Adverse Reactions
1. Central Nervous System Effects: sedation, dizziness, vertigo, headache are most frequently

nalbuphine hydrochloride
(continued)
seen. Others include: nervousness, depression, restlessness, extremes in emotions, hallucinations, dysphoria, feeling of heaviness, numbness, tingling, feeling of unreality, delusions.
2. Cardiovascular: hypertension, hypotension, bradycardia, tachycardia.
3. Gastrointestinal: cramps, dyspepsia, nausea, vomiting, bitter taste.
4. Respiratory: depression, dyspnea, asthma.
5. Dermatological: rashes, itching, burning and urticaria.
6. Miscellaneous: hypersensitivity, speech difficulty, urinary urgency, blurred vision, flushing and warmth.

Overdosage
Naloxone hydrochloride (Narcan) is a specific antidote that will reverse respiratory and CNS depression. Oxygen, assisted breathing, fluids, and vasopressors should be used as indicated. See Nursing Implications.

☐ **Nursing Implications**
1. Monitor closely for respiratory depression for 1 hour after an intravenous injection of this drug. If respiratory rate falls below 8 per minute, attempt to stimulate the patient to breath deeply at an adequate rate (10–12 times per minute). If the patient is too drowsy to respond, begin to assist breathing either by the mouth-to-mouth technique or with a manual breathing bag and mask with oxygen (one should be readily available). Notify the physician and have naloxone hydrochloride prepared for intravenous administration. The initial dose will be 0.1 to 0.4 mg. Fluids and vasopressors may also be needed. Do not leave the patient unattended until a full recovery is made.
2. Special preparations should be made for patients not on a respirator who have preexisting problems that will predispose them to respiratory depression; e.g., hypoxia, pulmonary infection, chest trauma, chest surgery, chest malformations, emphysema, asthma, postanesthesia patients, patients in shock or those who have received neuromuscular blocking agents. These patients should not be left alone. At the bedside have the following:
  a. Oxygen
  b. Oral-pharyngeal airways
  c. Suction equipment
  d. Endotracheal tubes and laryngoscope
  e. Manual breathing bag
Follow guidelines under No. 1 above. Peak depression will occur within 15–30 minutes after injection. Normal respirations will return in 2 hours.
3. In patients who may have or have the potential to develop a rise in intracranial pressure, monitor neurologic signs, blood pressure and heart rate every 30 minutes after injections.
4. Monitor for changes in mental status and take precautions to prevent undue anxiety and injury. Use siderails for all patients. If the patient becomes confused, close attendance and reassurance will be needed. Warn the patient about blurred vision and speech difficulties to decrease anxiety.
5. Monitor patients electrocardiographically who have preexisting arrhythmias, tachycardia, and bradycardias. Monitor blood pressure every 30 minutes for the first one to one and one half hours.
6. Be prepared to manage vomiting to prevent aspiration.
7. Monitor for signs of hypersensitivity.
8. If administration has been prolonged (several weeks) monitor for signs of withdrawal. Also monitor for withdrawal symptoms in patients who may be drug (narcotic) dependent at

the time of injection. Nalbuphine is a narcotic antagonist agent. See Precaution No. 5.

9. Monitor neonatal respiratory status if the mother received this drug during labor, especially if the infant is premature or has other problems. Be prepared for respiratory resuscitation.

10. Use with caution in outpatients; they should be fully recovered prior to discharge and should be accompanied home by a responsible adult. The patient should not drive or perform potentially hazardous tasks for the next 24 hours. Ambulate all patients carefully to prevent injury.

11. Administer successive doses when pain is just beginning to return. Do not wait until it returns to full intensity. Dosage intervals must be determined by patient response rather than time intervals. Notify the physician if pain is returning before the time interval he has prescribed is reached.

naloxone hydrochloride ■
(Narcan and Narcan Neonatal)

Actions/Indications
Narcotic antagonist.

Used to reverse narcotic depression, including respiratory depression, induced by natural and synthetic narcotics, i.e., opiates, opiate derivatives and synthetic opiates such as:
- Alphaprodine
- Anileridine
- Butorphanol
- Codeine
- Fentanyl
- Heroin
- Hydromorphone
- Meperidine
- Methadone
- Morphine
- Nalbuphine
- Oxycodone
- Oxymorphone
- Pentazocine

- Propoxyphene

Does not produce respiratory depression seen in other narcotic antagonists.

Exhibits no activity in the absence of a narcotic.

Onset of action is within 2 min.

Dosage
Adults:
Narcotic overdosage—0.4 mg (1 ml). Repeat at 2- to 3-min intervals as necessary.

Failure after 2–3 doses indicates non-narcotic source of depression.

Postoperative narcotic depression—titrate with 0.1–0.2 mg at 2–3 min intervals. Objective is return of respiratory adequacy without loss of analgesia.

Children and Neonates:
Narcotic overdosage—0.01 mg/kg; repeat at 2- to 3-min intervals. Lack of response after 2–3 doses indicates non-narcotic source of depression. Use only Neonatal Injection form.

Repeat doses may be necessary within 1 to 2 hours or more depending on the duration of action of the narcotic that the patient has received.

Preparation and Storage
Supplied in 1-ml vials.
Adult strength—0.4 mg/ml.
Neonatal strength—0.02 mg/ml.
Do not add to fluids.

Drug Incompatibilities
Do not mix with any other medication in any manner.

Modes of IV Administration

Injection
Yes
May be injected without further dilution directly into the vein (umbilical in neonates) or into the Y injection site of IV tubing. Slow injection avoids nausea and vomiting.

Intermittent Infusion
No
Pharmacologically inappropriate.

naloxone hydrochloride
(continued)
Continuous Infusion
No
Not recommended by manufacturer; some groups using this mode experimentally.

Contraindications; Warnings; Precautions; Adverse Reactions

Contraindications
Hypersensitivity

Warnings
1. Administer with caution to any patient thought to be an opiate addict, including newborns. This drug will induce acute withdrawal.
2. Keep patients under constant surveillance. The duration of some narcotics may exceed that of naloxone.
3. This agent is not effective against respiratory depression secondary to nonopioid drugs or other conditions.
4. Safety for use in pregnancy has not been established; must be used only when expected benefits outweigh the potential risks.

Precautions
1. All other supportive measures for respiratory and circulatory depression must be applied.
2. Ventricular tachycardia and fibrillation have been reported in patients with pre-existing ventricular irritability, or who were on isoproterenol or epinephrine for hypotension.
3. In rare cases, rapid reversal of narcotic anesthesia in cardiac patients has resulted in pulmonary edema.

Adverse Reactions
1. Nausea and vomiting (rarely seen)
2. Abrupt reversal of narcotic depression may result in diaphoresis, tachycardia, increased blood pressure, and tremulousness.

☐ Nursing Implications
1. Respiratory depression can return if the duration of depressive effects of the narcotic last longer than the effects of naloxone.
2. Place the following equipment at the bedside or nearby: oralpharyngeal airways, endotracheal tubes and laryngoscope, suction, oxygen, manual breathing bag (Ambu, Hope, Puritan), arterial blood gas sampling equipment.
3. The patient should be under constant observation.
4. Monitor respiratory status. Respiratory depression is the primary indication for the use of this drug and is diagnosed by the presence of hypercarbia (elevated pCO_2) and hypoxemia (reduced pO_2). Signs and symptoms of hypoxia include: tachycardia, pallor, hypotension, confusion, restlessness.
5. Assist respirations until naloxone is effective as indicated by an adequate spontaneous respiratory rate and return of gag, cough and swallow reflexes. (See No. 1 above.)
6. Examine frequently for signs of vomiting. Take precautions to prevent aspiration (position patient on one side, keep suction equipment ready to use, gastric intubation if abdominal distention is present).
7. Patients should be intubated if there is vomiting, if ventilation via airway and mask is ineffective (no improvement in arterial blood pO_2 or pCO_2) or if such support will be required for a prolonged period of time.
8. Monitor blood pressure and heart rate (apically or via ECG monitor) every 3–5 minutes until the patient has recovered and/or vital signs have reached desirable levels and stabilized (as determined by the physician).
9. Patients with pre-existing ventricular irritability, secondary to pathology or drugs, should be

placed on continuous ECG monitoring. Be prepared to treat ventricular tachycardia or fibrillation.

10. Be prepared to manage acute narcotic withdrawal symptoms in the narcotic addict. Use side rails at all times; restraints may be necessary.

11. Signs of acute withdrawal in the neonate:[1]
    a. Excessive irritability, crying, etc.
    b. Increased appetite, yet poor feeding ability
    c. Reduced sleeping periods
    d. Tremulousness
    e. Rarely seizures
    f. Diarrhea and vomiting
    g. Tachypnea
    h. Fever
    i. Sneezing
    Report the onset of any one of these signs to the physician.

12. Withdrawal of any form of support should be supervised by a physician.

Reference

1. Kandall, Stephen R.: Managing Neonatal Withdrawal. *Drug Therapy*, May 1976, p. 48.

Suggested Readings

Kandall, Stephen R.: Managing Neonatal Withdrawal. *Drug Therapy*, May 1976, pp. 47–58.

McCaffery, Margo, and Hart, Linda: Undertreatment of Acute Pain with Narcotics. *American Journal of Nursing*, 76(10):1586–1591, October 1976.

Rogers, Robert M., and Juers, John A.: Physiologic Considerations in the Treatment of Acute Respiratory Failure. *Basics of Respiratory Disease*, 3(4), March 1975.

neostigmine methylsulfate ■
(Prostigmin)

Actions/Indications

Cholinesterase inhibitor; enhances transmission of impulses at nerve-muscle junction. *Intravenous route* is indicated as an antidote for tubocurarine or curarelike drugs, e.g., pancuronium. Also can be used in emergency management of myasthenia gravis.

Dosage

Adults and Older Children Over 12 Years of Age:
0.5–2.0 mg. Do not exceed 5 mg. The heart rate should be increased pharmacologically (with atropine) to 80 beats/min before neostigmine is administered (see Precaution No. 2).

Do not administer in the presence of high concentrations of halothane or cyclopropane.

The ideal time to administer this drug is when the patient is being hyperventilated and the pCO_2 of the blood is low.

Children Under 12 Years of Age:
No dosage recommendation available from the manufacturer.

Preparation and Storage

Supplied in the following forms:
1-ml ampuls, 1:2000 (0.5 mg/ml)
1-ml ampuls, 1:4000 (0.25 mg/ml)
10-ml multidose vials, 1:1000 (1 mg/ml)
10-ml multidose vials, 1:2000 (0.5 mg/ml)
Do not add to fluids.

Drug Incompatibilities

Do not mix with any other medication.

Modes of IV Administration

Injection
Yes
May give undiluted *slowly* 0.5 mg/min.

Intermittent Infusion
No
Pharmacologically inappropriate.

Continuous Infusion
No
Pharmacologically inappropriate.

neostigmine methylsulfate
(continued)
Contraindications; Warnings; Precautions; Adverse Reactions

Contraindications
1. Mechanical intestinal or urinary obstruction
2. Hypersensitivity

Precautions
1. Use with caution in asthmatics.
2. Atropine (1 mg) should be at the bedside. Some groups administer 0.6–1.2 mg of atropine prior to neostigmine.
3. Atropine may be used to abolish or decrease gastrointestinal side effects of this drug but can mask overdosage and lead to inadvertent induction of a cholinergic crisis, and should therefore be given in small doses, carefully titrated with patient response.
4. Overdose may result in a cholinergic crisis characterized by increasing muscular weakness involving respiratory muscles; apnea may result. This may be difficult to distinguish from a myasthenic crisis. Such distinction *must* be made to avoid grave consequences. Tensilon test (edrophonium) may be used to differentiate between cholinergic and myasthenic crises. See page 144.

Adverse Reactions
1. Usually due to overdosage: nausea, vomiting, diarrhea, cramps, increased salivation, increased bronchial secretions, diaphoresis. These can be counteracted by *careful* use of atropine 0.5 mg (see Precautions Nos. 2–4). Other symptoms of overdosage are muscle cramps, muscle twitching, and weakness.
2. Bradycardia may also occur, and can be treated with atropine if necessary.

☐ **Nursing Implications**
1. Maintain an adequate airway and ventilation until recovery is complete and spontaneous respirations have returned.
2. Respiratory support equipment (airways, oxygen, suction, endotracheal tubes and laryngoscope, manual breathing bag [Ambu, Hope, Puritan]) should be readily available or in use until respiratory effort, rate, and effectiveness are appropriate and gag, cough, swallow reflexes have returned. (See care of the patient receiving tubocurarine, p. 343.)
3. Atropine 1.0 mg should be at the bedside. (See administration of atropine, p. 24.)
4. Monitor for adverse effects (see above).
5. Be prepared to manage vomiting to maintain airway and prevent aspiration. Keep the patient in lateral decubitus position if possible; keep suction equipment ready for use.

Suggested Readings
Guyton, Arthur C.: *Textbook of Medical Physiology* (5th ed.), Philadelphia, W. B. Saunders Company, 1976; Chapter 12, Neuromuscular Transmission, Function of Smooth Muscle, pp. 147–157; Chapter 15, The Autonomic Nervous System; The Adrenal Medulla, pp. 768–781.
Jones, LeAnna: Myasthenia and Me. *RN*, June 1976, pp. 50–55.
Smith, Dorothy W., and Germain, Carol P. Hanley: *Care of the Adult Patient,* (4th ed.), Philadelphia, J. B. Lippincott Company, 1977, pp. 382–384.

nitrofurantoin sodium ▧
(Ivadantin)

Actions/Indications
Synthetic antibacterial agent for urinary tract infections due to: *E. coli*, enterococci (e.g., *Streptococcus faecalis*), *Staphylococcus aureus*. Some strains of *Enterobacter* and *Klebsiella* species are resistant to this drug, as are most *Proteus* and *Serratia* species. There is no activity against *Pseudomo-*

nas organisms. Susceptibility tests must be performed.

This drug should only be used when oral therapy is impossible. Excretion is through the kidneys.

Dosage
In patient over 120 lbs—180 mg twice daily

In patients less than 120 lbs—3 mg/lb/day in 2 equal doses

Continue for at least 7 days, and for 3 days after sterile urine is obtained.

Preparation and Storage
Supplied in vials of 180 mg of drug powder. Dissolve just prior to administration. Add 20 ml of D5W or sterile water for injection (do not use any other diluent) to vial and shake. For final dilution add each ml of drug to 25 ml of intravenous fluid. For example, a 180 mg dose (in 20 ml of initial diluent) should be added to 500 ml of fluid for infusion (D5W, NS, etc.). Gently shake final solution prior to infusion. Use solutions immediately; infuse within 24 hours.

Drug Incompatibilities
Do not mix with any other medication in any manner.

Modes of IV Administration

Injection
No

Intermittent Infusion
Yes
Infuse at a rate of 2–3 ml/minute. (Avoid rapid administration)

Continuous Infusion
Yes
Infuse at a rate of 2–3 ml/minute. (Avoid rapid administration)

Contraindications; Warnings; Precautions; Adverse Reactions

Contraindications
1. Anuria, oliguria, or significant renal impairment (creatinine clearance under 40 ml per minute).

2. Pregnancy at term (may cause hemolytic anemia in infant).
3. Known hypersensitivity to this drug, or any nitrofurantoin preparation.

Warnings
1. Acute (pneumonitis), subacute and chronic (fibrosis) pulmonary reactions may occur. If this occurs, the drug must be discontinued. Onset may be insidious; monitor carefully. **Deaths have been reported.**
2. Hemolytic anemia (primaquine sensitivity type) can be induced by this drug. This may be linked to glucose-6-phosphate dehydrogenase deficiency. If this occurs, discontinue therapy, hemolysis will cease.
3. Superinfections have occurred secondary to *Pseudomonas* and other resistant organisms.
4. Hepatitis including chronic-active has occurred. This may be a hypersensitivity reaction. Monitor liver enzymes. Fatalities have been reported.

Precautions
1. Peripheral neuropathy may occur; this may become severe or irreversible. Fatalities have been reported. Predisposing conditions to this are: renal impairment, anemia, diabetes, electrolyte imbalance, vitamin B deficiency and other debilitating conditions.
2. Safety for use in pregnancy and lactation has not been established.
3. Safety for use in children under 12 has not been established.

Adverse Reactions
1. Gastrointestinal: anorexia, nausea, vomiting, abdominal pain, diarrhea (these can be avoided by proper infusion rate; see Modes of Intravenous Administration).
2. Hepatitis (hypersensitivity reaction).
3. Pulmonary hypersensitivity: see

nitrofurantoin sodium
(continued)

Warning No. 1. Acute reactions in the form of pneumonitis usually occur within the first week of therapy and are reversible with discontinuation of the drug. Subacute reactions, fever, and eosinophilia are seen less frequently; recovery is slower after withdrawal of the drug. Chronic reactions are more likely to occur in patients who have been on continuous therapy for 6 months or more. Pulmonary function may be permanently impaired secondary to fibrosis. The problem must be recognized early for prompt withdrawal of the drug and subsequent resolution of the problem. See Nursing Implications for symptomatology.

4. Dermatologic: maculopapular, erythematous, or eczematous eruption, pruritus, urticaria, and angioedema.
5. Other sensitivity reactions: anaphylaxis, asthmatic attack in asthmatic patients, cholestatic jaundice, drug fever, and arthralgia.
6. Hematologic: hemolytic anemia, granulocytopenia, leukopenia, eosinophilia, and megaloblastic anemia (blood counts return to normal after cessation of the drug).
7. Neurologic: peripheral neuropathy, headache, dizziness, nystagmus and drowsiness.
8. Miscellaneous: transient alopecia, superinfections by resistant organisms; this only occurs in the genitourinary tract.

☐ **Nursing Implications**
1. Monitor for the onset of an acute pulmonary hypersensitivity reaction. Symptoms:
   a. Fever
   b. Chills
   c. Cough
   d. Chest pain
   e. Dyspnea
   f. Increased respiratory rate

Chest x-ray changes will be infiltrates, with consolidation or pleural effusion. There will be eosinophilia. This will occur usually during the first week. Notify the physician of the onset of any symptom.
Chronic reactions may be more insidious in onset and should be watched for in any patient on prolonged therapy. There will be malaise, dyspnea, cough on exertion and altered pulmonary function studies. Chest x-ray will show diffuse interstitial pneumonitis or fibrosis. Fever is rare.

2. Monitor for the onset of hemolytic anemia; i.e., jaundice. Notify the physician.
3. Urine should periodically be sent for culture to detect effectiveness of therapy; i.e., sterile specimen, and the onset of a superinfection due to *Pseudomonas* or other resistant organism.
4. Monitor for signs and symptoms of peripheral neuropathy; e.g., numbness in fingers and toes, "pins and needles" sensations, difficulty in fine motor control of the hands.
5. Maintain correct infusion rate to prevent gastrointestinal disturbances. Use an infusion pump.
6. Take anaphylaxis precautions; see Appendix.
7. Monitor temperature every 8 hours for effectiveness of therapy (normal temperature) or for signs of drug fever or other adverse reactions. Notify the physician of an elevation or patterns in elevations.
8. Warn the patient that his urine will be brown. Inform him of the possibility of alopecia. Reassure him that this is transient, and that the hair will grow back.
9. Provide comfort measures for rashes; e.g., cool environment, topical care, frequent turning and skin care. Avoid plastic underpads on affected areas.
10. Take safety precautions if the patient experiences neurologic effects such as dizziness, nystagmus, or drowsiness.

nitroglycerin ■
Nitrostat IV, Tridil

Actions/Indications
Vasodilator. Relaxes smooth muscle
of blood vessels, dilating venous and
arterial beds; decreases venous return, reducing left ventricular end-
diastolic pressure; reduces arterial
pressure; decreases myocardial oxygen consumption.
Indicated for:
- control of blood pressure in
  perioperative hypertension
- congestive heart failure associated
  with acute myocardial infarction
- treatment of angina pectoris in
  patients who have not responded
  to organic nitrates or a beta-
  blocker
- production of controlled hypotension during surgical procedures

Dosage

*The dosage delivered to the patient
is affected by the type of container
and administration tubing used; see
warnings.*

Adults:
(Using non-absorbing tubing—
Nitrostat IV infusion set[1] or
Tridilset[2])
  Initial dose—5 mcg/ min using an
infusion pump. Titrate in 5 mcg/min
increments with increases every 3–5
minutes until a response is noted. If
no response is seen at 20 mcg/min,
use increments of 10 mcg/min, then
20 mcg/min. Once a partial response occurs, reduce the dose increases and lengthen the interval
between increases.
  If standard plastic (PVC) tubing is
used, as much as 25 mcg/min may
be required for the initial dose.

Children:
NOT RECOMMENDED

Preparation and Storage
Note: Several preparations of IV Nitroglycerin are available, differing in
concentration per ampul. BE SURE
OF THE PRODUCT BEING USED
AND FOLLOW MANUFACTUR-
ER'S INSTRUCTIONS FOR DILU-
TION, DOSAGE AND
ADMINISTRATION.
  Nitrostat[1]—supplied in 10 ml ampuls containing 8 mg of drug. Tridil
[2]—supplied in 10 ml ampuls containing 50 mg of drug.
  Both preparations may be diluted
in either D5W or NS. In selecting
the appropriate dilution it is necessary to consider the patient's fluid
requirements as well as the expected
duration of the infusion.
  For **Nitrostat IV**, the most convenient dilution for calculation is to
add 2, 10 ml ampuls (16 mg) to 250
ml D5W or NS **in glass bottles**. This
provides a concentration of 60
mcg/ml. Using a **microdrop set** (60
drops = 1 ml), the desired dose in
mcg/min will equal the number of
drops/min (and ml/hr); e.g., to obtain 5 mcg/min, adjust flow to 5
drops/min; to obtain 20 mcg/min,
adjust flow to 20 drops/min.
  A less concentrated solution can
be made by adding 1, 10ml ampul
(8 mg) to 250 ml D5W or NS, providing a concentration of approximately 30 mcg/ml. To achieve a
desired dose, double the number of
drops/min; e.g., to obtain 5
mcg/min, adjust flow to 10
drops/min; to obtain 20 mcg/min,
adjust flow to 40 drops/min.
  In patients for whom fluid restriction is required, a more concentrated solution can be made by adding
3, 10 ml ampuls (24 mg) to 250 ml
D5W or NS, to provide a concentration of approximately 85 mcg/ml.
The desired dose at this concentration can be achieved as follows:

With a Concentration of 85 mcg/ml (Nitrostat IV)

Dose (mcg/min)	Flow rate (microdrops/min)
5	3
10	7
15	10
20	14
50	35
80	56
100	70

nitroglycerin
(continued)
Whenever the concentration is changed, it is necessary to flush the tubing to avoid a delay in the delivery of the new concentration to the patient. (With very low flow rates it could take up to 3 hours for the new concentration to reach the patient.)

For **Tridil**, initial dilution add 1 ampul (50 mg) to 500 ml **glass** container of D5W or NS. This provides a concentration of 100 mcg/ml. For patients requiring high dosages or prolonged infusion and those on fluid restriction, more concentrated solutions can be made: Add 1 ampul (50 mg) to 250 ml (or 2 ampuls-100 mg to 500 ml) of D5W or NS to provide 200 mcg/ml or add 2 ampuls (100 mg) to 250 ml (or 4 ampuls 200 mg to 500 ml) D5W or NS to provide 400 mcg/ml. The concentration should not exceed 400 mcg/ml.

Using a **microdrop** set (60 microdrops = 1 ml) the desired dosage can be calculated as follows:

With a Concentration of 100 mcg/ml (Tridil)

Dose (mcg/ml)	Flow Rate (Microdrops/min)
5	3
10	6
20	12
40	24
80	48
120	72
160	96

With a Concentration of 200 mcg/ml (Tridil)

Dose (mcg/ml)	Flow Rate (Microdrops/min)
10	3
20	6
40	12
80	24
160	48
240	72
320	96

With a Concentration of 400 mcg/ml (Tridil)

Dose (mcg/ml)	Flow Rate (Microdrops/min)
20	3
40	6
80	12
160	24
320	48
480	72
640	96

Drug Incompatibilities
Do not mix with any other medication in any manner.

Modes of IV Administration

Injection
No
THIS IS A CONCENTRATED, POTENT DRUG THAT MUST BE HIGHLY DILUTED BEFORE ADMINISTRATION.

Intermittent Infusion
No
This drug must be highly diluted and administered by titration. See Continuous Infusion.

Continuous Infusion
Yes
Use D5W or NS. The type and volume of diluent used is determined by the patient's fluid requirements and expected duration of the infusion. See Preparation and Storage section for specific instructions regarding preparation of solution. Use an infusion pump and microdrop tubing. See Nursing Implications No. 1. Titrate as indicated under Dosage to achieve desired blood pressure or relief of symptoms.

Contraindications; Warnings; Precautions; Adverse Reactions

Contraindications
1. Known hypersensitivity to nitroglycerin or idiosyncratic reaction to organic nitrates.
2. Hypotension or uncorrected hypovolemia.

3. Increased intracranial pressure (head trauma or cerebral hemorrhage).
4. Constrictive pericarditis or pericardial tamponade.

Warnings

1. Use only glass intravenous solution bottles; nitroglycerin is absorbed by polyvinyl chloride (PVC) plastic containers. (Recent evidence suggests that semirigid polyolefin containers (Accumed[3]) may be used for nitroglycerin solution without loss of nitroglycerin[4]).
2. Avoid use of micropore filters if possible; some absorb nitroglycerin.
3. Forty to eighty percent of nitroglycerin in the final solution is absorbed by the standard intravenous tubing. Loss is minimal (<one percent) with special sets designed specifically for nitroglycerin administration (See Dosage). Calculation of dosage *must* consider which type of tubing is being used.

Precautions

1. Use the caution in severe hepatic or renal disease
2. Avoid excessive hypotension especially for prolonged periods; ischemia, thrombosis and malfunction of vital organs can result. Hypotension is more likely in patients with normal or low pulmonary capillary wedge pressure.
3. Safety for use in pregnancy and lactation has not been established; use in pregnancy and lactation only when clearly needed.
4. Safety and effectiveness in children has not been established.

Adverse Reactions

1. Headache
2. Tachycardia
3. Nausea, vomiting
4. Apprehension, restlessness
5. Muscle twitching

6. Retrosternal discomfort, palpitations
7. Dizziness
8. Abdominal pain

Overdosage

Overdosage may produce severe hypotension and reflex tachycardia. Treat by elevating legs; decrease or discontinue infusion until the condition stabilizes. On rare occasions use of an agent such as methoxamine or phenylephrine may be required.

☐ Nursing Implications

1. Since there is a marked variation in concentration among different preparations of this drug, it is essential to be certain which form is being used for accuracy in preparation and administration of infusion. Whenever possible, use an administration set designed for nitroglycerin (Nitrostat IV infusion set or Tridilset) to prevent absorption by the tubing. Volumetric infusion pumps requiring special tubing with volume control chambers cannot be used in conjunction with Nitrostat or Tridil tubing. If this tubing is used, the linear peristaltic type of pump must be used, with care taken to monitor dosage being delivered. An alternative is to use the standard PVC tubing provided with the volumetric pumps. (See Warning No. 3.) If standard plastic (PVC) tubing must be used, dosage must be increased accordingly to allow for the absorption. Highest rates of absorption occur during the early phase of infusion and whenever flow rates are low.
2. During administration, blood pressure and heart rate *must* be monitored in all patients to guide titration of this drug. When indicated, it is also desirable to monitor direct arterial blood pressure and pulmonary capillary wedge pressure. A fall in wedge pressure precedes a

nitroglycerin
(continued)
fall in arterial blood pressure.
3. Keeping in mind the patient's pretreatment blood pressure, begin the infusion at the prescribed rate. Obtain blood pressure (and other parameters) every 1–2 minutes. Titrate the infusion (increasing in 5 mcg increments) every 3–5 minutes until the blood pressure reaches the desired limits preset by the physician.
4. Prevent a sudden fall in blood pressure below the normal limits for the patient since severe hypotension can produce ischemia of the heart and other vital organs. Report hypotension or tachycardia to the physician. (See Overdosage.)
5. Instruct the patient to report, if possible, any chest pain or palpitations especially if the patient is receiving nitroglycerin for angina pectoris or congestive heart failure associated with a myocardial infarction. The physician must differentiate between chest pain caused by the pathology and by the drug and then discontinue or adjust the dosage as indicated.
6. Monitor urine output hourly, especially in patients with renal disease. Excessive reduction of arterial pressure will decrease the urinary output. Notify the physician if this occurs.
7. Nausea and vomiting may occur; be prepared to prevent aspiration.

References
1. Park-Davis, Division of Warner-Lambert Company, Morris Plains, NJ 07950
2. American Critical Care, Division of American Hospital Supply Corporation, McGaw Park, IL 60085
3. McGaw Laboratories, Inc., Irvine, CA 92714
4. Amann, A.H., et al: Plastic IV Containers for Nitroglycerin

(letter), *American Journal of Hospital Pharmacy*, 37: 618, May 1980.

nitroprusside, sodium ■
(Nipride)

Actions/Indications
Antihypertensive, potent and rapid-acting. Effect is immediate and ends on stopping infusion. Has direct action on blood vessel walls, both arterial and venous, to produce vasodilatation.

There are no direct effects on the central or autonomic nervous systems.

Used to control hypertensive crisis in essential and malignant hypertension, acute glomerulonephritis, eclampsia, and dissecting aortic aneurysm.

Also used by some groups for vasodilation in acute myocardial infarction and pump failure. (The use of this drug in this manner has not been approved by the FDA.)

Nitroprusside can also be used to produce controlled hypotension during surgery to decrease bleeding.

Dosage
Adults and Children:
Average dose in the absence of any other antihypertensive agent: 3 mcg/kg/min.
Range—0.5–10.0 mcg/kg/min.
Titrate With Arterial Blood Pressure.
Infusion rates greater than 10 mcg/kg/min should not be used. If at this rate an adequate reduction of BP is not obtained in 10 min, **stop** infusion.
Infusion is usually continued for 24–48 hours while oral antihypertensive therapy is initiated.

Preparation and Storage
Supplied in 5-ml vials containing 50 mg of drug. Reconstitute by adding 2–3 ml D5W to vial. Prepare for infusion by adding 50 mg of drug to 500 ml D5W *only*. This solution contains 100 mcg/ml (50 mg can also be added to 250 ml D5W to produce a solution of 200 mcg/ml).

Solutions of 100 mcg/ml are now considered to be stable for up to 24 hours. More concentrated solutions must still be replaced after 4 hours. Promptly wrap IV bottle with aluminum wrap provided by manufacturer to protect the solution from light.* Use within 4 hours of preparation. Discard solution that is any color besides light brown.
Use infusion pump and microdrop administration set.
With the 100 mcg/ml solution, there is 1.5 mcg/microdrop of solution.
*It is not necessary to wrap the IV tubing because the time spent by the drug in the tubing is minimal.

Drug Incompatibilities
Do not mix with any other medication in bottle or line.

Modes of IV Administration

Injection
No

Intermittent Infusion
No

Continuous Infusion
Yes
Use D5W only. See Preparation and Storage.
Use infusion pump and microdrop administration set.

Contraindications; Warnings; Precautions; Adverse Reactions

Contraindications
1. Compensatory hypertension in A-V shunt or coarctation of the aorta
2. For controlled hypotension, during surgery in patients with known inadequate cerebral circulation

Warnings
1. Use only dextrose 5% and water for reconstitution and infusion.
2. This drug is metabolized into thiocyanate. Excess infusion of nitroprusside, greater than 10 mcg/min., can result in thiocya-

nate toxicity (tinnitus, blurred vision, delirium, muscle spasm). Gross overdosage can produce *cyanide* toxicity.
When higher infusion rates are needed, blood acid-base balance must be carefully monitored, as metabolic acidosis is the earliest, most reliable evidence of cyanide toxicity. If acidosis occurs, alternate forms of therapy must be sought.
3. Thiocyanate inhibits uptake and binding of iodine. Use with caution in hypothyroidism.
4. Use with caution in severe renal or hepatic impairment. Therapy should be guided by serum thiocyanate levels (not to exceed 10 mg/100 ml).
5. Chronically hypertensive patients and those receiving other antihypertensive agents are more sensitive to the action of this drug. Careful titration with blood pressure will prevent overdosage.
6. Safety for use in pregnancy has not been established. Benefits to the mother must outweigh potential hazards to the fetus.
7. A rebound tachycardia may occur secondary to reduction in blood pressure. In patients where such a tachycardia could be detrimental (congestive heart failure, aortic aneurysm), pretreat with propranolol to reduce sinus rate (see page 298 for further information on propranolol).
8. Warnings that apply when this drug is used for controlled hypotension during surgery:
   a. Correct pre-existing anemia, and hypovolemia if possible.
   b. Hypotensive anesthetic techniques can alter pulmonary ventilation perfusion ratios, making some patients require higher oxygen partial pressure.
   c. *Extreme* caution should be used during this procedure on patients who are poor surgical risks.

nitroprusside, sodium
(continued)
Precautions
1. The patient must be under constant surveillance. Means by which to monitor direct arterial blood pressure (preferred) or indirect pressure (acceptable) must be employed.
2. Infusion rates greater than 10 mcg/kg are rarely required. If adequate reduction in blood pressure is not seen at this rate, stop the infusion.
3. Avoid extravasation.
4. Use with caution and in initially low doses in the elderly; they are more sensitive to the hypotensive effects of this drug.
5. This drug is thought to affect platelet function.

Adverse Reactions
1. Nausea, vomiting, diaphoresis, abdominal pain, chest pain, anxiety, headache, restlessness, muscle twitching, dizziness, are usually due to rapid infusion and disappear with decreased flow rate.
2. Cyanide toxicity; see Warnings No. 2, 3, 4.
3. Irritation of vein at infusion site.

Overdosage
1. First sign of overdosage (thiocyanate toxicity) is profound hypotension.
2. Metabolic acidosis may be an early indication of overdosage, and may be associated with dyspnea, headache, vomiting, dizziness, ataxia, loss of consciousness. Confirm the presence of acidosis with an arterial blood gas study.
3. Infusion must be stopped with the appearance of any of the above. In the patient with renal failure, hemodialysis may be required to remove thiocyanate from the body.
4. Massive overdosage may produce signs similar to those of cyanide poisoning: coma, imperceptible peripheral pulses, absent reflexes, widely dilated pupils, pink skin color, hypotension and shallow breathing.
5. Treatment of massive overdosage, i.e. cyanide accumulation in the tissues:
   a. Discontinue Nitroprusside.
   b. Administer amyl nitrite inhalations for 15–30 seconds each minute until a 3% sodium nitrite solution can be prepared for IV administration.
   c. Inject 3% sodium nitrite IV at a rate not to exceed 2.5–5.0 ml/minute up to a total dose of 10–15 ml with careful monitoring of blood pressure. Use vasopressors to correct hypotension.
   d. Following the above steps, inject sodium thiosulfate IV, 12.5 gm in 50 ml of D5W, over a 10-minute period.
   e. Signs of overdosage may reappear. If this occurs, repeat above therapy at 1/2 dosage.

☐ **Nursing Implications**
1. Be prepared to accurately monitor arterial blood pressure, preferably by arterial cannulation. If this type of monitoring is unavailable, indirect readings using a sphygmomanometer can be used.
2. Monitor the ECG continuously during therapy.
3. Weigh the patient for dosage calculation.
4. Keeping in mind the patient's pretreatment blood pressure, begin the infusion at 0.5–1.0 mcg/kg/minute (approximately 1 microdrop/kg/minute using 100 mcg/ml solution). A lower dosage will be prescribed for renal patients. Obtain blood pressure readings every 1–2 minutes. Do not allow the blood pressure to drop at too rapid a rate. The physician must determine the blood pressure goal to be reached by therapy. Increase the infusion every 5 minutes by 0.5–1.0 mcg/kg/min (or 5

microdrops) until the blood pressure goal has been reached.

5. Monitor for signs and symptoms of thiocyanate toxicity: ringing in the ears, blurring of vision, slurred speech, delirium, muscle spasms. If one or more of these effects occur, decrease the infusion rate immediately. Notify the physician, who may want to monitor serum acid-base balance and/or thiocyanate levels. (Toxic signs and symptoms appear at serum levels of 5–10 mg/100 ml.; fatalities have occurred at levels of 20 mg/100 ml.[2]) Continue close monitoring of blood pressure. (See Overdosage above.)

6. Monitor for the consequences of sudden severe elevation of blood pressure:
   a. Encephalopathy—confusion, stupor
   b. Cerebrovascular accident—muscle paralysis or weakness
   c. Myocardial ischemia and/or infarction—chest pain, ECG changes, arrhythmias
   d. Left ventricular failure—shortness of breath, orthopnea, elevated central venous pressure or pulmonary artery (wedge) pressure, tachycardia, rales, third and/or fourth heart sound
   e. Renal failure—oliguria, rising BUN and creatinine.[3]

   Prevent a sudden fall in blood pressure below normal levels for the patient. Hypotension can also produce the complications listed above. If the patient is receiving nitroprusside for hypertension associated with an acute myocardial infarction, the physician must differentiate between chest pain caused by the pathology and by the drug, and then order adjustment in drug dosage.[4]

7. Keep the patient on bed rest.

8. After allowing the first dose of the oral antihypertensive agent to take effect, the infusion of nitroprusside can be discontin-ued abruptly. Keep the infusion connected to the IV line, ready for reinitiation in the event the blood pressure has not been controlled by the oral agent.

9. Monitor urine output hourly. Excessive reduction of arterial pressure will decrease the urine output. If this occurs, reduce the infusion rate by 1 mcg every 5 minutes until urine output improves. Notify the physician. The drug may also increase urine output due to decreased renal vascular resistance. Monitor for signs of hypovolemia and electrolyte imbalances, e.g., hyponatremia.[5]

10. Avoid extravasation; see Appendix.

11. Provide instruction on hypertension self-care prior to the patient's discharge from the hospital.

References

1. Communication from Roche Laboratories, April, 1982.
2. Palmer, Roger F. and Lasseter, Kenneth C.: Sodium Nitroprusside. *New England Journal of Medicine*, 292(6):295, February 6, 1975.
3. Romankiewicz, J. A.: Pharmacology and Clinical Use of Drugs in Hypertensive Emergencies. *American Journal of Hospital Pharmacy*, 34(2):185, February 1977.
4. Ziesch, Susan and Franciosa, Joseph: Clinical Application of Sodium Nitroprusside. *Heart and Lung*, 6:102, January–February 1977.
5. Ginkus-O'Connor, Nancy: Intravenous Drugs Used in Treating Hypertensive Emergencies. *Heart and Lung*, 10(5):849, Sept.–Oct. 1981.

Suggested Readings

American Medical Association Committee on Hypertension: The Treatment of Malignant Hypertension and Hypertensive Emergencies. *JAMA*, 228:1673–1679, June 24, 1974.

Ginkus-O'Connor, Nancy: Intravenous Drugs Used in Treating Hy-

nitroprusside, sodium
(continued)

pertensive Emergencies. *Heart and Lung*, 10(5):848–855, Sept.–Oct. 1981.

Jones, L. N.: Symposium on Teaching and Rehabilitation of the Cardiac Patient. Hypertension: Medical and Nursing Implications. *Nursing Clinics of North America*, 11:283–295, June 1976 (references).

Keith, Thomas: Hypertensive Crisis, Recognition and Management. *JAMA*, 237(15):1570–1577, April 11, 1977.

Koch-Wiser, Jan: Hypertensive Emergencies. *New England Journal of Medicine*, 290:211–214, January 24, 1974.

Kohli, R. K., et al.: Treating Acute Hypertensive Crisis With Sodium Nitroprusside. *American Family Physician*, 15(1):141–145, January 1977.

Long, M. L., et al.: Hypertension: What Patients Need to Know. *American Journal of Nursing*, 76:765–770, May 1976.

Moskowitz, Lani: Vasodilator Therapy in Acute Myocardial Infarction. *Heart and Lung*, 4(6):939–942, November–December 1975.

Palmer, Roger F. and Lasseter, Kenneth C.: Sodium Nitroprusside. *New England Journal of Medicine*, 292:294–296, February 6, 1975.

Romankiewicz, J. A.: Pharmacology and Clinical Use of Drugs in Hypertensive Emergencies. *American Journal of Hospital Pharmacy*, 34(2):185–193, February 1977 (references).

Ziesch, Susan, and Franciosa, Joseph: Clinical Application of Sodium Nitroprusside. *Heart and Lung*, 6:99–103, January–February 1977.

norepinephrine bitartrate ■
(Formerly called levarterenol bitartrate)
(Levophed Bitartrate)

Actions/Indications
Alpha and beta adrenergic stimulant, norepinephrine, which produces the following effects:

- Increased myocardial contractility (increases cardiac output)
- Dilatation of coronary arteries (increases coronary blood flow)
- Increased systemic blood pressure
- Increased venous return to the heart

Used to restore normal blood pressure in these hypotensive states:
- Postpheochromocytomectomy
- Postsympathectomy
- Acute myocardial infarction
- Septicemia
- Anaphylaxis
- Idiosyncratic or toxic reactions to drugs or blood transfusions
- Cardiac arrest
- Poliomyelitis
- Spinal anesthesia

Dosage
Adults and Children:
(All indications)
Initial drip rate—8–12 mcg/min. *Maintenance drip rate*—0.5–1.0 ml/min (2–4 mcg/min). Up to 68 mg/day have been given in severe cases.

Titrate to maintain arterial blood pressure, adequate tissue perfusion, CVP, or pulmonary capillary wedge pressure at desired level.
Do Not Abruptly Stop Infusion; Taper dosage down over several hours.

Preparation and Storage
Supplied in 4 ml ampuls containing 4 mg of drug. Do not use if solution is brown in color or contains a precipitate

Standard infusion solution: 4 ml (4 mg) of drug in 1000 ml D5W or D5/NS. Concentration will be: 4 mcg/ml

A more dilute solution may be used for patients requiring large volumes of fluid.

For patients requiring fluid restriction, add 4 ml (4 mg) to 500 ml solution. Concentration will be: 8 mcg/ml
Use **Only** D5W or D5/NS for Infusion Fluid.

Drug Incompatibilities
Do not mix in any manner with:
Aminophylline

Amobarbital
Barbiturates
Any cephalosporin
Chlorothiazide
Chlorpheniramine
Lidocaine
Novobiocin
Phenytoin
Sodium bicarbonate
Sodium iodide
Streptomycin
Sulfadiazine
Sulfisoxazole
Thiopental

Modes of IV Administration

Injection
No

Intermittent Infusion
No
Administer by titration; see Continuous Infusion below.

Continuous Infusion
Yes
Using the 4 or 8 mcg/ml solution, begin the infusion at the lowest suggested dosage rate. Increase dosage as necessary to elicit a patient response.
Use a volumetric infusion pump.

Contraindications; Warnings; Precautions; Adverse Reactions

Contraindications
1. Untreated hypovolemia, except as an initial emergency measure until blood replacements given.
2. Mesenteric or peripheral vascular thrombosis, unless given as a lifesaving measure.
3. During cyclopropane and halothane anesthesia and in profound hypoxia and hypocarbia, may precipitate ventricular tachycardia and/or fibrillation.

Warnings
Use with extreme caution in the presence of MAO inhibitors or antidepressants of the triptyline or imipramine types; concomitant use with norepinephrine may precipitate severe hypertension.

Precautions
1. Avoid producing hypertension with excessive administration of this drug. In previously hypertensive patients, it is recommended that the blood pressure be increased no higher than 40 mm Hg below the preexisting systolic pressure.
2. Use a large vein such as an antecubital for infusion. Avoid use of a cutdown site and use of lower extremity veins especially in the elderly or patients with occlusive vascular disorders.
3. Prevent extravasation; this drug's intense vasoconstrictive action will cause tissue necrosis and sloughing. Should extravasation occur, the area must be infiltrated with phentolamine (5–10 mg) *as soon as possible*. See Nursing Implication No. 7.

Adverse Reactions
1. Sinus bradycardia.
2. Overdosage can produce severe hypertension, reflex bradycardia, increased peripheral vascular resistance and decreased cardiac output.
3. Prolonged administration of any vasopressor may produce plasma volume depletion. Unless continuously corrected, hypotension or poor tissue perfusion could recur when drug is discontinued.
4. Ischemia and gangrene of fingers or toes can occur with large doses.

☐ Nursing Implications
1. At a minimum, the following parameters must be monitored to guide titration of this drug: heart rate, ECG, central venous pressure (CVP), blood pressure (BP), and urinary output. When possible, direct arterial BP and pulmonary capillary wedge pressure (PCWP) should also be monitored. Because of this drug's vasoconstrictive actions, the indirectly obtained BP may be significantly different from the intra-arterial BP. The ac-

norepinephrine bitartrate
(continued)

ceptable limits for these parameters must be set by the physician.

2. Record heart rate and BP (direct or indirect) prior to therapy and every 2–3 minutes until the desired BP is reached, then every 5–15 minutes during the remainder of administration, as indicated by the patient's condition.
3. Record CVP or PCWP prior to and every 30 minutes during titration. A continuous oscilloscopic display of the arterial pressure and PAP is ideal.
4. Maintain continuous ECG monitoring to detect arrhythmias particularly premature ventricular contractions (due to myocardial irritability) and sinus bradycardia. Report these to the physician and be prepared to treat them.
5. Initially, record urinary output hourly, then as indicated. Since it indirectly reflects kidney perfusion, decreased urine flow may indicate the need to increase the infusion rate or to discontinue it and initiate another agent. Notify the physician if urinary output falls below 30 ml/hour for 2 consecutive hours in adult patients.
6. Use an infusion pump, preferably the volumetric type; use the infiltration alarm with models so equipped. When a pump is unavailable, use microdrop administration set and check the flow rate frequently.
7. Avoid extravasation, see Appendix for guidelines. Check the infusion site frequently for blood return and free flow of fluid. Observe for blanching of the skin along the course of the vein; if this occurs, change the infusion site. Some physicians recommend the addition of the vasodilator phentolamine (Regitine) 5–10 mg to each 1000 ml of norepinephrine solution to decrease tissue damage in the event of extravasation.[1] If extravasation does occur, the affected area must be infiltrated with a solution of phentolamine 5–10 mg in saline 5–10 ml, using a 25 gauge needle. This procedure should be carried out *immediately* upon discovery of the infiltration. Involved areas of tissue will be severely blanched and cold. After the phentolamine treatment, protect the area from additional trauma.

8. Observe for signs and symptoms of overdosage (too rapid an infusion rate): headache, tachycardia, premature ventricular contractions, diaphoresis, pallor (if not already present), chest pain. If any one of these appears, slow the infusion and notify the physician.
9. Patients receiving therapy with this drug frequently require respiratory support. Monitor respiratory rate, effort and blood gases with other parameters. Be prepared to initiate manual ventilation.

Reference
1. Tarazi, Robert C.: Sympathomimetic Agents in the Treatment of Shock. *Annals of Internal Medicine*, 81:369, September 1974.

Suggested Readings
Amsterdam, Ezra A. et al.: Evaluation and Management of Cardiogenic Shock. Part I. Approach to Patient. *Heart and Lung*, 1(3):402–408, May–June 1972 (references).
————Evaluation and Management of Cardiogenic Shock. Part II. Drug Therapy. *Heart and Lung*, 1(5):663–671, September–October 1972 (references).
Tarazi, Robert C.: Sympathomimetic Agents in the Treatment of Shock. *Annals of Internal Medicine*, 81:364–371, September 1974 (references).
Woods, Susan L.: Monitoring Pulmonary Artery Pressures. *American Journal of Nursing*, 76:1765–1771, November 1976 (references).

Intravenous Infusion of Vasopressors—Programmed Instruction. *American Journal of Nursing,* 65(11):129–152, November 1965. (Useful information on the theory behind titration)

orphenadrine citrate ■
(Norflex Injectable)

Actions/Indications
Centrally acting skeletal muscle relaxant and anticholinergic, sedative. Used as an adjunct to rest and physical therapy to relieve pain associated with acute, painful musculoskeletal conditions.

Dosage
Adults:
60 mg (1 ampul)
   Repeat every 12 hrs. Use oral form for maintenance.
Children:
Not recommended.

Preparation and Storage
Supplied in 2-ml ampuls, 30 mg/ml.

Drug Incompatibilities
Do not mix with any other medication in any manner.
   Do not add to IV fluids.

Modes of IV Administration

Injection
Yes
Undiluted at a rate of 30 mg/min.

Intermittent Infusion
No

Continuous Infusion
No

Contraindications; Warnings; Precautions; Adverse Reactions

Contraindications
  1. Glaucoma
  2. Pyloric or duodenal obstruction
  3. Stenosing peptic ulcers
  4. Obstruction of bladder neck
  5. Cardiospasm (megaesophagus)
  6. Myasthenia gravis
  7. Hypersensitivity

Warnings
  1. Dizziness and syncope may occur following injection.
  2. Safety for use in pregnancy, lactation, or children has not been established.
  3. If prolonged use is planned, monitor hepatic and renal function.

Precautions
  1. Confusion, anxiety and tremors may occur in patients also receiving propoxyphene.
  2. Use with caution in patients with cardiac arrhythmias or decompensation. See Adverse Reaction No. 2.

Adverse Reactions
  1. Dryness of mouth
  2. Larger doses: tachycardia, urinary retention, blurred vision, increased intraocular pressure, nausea, weakness, vomiting, headache
  3. Hallucinations, anxiety, agitation
  4. Hypersensitivity
  5. Rarely—aplastic anemia

☐ Nursing Implications
  1. Keep the patient in a recumbent position during the injection of this drug and for at least one hour following. See Warning No. 1. Monitor heart rate and blood pressure every 15 minutes following injection, for one hour.
  2. Monitor for signs of increased intraocular pressure: severe ocular pain, nausea and vomiting, decreasing vision, patient sees rainbows around lights.[1]
  3. Palpate bladder size every 4 hours and measure urine output every 8 hours to detect urinary retention.
  4. Observe for mental confusion and hallucinations. Reassurance and safety precautions such as restraints and side rails may be needed.
  5. Ambulate with caution one hour after injection if appropriate. There may be mild dizziness, blurred vision and weakness.

orphenadrine citrate
(continued)
6. Take anaphylaxis precautions, see Appendix.

Reference
1. Newell, Frank W., and Ernest, J. Terry: *Ophthalmology — Principles and Concepts* (3rd ed.), St. Louis: C. V. Mosby Company, 1974, p. 337.

ouabain ■
(Strophanthin-G)

Actions/Indications
Short-acting cardiac glycoside, with the same effects as digitalis.

Used to produce rapid digitalization in acute congestive heart failure and in the management of atrial tachyarrhythmias.

This is the most rapid-acting digitalis preparation available. Full effect is seen within 2 hours of injection.

Dosage
Adults:
Initially: Nonemergency situations — 0.25 mg; emergencies — 0.5 mg.

Then, 0.1 mg increments hourly until digitalization is reached or when 1.0 mg has been given.

Maintenance is obtained with digoxin or digitoxin.

Children:
0.3 mg/M^2/dose (0.01 mg/kg/dose), one-half dose immediately then fractions of the dose every 30 min. until response is seen or total dose given.[1]

Preparation and Storage
Supplied in 2-ml ampuls, 0.25 mg/ml.

Do not add to IV fluids other than that in the IV tubing; this drug is unstable when diluted.

Drug Incompatibilities
Do not mix with any other medication in syringe.

Modes of IV Administration

Injection
Yes
Over 1–2 minutes.

Intermittent Infusion
No
Cannot be mixed with fluids.

Continuous Infusion
No
Cannot be mixed with fluids.

Contraindications; Warnings; Precautions; Adverse Reactions

Contraindications
Digitalis toxicity

Warning
Administration should be discontinued if nausea, vomiting, or arrhythmia occurs. These are signs of digitalis toxicity.

Precautions
1. The patient must be monitored electrocardiographically during therapy to detect the onset of arrhythmias due to toxicity (usually premature ventricular contractions, conduction defects, and sinus bradycardia).
2. Administer with caution to patients who have received digitalis preparations in the past 2–3 weeks. These patients will require lower dosage of ouabain.
3. Arrhythmias that this drug is used to treat may be produced by digitalis toxicity. Discontinue injections if arrhythmias become more severe.
4. Reduce the dosage in the presence of hypokalemia, hypothyroidism, myocardial damage, coronary disease, conduction disorders, or in the elderly.

Treatment of Digitalis Toxicity
1. Discontinue the drug at the first suspicion of toxicity, and do not reinitiate until signs and symptoms of toxicity subside.

2. Initiate continuous ECG monitoring if not already present.
3. Maintain a normal serum potassium (3.5–5.5 mEq/liter), but do *not* administer intravenous potassium in the presence of advanced or complete heart block secondary to digitalis toxicity; the block may increase.[2]
4. Pharmacologic treatment of toxicity should be guided by the arrhythmia produced. Phenytoin (Dilantin) is usually the drug of choice. Quinidine, lidocaine, procainamide, and propranolol can also be used depending on the clinical situation. (If propranolol is used, monitor atrioventricular conduction closely. This drug may cause increasing A-V block.) Atropine can be used to treat bradyarrhythmias. See entries for each drug for further details on their use.
5. If profound bradycardia and/or complete A-V block occur, temporary transvenous pacing may be necessary until toxicity resolves.

☐ Nursing Implications

1. Patients receiving this medication intravenously should, in most instances, be observed for arrhythmias via continuous ECG monitoring. Observe for improvement if the drug is given to treat an arrhythmia, and observe for arrythmias which may be produced by the drug (see Precaution No. 1). Some of the more common arrhythmias produced by toxic levels of ouabain are sinus bradycardia, premature ventricular and atrial contractions, atrioventricular block of all degrees, and paroxysmal atrial tachycardia. Notify the physician of improvement in the arrhythmia being treated and document with an ECG tracing. If arrhythmias of toxicity appear, notify the physician, document with an ECG tracing, and hold the next dose of ouabain until the physician decides what course of action is appropriate.
2. Be prepared to administer immediate care in the event of arrhythmias due to toxicity. (See Treatment of Digitalis Toxicity above.) Atropine 0.5–1.0 mg can be given for a heart rate less than 50–60/minute. (In units where registered nurses are expected to administer drugs in such an event, the unit physician should decide at what heart rate the atropine should be administered and in what amount.) See page 24 for details on atropine.

   For premature ventricular contractions or ventricular tachycardia, lidocaine 50–100 mg can be given by intravenous injection. Again, unit policy should dictate when and how much drug is given. See page 186 for details on lidocaine.
3. Observe for noncardiac symptoms of digitalis toxicity: anorexia; nausea; vomiting and diarrhea; visual disturbances, e.g., rainbow vision or yellow vision (rare); in children poor feeding and irritability; headache (rare); confusion; severe fatigue.[3]
4. Monitor for signs of improvement if the patient is being treated for congestive heart failure:
   a. Reduction in weight (weigh the patient daily)
   b. Reduction in peripheral edema
   c. Increased urine output (measure every 8 hours)
   d. Decreased resting heart rate to normal limits (record every 4–8 hours)
   e. Decreased respiratory rate, disappearance of rales
   f. Increased exercise tolerance
   g. Increased cardiac output.
   Note that worsening congestive failure despite digitalis administration may be a sign of digitalis toxicity.
5. Be aware of the patient's serum

ouabain
(continued)

potassium. Hypokalemia can precipitate digitalis toxicity. Administer potassium supplements as ordered. These may produce nausea and vomiting (liquid preparations especially) usually soon after administration. The nurse's observations will be needed to differentiate between potassium-induced nausea and vomiting and that due to digitalis toxicity. (Normal serum potassium: 3.5–55 mEq/liter.)

6. Rarely, elderly patients experience hallucinations, anxiety, and delusions secondary to toxic levels of digitalis preparations. Monitor for onset of this complication; notify the physician and initiate safety measures.

7. Patients who will require a digitalis preparation on a chronic basis must be instructed on safe self-administration of the digitalis.

References
1. Shirkey, Harry C.: *Pediatric Drug Handbook*, Philadelphia: W. B. Saunders Company, 1977, p. 135.
2. Davis, Richard H., and Risch, Charles: Potassium and Arrhythmias. *Geriatrics*, November 1970, p. 110.
3. Lely, A. H., and van Enter, C. H. J.: Noncardiac Symptoms of Digitalis Intoxication. *American Heart Journal*, 83(2):150, February 1972.

Suggested Readings
Amsterdam, Ezra A., et al.: Systemic Approach to the Management of Cardiac Arrhythmias. *Heart and Lung*, 2(5):747–753, September–October 1973 (references).
Arbeit, Sidney, et al.: Recognizing Digitalis Toxicity. *American Journal of Nursing*, 77(12):1936–1945, December 1977 (references).
Lely, A. H., and van Enter, C. H. J.: Noncardiac Symptoms of Digitalis Intoxication. *American Heart Journal*, 83(2):149–152, February 1972.
Rosen, Michael R., Wit, Andrew, and Hoffman, Brian F.: Electrophysiology and Pharmacology of Cardiac Arrhythmias. IV Cardiac Antiarrhythmic and Toxic Effects of Digitalis. *American Heart Journal*, 89(3):391–399, March 1975 (references).
Treatment of Cardiac Arrhythmias. *Medical Letter on Drugs and Therapeutics*, 16(25):101–108, December 6, 1974.
Tanner, Gloria: Heart Failure in the MI Patient. *American Journal of Nursing*, 77:230–234, February 1977.

oxacillin sodium ■
(Prostaphlin, Bactocill)

Actions/Indications
Antibiotic, penicillinase-resistant penicillin.

Used to treat infections due to penicillinase-producing staphylococci. Sensitivity tests must be performed. Also may be effective in infections caused by *Strep. pneumoniae*, group A beta-hemolytic streptococci, pneumococci, and nonpenicillinase-producing staphylococci.

Dosage
Adults and Children Over 40 KG:
Mild to moderate infections of upper respiratory tract, skin, and soft tissue— 250–500 mg every 4–6 hrs.
Severe infections of lower respiratory tract or disseminated infections— 1 gm or more every 4–6 hrs.
Children Less Than 40 KG, Over 2 Weeks of Age:
*Mild to moderate infections—*50 mg/kg/24 hrs in equally divided doses every 6 hrs.
*Severe infections—*100 mg/kg/day given in equally divided doses every 6 hrs. Infections due to group A beta-hemolytic streptococci must be treated for at least 10 days to prevent rheumatic fever.
Neonates Under 2 Weeks of Age:
50 mg/kg/24 hrs in equally divided doses every 6 hrs.

Renal Impairment:
In mild impairment, no change in dosage is necessary. In uremia the dosage should be reduced to 1 gm every 6 hours for *adults*. Administer after dialysis.[1]

Preparation and Storage
Reconstitute with: sterile water for injection or sodium chloride injection as follows:

Vial Size	Vol. Diluent
250 mg	5 ml
500 mg	5 ml
1 gm	10 ml
2 gm	20 ml
4 gm	40 ml

Piggyback bottles of 1, 2 and 4 gm are also available. See directions on bottles for dilution. Shake well until a clear solution is obtained.

Discard reconstituted solutions after 7 days if refrigerated.

Drug Incompatibilities
Do not mix with any other medication in an IV bottle and do not inject into an IV line containing:
Penicillin
Aminoglycoside antibiotics
Tetracycline

Modes of IV Administration

Injection
Yes
Dilute the reconstituted solution further with an equal amount of NS. Inject over 10 min.

Intermittent Infusion
Yes
Dilute each gm of drug with 50 ml. Infuse over 20 min. Use any fluid listed under Continuous Infusion.

Continuous Infusion
Yes
Add 6-hr dose to any of the following IV solutions:
NS
D5W
D5/NS 10% Fructose in Water
10% Fructose in Saline
RL

10% Invert Sugar in Water
10% Invert Sugar in Saline
Travert 10% #1, #2, and #3
Use enough volume to produce a drug concentration of 0.5–2.0 mg/ml and infuse over 6 hrs.

Contraindications; Warnings; Precautions; Adverse Reactions

Contraindications
Hypersensitivity to any penicillin

Warnings
There may be cross-allergenicity to cephalosporins. Use with caution in patients with this hypersensitivity.

Precautions
1. There can be bacterial or fungal overgrowth secondary to organisms resistant to this drug.
2. Renal, hepatic, and hematopoietic systems should be monitored during therapy.
3. Use with caution in premature and newborn infants.
4. Safety for use in pregnancy has not been established.
5. This drug contains 3.1 mEq. of sodium per gram.[2] This should be considered when giving this drug to patients with congestive heart failure or any patient in whom sodium intake should be limited.
6. Can cause acute interstitial nephritis which is preceded by fever, eosinophilia and a rash. Urinalysis will show white cells, casts and proteinuria. There may also be oliguria and azotemia. If this occurs, the drug should be discontinued. Some groups then treat with steroids.

Adverse Reactions
1. Hypersensitivity reactions ranging from rash to anaphylaxis have been reported; increased SGOT and SGPT may also be manifestations of hypersensitivity
2. Oral lesions: glossitis (inflammation of the tongue) and stomatitis (inflammation of oral membranes)

oxacillin sodium
(continued)
3. Fever
4. Oral (thrush) and perineal (monilia) *Candida albicans* infections
5. Blood dyscrasias
6. Nephrotoxicity (oliguria, albuminuria, hematuria, pyuria) especially in infants

☐ **Nursing Implications**
1. Take anaphylaxis precautions; see Appendix.
2. Monitor for signs and symptoms of overgrowth infections:
   a. Fever (take rectal temperature at least every 4–6 hours in all patients)
   b. Increasing malaise
   c. Newly appearing localized signs and symptoms: redness, soreness, pain, swelling, drainage (increased volume or change in character of preexisting drainage)
   d. Monilial rash in perineal area (reddened areas with itching), or reddened areas on oral membranes (thrush)
   e. Cough (change in preexisting cough or sputum production)
   f. Diarrhea
3. Monitor renal status for onset of nephrotoxicity:
   a. Measure urine output every 8 hours (or more frequently if the patient's condition warrants). Notify the physician as to the onset of oliguria (urine output less than 240 ml in 8 hours for adults.
   b. Observe for hematuria.
   c. Collect urine for analysis at least every other day to be examined for white cells, casts, proteinuria.
4. Examine oral membranes and tongue daily for signs of stomatitis and glossitis. Notify the physician of findings and begin therapeutic oral care as ordered.
   Place the patient on a bland, soft diet. Patients with severe reactions may be placed on NPO status by the physician.

Those who can tolerate oral intake may benefit from the use of Xylocaine Viscous or acetaminophen elixir mouthwashes before meals.
Keep the patient hydrated.
Administer parenteral analgesics as needed.

References
1. Appel, Geral B. and Neu, Harold C.: The Nephrotoxicity of Antimicrobial Agents. *New England Journal of Medicine,* 296(12):667, March 24, 1977.
2. Ibid, p. 664.

oxytetracycline hydro-chloride ■
(Terramycin Intravenous)

Actions/Indications
Antibiotic used to treat infections caused by the following organisms:
• Rickettsiae
• *Mycoplasma pneumoniae*
• Agents of psittacosis and ornithosis
• Agents of lymphogranuloma venereum and granuloma inguinale
• Agent of relapsing fever
• Other gram-positive, gram-negative and anaerobic organisms as determined by sensitivity testing

Dosage
Adults:
250–500 mg every 6 to 12 hrs. Do not exceed 500 mg. every 6 hrs.
Children:
(over 8 years of age): 10–15 mg/kg/day divided into 2 equal doses. Up to 20 mg/kg/day can be given in severe infections. See Warning No. 1.
Not usually recommended for newborn infants. However, 10 to 15 mg/kg every 12 hours has been used.[1] See Warning No. 1.
In patients with renal impairment, dosage should be decreased or time interval between doses increased.

Preparation and Storage
There are separate oxytetracycline preparations for IM and IV use. Be

certain to use *IV form.* IV form should not be used for IM.

Reconstitute from powder by adding 10 ml of sterile water for injection to both 250-mg and 500-mg vials. Concentrations produced are 25 mg/ml and 50 mg/ml, respectively.

Store in refrigerator and discard after 48 hours.

Drug Incompatibilities
Do not mix with any other medication.

Modes of IV Administration

Injection
No

Intermittent Infusion
Yes
Preferred mode. Use D5W, NS or RL, at least 100 ml. Infuse over 1 hour.

Continuous Infusion
Yes
Use D5W, NS or RL in desired volume. Infuse over 6–12 hours.

Contraindications; Warnings; Precautions; Adverse Reactions

Contraindications
Hypersensitivity to any tetracycline

Warnings
1. Use during tooth development may cause permanent discoloration of the child's teeth. Enamel hypoplasia has also been reported. Use should be limited to situations where no other drug may be effective.
2. If renal impairment exists, even at normal doses, accumulation may occur and lead to liver toxicity. Avoid use of this drug in such patients, and in postpartum patients with pyelonephritis.
3. Monitor liver function. Do not use other hepatotoxic drugs concomitantly. Liver failure and death have been reported in the presence of renal failure espe-

cially during pregnancy, when daily doses exceeded 2 gm.
4. Exposure to ultraviolet radiation may produce exaggerated sunburn.
5. There may be an increase in BUN secondary to an anabolic effect. This is not a problem in the presence of normal renal function, but may lead to azotemia, hyperphosphatemia and acidosis in the presence of renal impairment.
6. Use in pregnancy can cause retardation in fetal bone development.
7. This drug is secreted in breast milk.

Precautions
1. Overgrowth of nonsusceptible organisms, including fungi, may occur. If a significant superinfection develops, discontinue oxytetracycline and initiate appropriate therapy.
2. Patients concomitantly receiving anticoagulants may require lower doses of the anticoagulant.
3. All infections secondary to group A beta-hemolytic streptococcus must be treated for at least 10 days to prevent rheumatic fever.
4. Do not administer concomitantly with penicillin. Penicillin activity may be reduced by this drug.

Adverse Reactions
1. Gastrointestinal: anorexia, nausea, vomiting, diarrhea, glossitis (inflammation of the tongue — rare)
2. Skin: rashes, photosensitivity
3. Renal toxicity: rise in BUN secondary to an anabolic effect
4. Hypersensitivity: urticaria and anaphylaxis, exacerbation of lupus erythematosus. Bulging fontanels have been reported in young infants with full therapeutic dosage. This disappeared on discontinuation of the drug. (See Contraindications.)
5. Hematologic: hemolytic anemia,

oxytetracycline hydrochloride
(continued)
thrombocytopenia, neutropenia, eosinophilia.

6. Overgrowth infection secondary to nonsusceptible organisms.

□ **Nursing Implications**

1. Take anaphylaxis precautions; see Appendix.

2. If gastrointestinal disturbances occur, notify the physician; if nausea, vomiting or diarrhea are pronounced, the drug will probably be discontinued. Antiemetics, antacids, and constipating agents can be ordered to control symptoms. Monitor intake and output to assist the physician in planning for parenteral fluid replacement. Maintain hydration orally when possible.

3. If the patient will be taking the oral form of this drug as an outpatient, instruct him/her on the possibility of photosensitivity and the advisability of avoiding exposure to the sun (sun-block lotions may be of help if exposure cannot be avoided).

4. Women of childbearing age and potential and mothers of children who may receive this drug should be informed of Warnings No. 1, 2, 3, 6 and 7 by the physician. Assist in the interpretation of these warnings to the patient.

5. Even though blood dyscrasias are infrequently caused by this agent, be aware of the patient's complete blood cell count during therapy. If the platelet count begins to fall, the drug will probably be discontinued. Bleeding secondary to a low platelet count usually begins only after the count falls below 100,000 cu mm.

6. Monitor for signs and symptoms of overgrowth infections:
   a. Fever (take rectal temperature at least every 4–6 hours in all patients)
   b. Increasing malaise
   c. Newly appearing localized signs and symptoms: red-

ness, soreness, pain, swelling, drainage (increased volume or change of pre-existing drainage)
   d. Monilial rash in perineal area (reddened areas with itching)
   e. Cough (change in pre-existing cough or sputum production)
   f. Diarrhea

7. Report the onset of any rash to the physician. Keep the patient's environment comfortably cool and the skin clean. Diphenhydramine (Benadryl) may be ordered to relieve itching.

8. Report the onset of jaundice to the physician.

9. Report the onset of bulging fontanels and other signs of increasing intracranial pressure to the physician.

10. Be aware of this drug's relationship with renal function. Tetracyclines are usually not given to patients with renal impairment because:
   a. The drug accumulates in the body owing to decreased excretion.
   b. The presence of the drug may cause further deterioration in renal function.
   c. It may cause a catabolic state with metabolic acidosis, increasing BUN and possibly death due to uremia.[2]
   If it is given, know what the patient's pretreatment BUN and creatinine levels are. Monitor for change in these values with initiation of treatment.
   Monitor urine output in renal patients receiving this drug. Report increasing oliguria to the physician. Send urine for analysis at least every other day.

References

1. American Society of Hospital Pharmacists. *American Hospital Formulary Service*, 8:12.24. 1981.
2. Barza, Michael, and Schiefe, Richard T.: Antimicrobial Spec-

trum, Pharmacology and Therapeutic Use of Antibiotics. Part I: Tetracyclines. *American Journal of Hospital Pharmacy*, 34:51, January 1977.

oxytocin citrate ■
(Pitocin, Syntocinon)

Actions/Indications
Synthetic oxytocic hormone. Increases uterine contractility. Used to initiate or improve uterine contractions. Can also be used to control postpartum uterine bleeding and in the treatment of incomplete or inevitable abortion.

Dosage
Induction or Stimulation of Labor:
Dosage is determined by uterine response titration, using a solution of 10 milliunits/ml.
Initial dose—1–2 milliunits/min. At 15-to 30-min intervals, increase dose by 1–2 milliunits/min until desired contraction pattern is seen.
Control of Uterine Bleeding:
10–40 units in 1000 ml D5W titrated with uterine firmness and bleeding rate; usually begin with 1–2 milliunits/min and increase by 1–2 milliunits/min until desired results are seen.
Incomplete or Inevitable Abortion:
Use a solution of 10 units in 500 ml NS (20 milliunits/ml), infuse at a rate of 2–4 ml/minute.

Preparation and Storage
Availability: 0.5-ml ampul containing 5 units; 1-ml ampul containing 10 units; 10-ml vial containing 100 units; disposable syringe containing 10 units in 1 ml.

Drug Incompatibilities
Do not mix with any other medication in IV bottle, and do not mix in an IV line with warfarin.

Modes of IV Administration

Injection
Yes
Only for *extreme* emergencies. Dilute dose in 5 ml NS and inject slowly.

Intermittent Infusion
No

Continuous Infusion
Yes
Add 10 units to 1000 ml D5W or NS. Solution will contain 10 milliunits/ml. Mix well. More concentrated solutions can be used for fluid-restricted patients. For example, add 10 units to 500 ml of fluid for a 20-milliunit/ml solution. Solutions (units/ml) should be made for easy dose calculation.
Use infusion pump. Attach as a secondary bottle to enable infusion to be discontinued when necessary. If no pump is available, use microdrip infusion set.
Titrate with desired uterine response.

Contraindications; Warnings; Precautions; Adverse Reactions

Contraindications
1. Significant cephalopelvic disproportion
2. Unfavorable fetal positions
3. In emergencies where the benefit-to-risk ratio for fetus or mother favors surgical intervention
4. In fetal distress where delivery is not imminent
5. Prolonged use in uterine inertia or severe toxemia
6. Hypertonic uterine patterns
7. Allergic and functional hypersensitivity
8. In cases where vaginal delivery is contraindicated such as cervical carcinoma, cord presentation or prolapse, placenta previa, and vasa praevia

Warnings
1. Must be used only in a hospital under adequate medical supervision.
2. Use only one route at a time to administer.

Precautions
1. When properly administered, the drug should stimulate normal contractions.

oxytocin citrate
(continued)
2. Overstimulation can endanger the mother and the fetus. Hypertonic contractions can occur, leading to fetal distress and possible uterine rupture.
3. Probably should not be administered in fetal distress, prematurity, placenta previa, abruptio placentae, borderline disproportion, any situation with predisposition for uterine rupture (previous C-section or uterine surgery, overdistention of the uterus, grand multiparity, traumatic delivery, or sepsis).
4. Hypertensive episodes have been reported and have led to cerebrovascular accident. (Usually only seen in large doses.)
5. This drug increases water reabsorption; water intoxication may occur.

Adverse Reactions
Mother:
1. Tetanic uterine contractions
2. Uterine rupture, pelvic hematomas
3. Hypotension
4. Arrhythmias (sinus tachycardia, premature ventricular contractions)
5. Water intoxication
6. Hypertensive episodes leading to CVA or subarachnoid hemorrhage
7. Rarely—chest pain, anxiety, dyspnea
8. Hypersensitivity
Fetus:
1. Death
2. Arrhythmias (premature ventricular contractions, bradycardia, tachycardia)
3. Hypoxia
4. Intracranial hemorrhage.

☐ **Nursing Implications**
1. Physician should be in attendance or readily available during the administration of this drug.
2. Monitor uterine contractions constantly: number per minute, strength (use contraction meter

if available; report if exceeds 50 mm Hg), duration, and resting tone. In the event of overstimulation, *stop infusion*; report to the physician. Administer oxygen to the mother as ordered.
3. Monitor maternal vital signs every 15 minutes or according to hospital policy. Report rising blood pressure, cardiac irregularities. Patients with a history of arrhythmia or other cardiac problems should be connected to a cardiac monitor to detect arrhythmias.
4. Monitor the mother for signs of water intoxication: fall in urine output, rise in weight, edema (lower extremities, sacral area, face).
5. Monitor fetal heart rate every 5 to 10 minutes or use continuous fetal ECG. Report arrhythmias immediately and discontinue infusion.

pancuronium bromide ■
(Pavulon)

Actions/Indications
Nondepolarizing (competitive) neuromuscular blocking agent.
Used as an adjunct to anesthesia to induce skeletal muscle relaxation and paralysis. Also used to control patients on mechanical ventilation; to increase muscle relaxation during electroconvulsive therapy, tetanus and status epilepticus.
Onset and duration of action are dose-dependent. With an average adult or pediatric dose, onset will be within 30 seconds, with the peak effect after 3 minutes. Recovery is nearly complete after 1 hour with a single dose. Repeated doses will prolong recovery time.

Dosage
Dosage must be individualized in relation to anesthetic used and patient's condition. See Nursing Implication No. 6 and Precaution No. 1 for situations which require reduction in dosage.

Adults:
Initial dose range—0.04–0.1 mg/kg followed by 0.01 mg/kg titrations based on patient response, at 25- to 60-minute intervals.
Children Over 1 Month of Age:
0.04–0.1 mg/kg, with 0.01 mg increments titrated with patient response (same as adult).
Neonates:
Test dose of 0.02 mg/kg; evaluate responsiveness (infants are sensitive to this type of neuromuscular blocking agent), then titrate as with adult.

A reversal agent is administered at the end of surgery or at any time when the effects of this drug are no longer needed or are undesirable. See Precaution No. 2.

A peripheral nerve stimulator can be used for dosage titration, especially in patients who require a reduction in dosage.

Preparation and Storage
Supplied in 2-ml and 5-ml ampuls (2 mg/ml) and in 10-ml vials (1 mg/ml).
Refrigerate unopened and opened vials.

Drug Incompatibilities
Do not mix with any other medication in any manner.

Modes of IV Administration

Injection
Yes
Over 1–2 minutes, while airway and ventilation are maintained. No further dilution needed.

Intermittent Infusion
No

Continuous Infusion
No

Contraindications; Warnings; Precautions; Adverse Reactions

Contraindications
Hypersensitivity to this drug or the bromide ion contained in the compound.

Warnings
1. Must be administered only by clinicians thoroughly experienced in its use (usually an anesthesiologist or anesthetist).
2. Should not be administered unless facilities for endotracheal intubation, assisted ventilation, oxygen and reversal agents are immediately available. Be prepared to assist and control ventilation.
3. Use with caution in patients with myasthenia gravis.
4. May have adverse effects on fetal development. Benefits must be weighed against risks to the fetus.
5. May be used during cesarean section. Reversal may be unsatisfactory in patients receiving magnesium sulfate for toxemia (magnesium salts enhance the blockade produced by this drug). Reduce the dosage in these cases. Pancuronium does not cross the placental barrier.

Precautions
1. Use with caution in patients with pre-existing pulmonary, hepatic or renal disease. This is particularly true of patients with renal disease since the drug is partially excreted in the urine. These patients can experience a prolongation of the neuromuscular blockade (20–40 minutes longer than normal, after a single dose).[1]
2. Neostigmine 0.5–2.0 mg reverses the actions of this drug. Atropine 0.5–1.0 mg should be administered a few minutes prior to neostigmine. See page 239 for detailed information on neostigmine.
3. Histamine release and resultant bronchospasm are rarely seen.
4. Prior administration of succinylcholine should warrant that the dose of pancuronium be delayed until the effects of succinylcholine have worn off.
5. See Nursing Implications for information on elements which

pancuronium bromide
(continued)
alter the duration and intensity of this drug's effects.

Adverse Reactions

1. Neuromuscular: extension and intensification of the drug's effects beyond the usual times
2. Cardiovascular: slight increase in heart rate
3. Gastrointestinal: increased salivation especially if an anticholinergic agent has not been given prior to pancuronium or anesthesia.
4. Skin: transient rash

☐ Nursing Implications

Be aware of institutional policies concerning the administration of this drug, e.g., who may administer it and under what circumstances.
Postanesthesia Care:

1. Equipment that should be readily available: suction, manual breathing bag, endotracheal tubes and laryngoscope, oxygen.
2. Patients receiving this agent must be intubated to assist in maintaining an adequate airway and ventilation. Monitor for adequacy of ventilation by presence or absence of cyanosis and arterial blood gases.
3. Be aware of the onset and duration of action of this drug (see Actions/Indications section), and when the patient received the last dose.
4. Be aware of the sequence of progression of the paralytic effects as they will occur after an injection of this drug:
   a. Loss of eye movement
   b. Eyelid droop
   c. Stiffness of jaw muscles
   d. Paralysis of trunk muscles
   e. Paralysis of pharyngeal muscles (tongue, swallowing, etc.)
   f. Respiratory paralysis, intercostal muscles and finally diaphragm
      Recovery will be a complete reverse of this sequence.[2]

5. During recovery, observe for rebound of the paralytic effects and for incomplete reversal of the paralytic effects by the antagonist agent (neostigmine). Keep reversal agent and atropine at the bedside or readily available (see Precaution No. 2).
6. Be aware of elements which may *prolong* the effects of this drug:
   a. Decreased circulation time, e.g., as in the presence of congestive heart failure or shock
   b. Decreased body temperature
   c. Dehydration
   d. Low blood pH[3]
   e. Hepatic or renal insufficiency (drug is excreted in bile and urine)
   f. Concomitant use of aminoglycoside antibiotics, polymyxin B, or bacitracin
   g. Other drugs, e.g., diazepam, halothane, quinidine, quinine, enflurane, methoxyflurane, magnesium salts, other neuromuscular blocking agents
   h. Age, e.g., the elderly
   i. The presence of myasthenia gravis
   j. Hypokalemia
   Patients under the influence of any one of these elements will require reduced dosage (in some cases), monitoring as described in Nursing Implication No. 7, and possibly prolonged respiratory support.
7. Discharge from the recovery room will depend on the following criteria:
   a. Grip strength
   b. Ability to lift the head
   c. Ability to open the eyes
   d. Respiratory status, e.g., vital capacity and tidal volume (preoperative values of these parameters are useful for comparison)

Maintenance Care for Controlled Ventilation:

1. This drug is usually administered on a p.r.n. basis for control of ventilation. The criteria

for administering the drug (by the anesthesiologist, qualified physician or, in some institutions, registered nurse) are determined by the physician. The criteria will include:

a. A respiratory rate
b. When the patient's respiratory effort is out of phase with the respirator
c. When the patient is struggling against the respirator
d. When positive end-expiratory pressure (P.E.E.P.) is in use

Monitor for the onset of any of the criteria and administer (or have administered) the prescribed amount of the drug.

2. Make certain that the endotracheal or tracheostomy tube is securely taped and correctly inserted. Check the connection between the tube and the respirator; it must be tight. KEEP RESPIRATOR ALARM SYSTEMS FUNCTIONING AT ALL TIMES.

3. This drug paralyzes skeletal muscles; it does not alter consciousness or relieve pain and anxiety. Therefore, the patient must be adequately sedated and given analgesics as needed to relieve anxiety and pain. He will not be able to make his needs known to those caring for him; needs must be anticipated. Many institutions assign one or more RNs to stay in constant attendance with these patients. Explain the paralysis to the patient and family as indicated.

4. Monitor vital signs before administration and every 5 minutes after until stabilization is seen, then every 15–30 minutes. Repeat the cycle with each dose. A slight increase in heart rate may be seen. Patients with a history of cardiac arrhythmias should be observed for exacerbation of those arrhythmias via a continuous ECG monitor.

5. Because this agent produces muscle paralysis, handle the patient with care to prevent trauma to joints and muscles during turning and positioning. The patient's position should be changed hourly to prevent skin breakdown. Use water-mattresses, flotation pads and similar devices as needed.

6. When this drug is discontinued, proceed with the nursing management as described under *Postanesthesia Care.*

References
1. Miller, Ronald D., Stevens, Wendell C., and Way, Walter L.: The Effect of Renal Failure and Hyperkalemia on the Duration of Pancuronium Neuromuscular Blockade in Man. *Anesthesia and Analgesia*, 52(4):663, July–August 1973.
2. Wylie, W. D., and Churchill-Davidson, H. C. (editors): *A Practice of Anesthesia* (3rd ed.), Chicago: Year Book Medical Publishers, 1972, p. 816.
3. Ibid., p. 833.

Suggested Reading
Hartridge, Virginia: Pancuronium Bromide (Pavulon). *American Association of Nurse Anesthetists Journal*, 42(4):301–310, August 1974, (references).

papaverine hydrochloride ▓

Actions/Indications
Smooth muscle relaxant and antispasmodic, causes vasodilatation and depresses speed of conductivity in myocardial conduction system.

Used in the following conditions:
Vascular spasm in
• Acute myocardial infarction
• Angina pectoris
• Peripheral and pulmonary embolism
• Peripheral vascular disease with spasm
• Cerebral angiospastic conditions
Visceral spasm in
• ureteral colic
• biliary colic
• gastrointestinal colic
Premature ventricular contractions

papaverine hydrochloride
(continued)

Dosage
Adults:
Vascular and visceral spasm—1–4 ml (30–120 mg) repeated every 3 hours as needed.
Management of premature ventricular contractions—30 mg every 10 min for 2 doses.
Children:
6 mg/kg day, given in 4 divided doses, as needed.

Preparation and Storage
Supplied in ampuls of 30 mg/ml.
Do not add to Ringer's Lactate; a precipitate will form.

Drug Incompatibilities
Do not mix with any other medication.

Modes of IV Administration

Injection
Yes
Slowly over 1–2 min.

Intermittent Infusion
Yes
In any fluid, except Ringer's Lactate.
Titrate with patient response.

Continuous Infusion
No

Contraindications; Warnings; Precautions; Adverse Reactions

Contraindications
IV injection, in presence of complete (third degree) atrioventricular heart block

Warnings
1. Injection of this drug should be performed by or under the supervision of a physician.
2. Rapid injection has been associated with cardiac arrhythmias and fatal apnea.
3. Administer with extreme caution in the presence of myocardial depression; arrhythmias are more likely to occur in this situation.

4. The effects of this drug may be potentiated by CNS depressants and synergism may result from combination with morphine.
5. Administer with caution to patients with glaucoma; intraocular pressure may be increased by this drug.

Adverse Reactions
1. Intensive flushing of the face
2. Diaphoresis
3. Increased depth of respirations
4. Increased heart rate
5. Slight rise in blood pressure
6. Sedation

☐ Nursing Implications
1. Monitor vital signs at least hourly.
2. Patients with first or second-degree atrioventricular heart block should be observed for intensification of the block and for other arrhythmias via continuous ECG monitoring. Atropine 1.0 mg will be used to treat bradycardia or increasing heart block.
3. Keep patient on bed rest during administration.
4. Monitor for signs and symptoms of increased intraocular pressure: increasing eye pain, blurred vision, reddening of the sclera, rainbow vision. Notify the physician at the onset of any one problem.

penicillin G, potassium and sodium ■

Actions/Indications
Antibiotic.
Used to treat infections caused by susceptible strains of the following organisms or conditions:
· Streptococcus
· *Strep. pneumoniae*
· Susceptible Staphylococcus
· Anthrax
· Actinomycosis
· Clostridial infections
· Diphtheria
· Erysipeloid endocarditis
· Fusospirochetosis (Vincent's gingivitis)

- Gram-negative organisms, if sensitive (many are not): *E. coli, Enterobacter aerogenes, A. faecalis, Salmonella, P. mirabilis*
- *Listeria*
- *Pasteurella* infections
- *N. gonorrhoeae*
- Syphilis (*T. pallidum*)
- *Meningococcus*

For prevention of bacterial endocarditis in susceptible patients, this drug is administered by the IM route.

Dosage

Dosage varies greatly with organism, general condition of the patient, and the severity of the infection.

Ranges:
Adults:
1–20 million units/day, in divided doses as often as every 2 hours or as a continuous infusion. In the presence of renal failure, increase the time interval between usual doses as follows based on glomerular filtration rate (GFR):

GFR (ml/min)	Time Interval for Doses
> 50	every 8 hours
50–10	every 8–12 hours
< 10	every 12–18 hours

No dosage adjustment is needed with dialysis.[1]
Children:
50,000–400,000 units/kg/day (Follow above schedule in the presence of renal failure.)
Neonates and Children:
0–7 days of age—50,000 units/kg/day, 100,000–150,000 units/kg/day in meningitis.
Over 7 days of age—75,000 units/kg/day, 150,000–250,000 units/kg/day in meningitis. (Larger doses for group B streptococcal meningitis than for pneumococcal meningitis are appropriate.) Avoid doses over 250,000 units/kg/day because of likelihood of CNS toxicity. Administer at 12-hour intervals for neonates 0–7 days of age; every 8 hours for children over 7 days of age, and every 6 hours in meningitis regardless of age.[2]

Preparation and Storage

Penicillin G *Sodium:*
Available in 5 million unit vials, and may be diluted as follows:

Vol Diluent (ml)	Concentration (units/ml)
23	200,000
18	250,000
8	500,000
3	1,000,000

Penicillin G *Potassium:*
Available in vials containing 1, 5, 10 and 20 million units, and may be diluted as follows:

Vial Size	Vol Diluent (ml)	Concentration (units/ml)
1,000,000 units	9.6	100,000
	4.6	200,000
	3.6	250,000
5,000,000 units	23	200,000
	18	250,000
	8	500,000
	3	1,000,000
10,000,000 units	15.5	500,000
	5.4	1,000,000
20,000,000 units	31.6	500,000

To reconstitute, loosen powder by shaking vial. Using sterile water for injection, NS or D5W, add the amounts shown in the tables above to make required concentrations. Hold vial horizontally and rotate while slowly directing stream of diluent against vial wall. Shake vigorously.

Storage: Penicillin G *Potassium* dry powder may be stored at room temperature. After reconstitution, store in the refrigerator and discard after 1 week (Squibb brand) or after 3 days (Lilly brand).

Penicillin G *Sodium* dry powder may be stored at room temperature. After reconstitution, refrigerate and discard after 1 week.

penicillin G, potassium and sodium
(continued)

Drug Incompatibilities
Do not mix in any manner with:
Metaraminol
Ascorbic acid
Tetracyclines
Aminophylline
Sodium Bicarbonate
THAM
Vancomycin
Cephalosporins
Heparin
Lincomycin
Phenothiazines
Thiopental
Vitamins
Aminoglycoside antibiotics

Modes of IV Administration

Injection
No

Intermittent Infusion
Yes
Use D5W or NS for infusion, at least
100 ml, infuse over 30–60 min.

Continuous Infusion
Yes
Use D5W or NS for infusion, at least
100 ml.
   Entire daily dose can be given in
one 24–hour infusion.

Contraindications; Warnings; Precautions; Adverse Reactions

Contraindications
Hypersensitivity to any penicillin

Warnings
1. Anaphylaxis can occur.
2. There may be cross-allergenicity
   with cephalosporins.

Precautions
1. Use with caution in patients
   with significant allergy history.
2. Monitor renal and hematopoietic systems during prolonged administration or with high dosage
   therapy.
3. Streptococcal infections must be
   treated for at least 10 days. Follow-up cultures must be
   obtained.

4. Reduction of dosage may be required in patients with renal or
   cardiac dysfunction because of
   sodium or potassium content of
   the drug and systemic accumulation of the drug (sodium or
   potassium content: 1.7 mEq/1
   million units). See Dosage section.
5. Overgrowth of nonsusceptible
   organisms may occur. Discontinue this drug if possible and
   initiate appropriate therapy in
   this situation.

Adverse Reactions
1. Most frequent is hypersensitivity
   ranging from rash or drug fever
   to anaphylaxis
2. Congestive heart failure secondary to high sodium content (See
   Precaution No. 4, above)
3. Minor hypersensitivity reactions
   may be controlled by antihistamines and corticosteroids if
   continued use of the penicillin
   cannot be avoided
4. Jarisch-Herxheimer reaction has
   been reported in patients being
   treated for syphilis
5. Hyperkalemia (elevated serum
   potassium) in patients with compromised renal function
6. Positive Coombs' test
7. Diarrhea
8. Seizures, usually seen in patients with renal impairment
   who are on high doses of penicillin
9. Overgrowth infections

☐ Nursing Implications
1. Take anaphylaxis precautions;
   see Appendix.
2. Monitor for signs of fluid overload and congestive heart failure:
   a. Increased weight (weigh
      daily)
   b. Peripheral edema
   c. Increased heart rate, CVP
      (engorged external jugular
      veins), and respiratory rate
   d. Rales in lung bases
   e. Decreased exercise tolerance
3. Monitor for signs and symptoms
   of overgrowth infection:

a. Fever (take rectal temperature at least every 4–6 hours)
b. Increasing malaise
c. Localized signs and symptoms of an infection: redness, soreness, pain, swelling, drainage
d. Cough
e. Diarrhea
f. Infection due to *Candida albicans,* oral (thrush) or perineal (monilia).

References
1. Bennett, William M., et. al.: Drug Therapy in Renal Failure: Dosing Guidelines for Adults. Part I: Antimicrobial Agents and Analgesics. *Annals of Internal Medicine,* 93:73, 1980.
2. McCracken, George H. and Nelson, John D.: *Antimicrobial Therapy for Newborns: Practical Application of Pharmacology to Clinical Usage.* New York: Grune and Stratton, 1977, p. 9.

pentobarbital, sodium ■
(Nembutal)

Actions/Indications
Short-acting barbiturate, CNS depressant. Used as a sedative and hypnotic; for preoperative sedation and to control seizures.

Dosage
Adults:
Average dose— 100 mg (70-kg patient).
Titrate in small increments to obtain desired effect* A total dose of 200–500 mg may be used.
Keep dose at a minimum in convulsive states to prevent overdepression.
Children:
Inject at a rate of 30 mg/M²/min. Titrate with response.*
*At least 1 minute is necessary to determine the full effect.

Preparation and Storage
Available in 2-ml ampuls and 20- and 50-ml multidose vials of 50 mg/ml; multidose vials of 12 mg/ml; and prefilled syringes of 1 and 2 ml of a 50 mg/ml solution.
Do not use a solution that is not clear and colorless.
Do not mix with fluids except to inject into the tubing of a running IV. See under Injection below.
This is a Schedule II drug under the Controlled Substances Act of 1970. Maintain hospital or institutional regulations guiding its use.

Drug Incompatibilities
Do not mix with other medications in any manner.

Modes of IV Administration

Injection
Yes
Dilute every 50 mg of drug in 9 cc NS. Inject at a rate of 50 mg/min.
(In children, inject at a rate of 1 mg/min or 30 mg/M²/min.)

Intermittent Infusion
No
Pharmacologically inappropriate.

Continuous Infusion
No
Pharmacologically inappropriate.

Contraindications; Warnings; Precautions; Adverse Reactions

Contraindications
1. Hypersensitivity to any barbiturate
2. Porphyria (confirmed or familial history)

Warnings
1. May antagonize some drugs by increasing liver enzyme activity, especially narcotic drugs.
2. Decreases potency of coumarin anticoagulants.
3. May produce psychic dependence with prolonged use.
4. May cause respiratory and circulatory depression, especially after rapid injection.
5. Safety for use in pregnancy has not been established insofar as

pentobarbital, sodium
(continued)
the effects on fetal development.
6. May cause respiratory depression in newborn infants when it is used during labor and delivery. Premature infants are more susceptible to this.
7. This drug may impair the mental and physical abilities required for the performance of potentially hazardous tasks, such as driving a car, for several hours after the obvious effects of the drug have disappeared.

Precautions
1. Use with caution in patients with impaired liver function. This drug is detoxified in the liver.
2. Administer with **extreme caution** in the presence of status asthmaticus, any respiratory depression, shock, uremia or after other respiratory depressants have been given. Be prepared to provide artificial ventilation.
3. Avoid extravasation and intra-arterial injection. Extravasation can lead to tissue necrosis. Intra-arterial injection can cause pain in the extremity and possibly gangrene. Signs and symptoms of accidental intra-arterial injection include:
   a. Pain in extremity
   b. Delayed onset of sedation
   c. Pallor and cyanosis of the extremity
   d. Patchy discoloration of the skin
   Any IV injection causing pain in the limb must be stopped.
4. Hypotension can occur, especially in hypertensive patients. Slow injection can prevent this.

Adverse Reactions
1. Respiratory depression, apnea
2. Circulatory collapse (hypotension)
3. Hypersensitivity; rashes and anaphylaxis

4. Central nervous system depression (excessive)
5. Residual sedation
6. Nausea, vomiting
7. Paradoxical excitement
8. Coughing, hiccoughs, laryngospasm, chest wall spasm, bronchospasm
9. Most reactions can be avoided by slow injection.

☐ **Nursing Implications**
1. Strictly adhere to maximum injection rate suggestions and maximum dose limits. Patients with liver impairment should receive smaller doses and should be monitored more closely and for a longer period of time than usual.
2. Keep the patient supine during and after injection. Monitor blood pressure, heart rate and respiratory rate every 5 minutes for 1 hour following an injection. This includes fetal heart rate monitoring. Do not leave the patient unattended. See Implication No. 7 for management of overdosage.
3. Patients with porphyria are sensitive to barbiturates in that they may experience an acute attack of the disease secondary to the administration of a barbiturate (see Contraindications). The onset of an acute attack is indicated by severe colicky abdominal pain radiating to the back. There is usually severe vomiting, fever and leukocytosis in addition.[1]
4. Avoid extravasation; see Appendix. Extravascular or intra-arterial injection of this drug can cause tissue necrosis and gangrene of the affected extremity, respectively. Thrombophlebitis can also occur. Examine for redness and pain along the vein tract. See Precaution No. 3.
5. Take anaphylaxis precautions; see Appendix.
6. Monitor for symptoms of acute overdosage (listed in order of progression):

a. Respiratory depression, i.e, decreased respiratory rate and depth
b. Peripheral vascular collapse, i.e., fall in blood pressure, pallor, diaphoresis, tachycardia
c. Pulmonary edema (rare)
d. Decreased or absent reflexes, pupillary constriction
e. Stupor
f. Coma
Stop the injection immediately upon noting one of these symptoms. Notify the physician.
7. Management of acute overdosage:
 a. Continue to stay with the patient and monitor vital signs
 b. Maintain an open airway and adequate ventilation
 c. Keep the patient as alert as possible by verbal and physical stimuli. Encourage the patient to breathe at an adequate rate (12–14 breaths/minute for an adult). If necessary, initiate artificial ventilation with a manual breathing bag (Puritan, Hope, Ambu, etc.) or mouth-to-mouth breathing at a rate of 12–14 breaths/minute
 d. Circulatory support in the form of fluids and drugs may be ordered
8. The sedation produced by this drug may be preceded by transient changes in mental status, such as feelings of euphoria and confusion. If this occurs, attempt to calm the patient and take measures to prevent injury until the patient returns to his normal status.
9. If a patient is to be ambulatory following an injection, ambulate with assistance; there may be transient dizziness. Obtain lying, then sitting and standing blood pressures to detect postural hypotension. If this drug has been used for an outpatient procedure, a responsible adult should accompany the patient home. The patient should not drive, consume alcohol or any other CNS depressant, for at least the next 8 hours. See Warning No. 7.

Reference
1. Beeson, Paul B., and McDermott, Walsh (editors): *Cecil-Loeb Textbook of Medicine* (14th ed.), Philadelphia: W. B. Saunders Company, 1975, p. 1873.

phenobarbital sodium ■
(Sodium Luminal)

Actions/Indications
Sedative, anticonvulsant, hypnotic, long-acting barbiturate.
Used in the intravenous mode for relief of severe anxiety, as an anticonvulsant, and as an antispasmotic, alone or in combination with other drugs.
Onset of action is 5 minutes, with maximum effects seen in 30 minutes.

Dosage
Adults:
Sedative— 16–32 mg 2–4 times a day.
 Hypnotic— 100–300 mg.
 Seizures—30–120 mg repeated as needed depending on patient response.
 Status epilepticus, delirium tremens— up to 600 mg may be needed depending on patient response.
 Do not exceed 600 mg in 24 hours.
Children:
Status epilepticus—5 mg/kg followed by 2.5 mg/kg every 5 min until seizures stop.

Preparation and Storage
Available in a premixed form in 1-ml ampuls of 130 mg/ml, and prefilled syringes of 60 and 130 mg/ml.
 Protect ampuls from light.
 This is a Schedule IV drug under the Controlled Substances Act of 1970. Maintain hospital or institutional regulations guiding its use.

phenobarbital sodium
(continued)

Drug Incompatibilities
Do not mix with any other medication, in any manner

Modes of IV Administration

Injection
Yes
Slowly, at a rate not to exceed 60 mg/minute, into the tubing of a running IV.

Intermittent Infusion
No

Continuous Infusion
No

Contraindications; Warnings; Precautions; Adverse Reactions

Contraindications
1. Hypersensitivity to any barbiturate
2. Porphyria (confirmed or familial history)
3. In children with renal or hepatic dysfunction

Warnings
1. May cause respiratory depression.
2. Administer with extreme caution in patients with nephritis. See Contraindication No. 3.
3. Physical and psychological dependence can occur as can withdrawal symptoms.
4. Signs of intoxication are: ataxia, slurred speech, vertigo, excessive sedation.
5. Safety for use in pregnancy has not been established.
6. Withdrawal symptoms can occur in newborns when the mother has received this drug (even in low doses as used for anticonvulsant therapy).
7. Status epilepticus has occurred with withdrawal of this drug from epileptic patients, after prolonged use.
8. Concomitant use with other central nervous system depressants will result in additive effects.
9. May lower blood levels of coumarin anticoagulants, dosage may need to be increased to maintain therapeutic prothrombin time. Conversely, phenobarbital withdrawal may lead to rise in prothrombin time and possible bleeding.
10. Accelerates metabolism of antihistamines, steroids and anticonvulsants.
11. May increase vitamin-D requirements, usually only in long-term oral therapy.

Precautions
1. Careful adjustment of dosage (usually lower doses) is needed in patients with hepatic, renal, cardiac and respiratory impairment, and in patients with myasthenia gravis and myxedema.
2. Lower doses are also required in elderly and debilitated patients to prevent oversedation.

Adverse Reactions
1. Central nervous system: dizziness, headache, confusion (especially in elderly), paradoxical excitation
2. Gastrointestinal: nausea, vomiting, epigastric pain
3. Allergy: facial edema, rashes, purpura, rarely exfoliative dermatitis, liver degeneration, anaphylaxis

☐ Nursing Implications
1. Strictly adhere to maximum injection rate suggestions and maximum dose limits to insure optimal benefit from the drug and to prevent overdosage. Patients with liver impairment should receive smaller doses and should be monitored more closely and for a longer period of time than usual.
2. Keep the patient supine during and after injection. Monitor blood pressure, heart rate and respiratory rate every 5 minutes for 1 hour following injection.

This includes fetal heart rate monitoring. Do not leave the patient unattended.
3. Patients with porphyria are sensitive to barbiturates in that they may experience an acute attack of the disease secondary to the administration of a barbiturate (see Contraindications). The onset of an acute attack is indicated by severe colicky abdominal pain radiating to the back. There is usually severe vomiting, fever and leukocytosis in addition.[1]
4. Avoid extravasation; see Appendix. Extravascular or intra-arterial injection of this drug can cause tissue necrosis and gangrene of the affected extremity, respectively. Thrombophlebitis can also occur. Examine for redness and pain along the vein tract.
5. Take anaphylaxis precautions; see Appendix.
6. Monitor for symptoms of acute overdosage (listed in order of progression):
   a. Respiratory depression, i.e., decreased respiratory rate and depth
   b. Ataxia, slurred speech, vertigo, excessive sedation
   c. Peripheral vascular collapse, i.e., fall in blood pressure, pallor, diaphoresis, tachycardia
   d. Pulmonary edema (rare)
   e. Decreased or absent reflexes, pupillary constriction
   f. Stupor
   g. Coma
   The injection should be stopped immediately upon noting one of these symptoms.
7. Management of acute overdosage:
   a. Continue to stay with the patient and monitor vital signs
   b. Maintain an open airway and adequate ventilation
   c. Keep the patient as alert as possible by verbal and physical stimuli. Encourage the patient to breathe at an adequate rate (12–14 breaths/minute for an adult). If necessary, initiate artificial ventilation with a manual breathing bag (Puritan, Hope, Ambu, etc.) or mouth-to-mouth breathing at a rate of 12–14 breaths/minute
   d. Circulatory support in the form of fluids and drugs may be ordered
8. The sedation produced by this drug may be preceded by transient changes in mental status, such as feelings of euphoria and confusion. If this occurs, attempt to calm the patient and take measures to prevent injury until the patient returns to his normal status.
9. If a patient is to be ambulatory following an injection, ambulate with assistance; there may be transient dizziness. Obtain lying, then sitting and standing blood pressures to detect postural hypotension. If this drug has been used for an outpatient procedure, a responsible adult should accompany the patient home. The patient should not drive for at least the next 8 hours.
10. If this drug is given for seizures, monitor effectiveness and initiate seizure precautions if not already in effect.

Reference
1. Beeson, Paul B., and McDermott, Walsh (editors): *Cecil-Loeb Textbook of Medicine* (14th ed.), Philadelphia: W. B. Saunders Company, 1975, p. 1873.

phentolamine mesylate ■
(Regitine)

Actions/Indications
Alpha adrenergic blocking agent. Produces vasodilatation. Used to prevent or control hypertensive episodes in pheochromocytoma. Diagnostic agent for pheochromocytoma.

phentolamine mesylate
(continued)
Prevention and treatment of tissue necrosis and sloughing caused by extravasation of sympathomimetic agents that produce vasoconstriction.

Dosage
Adults:
Prevention and control of hypertensive crisis in pheochromocytoma— 5 mg every 6 hrs., or 1–2 hours prior to surgery. During surgery an additional dose of 5 mg can be given as needed to control hypertension and tachycardia.
   Diagnosis of pheochromocytoma— 5 mg. See Nursing Implication No. 1 for test procedure.
   Prevention of dermal necrosis— 10 mg added to each 1000 ml norepinephrine.
   Treatment of dermal necrosis— 5–10 mg diluted in 10–15 ml NS for *subcutaneous injection*. See Nursing Implication No. 3 for procedure.
Children:
Prevention and control of hypertensive crisis in pheochromocytoma— 1 mg every 6 hrs., 1–2 hours prior to surgery.
   Diagnosis of pheochromocytoma— 1 mg. See Nursing Implication No. 1 for test procedure.
   Prevention and treatment of dermal necrosis is the same as for adults.

Preparation and Storage
Supplied in ampuls of 5 mg accompanied by an ampul of 1 ml sterile water for injection for reconstitution of the drug powder. Resulting solution will contain 5 mg/ml.
   Discard unused portions of solution; do not store.

Drug Incompatibilities
Do not mix with any other medications, except levarterenol.

Modes of IV Administration

Injection
Yes
No further dilution required after reconstitution.

Intermittent Infusion
No

Continuous Infusion
Yes
5 mg can be added to each liter of norepinephrine solution, for prevention of dermal necrosis.

Contraindications; Warnings; Precautions; Adverse Reactions

Contraindications
1. Acute myocardial infarction
2. History of myocardial infarction, coronary insufficiency, angina
3. Hypersensitivity

Warnings
1. Myocardial infarction, cerebrovascular spasm, and occlusion have occurred after an injection of phentolamine in association with marked lowering of blood pressure.
2. The phentolamine test for pheochromocytoma should be done only when other simpler tests have been positive.
3. Safety for use during pregnancy and lactation has not been established.

Precautions
1. Tachycardias and other cardiac arrhythmias may occur, monitor ECG during use.
2. If arrhythmias occur, defer the administration of any cardiac glycoside until the problem is resolved.

Adverse Reactions
1. Acute prolonged hypotensive episodes, with tachycardia and other arrhythmias after IV injection
2. Weakness
3. Dizziness
4. Flushing
5. Orthostatic hypotension
6. Nasal stuffiness
7. Nausea, vomiting, diarrhea

☐ Nursing Implications
1. Phentolamine test for pheochromocytoma:
   a. Discontinue all nonessential

medications at least 24 hours before the test, especially antihypertensives.

b. This test is usually not performed on normotensive patients.

c. Place the patient recumbent in a quiet, dark room, and begin taking his blood pressure every 10 minutes.

d. When the blood pressure has stabilized, notify the physician and prepare the phentolamine. Combine 5 mg of drug (1 mg in children) with 1 ml sterile water for injection.

e. The needle should then be inserted into the vein, and after a waiting period of 2 to 3 minutes, the phentolamine is injected rapidly.

f. Monitor blood pressure immediately after the injection and every 30 seconds for the first 3 minutes, and at 60-second intervals for the next 7 minutes.

g. A positive test consists in a drop in blood pressure more than 35 mm Hg systolic and 25 mm Hg diastolic. Maximal fall in pressure should occur in 2 minutes after the injection. The suspicion of pheochromocytoma should be confirmed by other diagnostic techniques.

2. Care of the patient receiving the phentolamine test:

a. Be prepared to manage hypotension; vasopressors should be readily available.

b. Monitor for cardiac arrhythmias either by frequent pulse readings in patients without a history of cardiac disease, or by continuous ECG monitoring in patients with cardiac disease. Lidocaine and atropine should be readily available.

c. After one hour of bed rest, the patient can be ambulated, but with caution. Evaluate for postural hypotension by taking lying and standing blood pressures. If there is a significant drop in blood pressure on standing, notify the physician and keep the patient at rest.

d. Assist in interpreting the test to the patient.

3. Infiltration therapy for extravasation of vasoconstrictor agents (e.g., dopamine, norepinephrine):

a. The affected area should be infiltrated with phentolamine as soon after the extravasation has occurred as possible. The affected area will be blanched and cool to touch.

b. Follow hospital policy as to who performs this physician-ordered treatment, i.e., nurse or physician.

c. A 25- or 26-gauge needle should be used with a 20 ml syringe. A solution of 5–10 mg of phentolamine in 10–15 ml of normal saline is recommended.

d. Infiltrate the area thoroughly. Monitor for hypotension secondary to the phentolamine for the next 2 hours. See No. 2 above for after-care.

e. The affected area will become reddened secondary to the vasodilatation produced by the phentolamine.

f. Protect the area from further trauma, and examine daily for the onset of tissue necrosis and sloughing. If these occur, the area should be cared for as a burn, to prevent infection and further damage.

g. Do not use the affected extremity for injections or blood pressure readings until healing has occurred.

phenylephrine hydrochloride ■
(Neo-Synephrine Injection)

Actions/Indications
Vasopressor, sympathomimetic amine.

phenylephrine hydrochloride
(continued)

This agent stimulates alpha receptors and produces the following effects either directly or indirectly through reflex action:

- Decreased heart rate (indirect)
- Increased cardiac output (direct)
- Vasoconstriction (direct)
- Does not usually produce arrhythmias

Indicated in:

- Maintenance of blood pressure during spinal or general anesthesia
- Treatment of shock due to vascular collapse, anaphylaxis or drug-induced hypotension
- Conversion of paroxysmal supraventricular tachycardia to normal sinus rhythm.

Dosage
Adults:

Mild to moderate hypotension—injection of 0.2 mg (range: 0.1–0.5 mg). Repeat no more frequently than every 10–15 min as needed; do not exceed 0.5 mg in one injection. Duration of action of one dose is 15 min.

Severe hypotension and shock—By infusion, start with 0.1–0.2 mg/min using a 0.02 mg/ml solution (10 mg in 500 ml of fluid). Titrate with blood pressure. Average maintenance dosage is 0.05–0.08 mg/min.

See Preparation section for solutions.

Higher doses may be required for hypotension produced by powerful peripheral adrenergic blocking agents or chlorpromazine.

Paroxysmal supraventricular tachycardia—*rapid* injection (over 20–30 seconds) initially of 0.5 mg (0.5 ml of a 1% solution). Subsequent doses which are determined by the initial blood pressure response should not exceed the preceding dose by more than 0.1–0.2 mg.

Do Not Exceed a Dose of 1 Mg.
Children:
Intravenous administration in any mode is not recommended. Use subcutaneous or intramuscular routes.

Preparation and Storage
Available in 1-ml ampuls, 10 mg/ml (1% solution).
Dosage Calculations for the 1% Solution:

Dose Required	Volume of 1% Solution to Use
10 mg	1.0 ml
5 mg	0.5 ml
1 mg	0.1 ml

To prepare an 0.1% solution, dilute 1 ml of a 1% solution (10 mg) in 9 ml sterile water for injection.
Dosage Calculations for a 0.1% Solution:

Dose Required	Vol. of 0.1% Solution to Use
0.1 mg	0.1 ml
0.2 mg	0.2 ml
0.5 mg	0.5 ml

For continuous infusion use an 0.02% solution. Prepare by adding 10 mg of drug to 500 ml of D5W or NS. This solution will contain 0.02 mg/ml.

Drug Incompatibilities
Do not add any other agent to IV bottle.

Do not inject into an IV line containing:
Sodium bicarbonate or Aminophylline.

Modes of IV Administration

Injection
Yes
Using a 1% or 0.1% solution as stated in Dosage section.

Intermittent Infusion
Yes
Using an 0.02 mg/ml solution as stated in Dosage and Preparation sections.
Use an infusion pump.

Continuous Infusion
Yes
Using an 0.02 mg/ml solution as stated in Dosage and Preparation sections. Begin with a rate of 0.1–

0.2 mg/min; titrate with blood pressure.
   Use an infusion pump.

Contraindications; Warnings; Precautions; Adverse Reactions

Contraindications
1. Uncontrolled hypertension
2. Ventricular tachycardia

Precautions
1. Use with extreme caution in:
   a. The elderly
   b. Hyperthyroidism
   c. Bradycardia
   d. Heart block of any degree
   e. Myocardial disease (coronary insufficiency, myocardial fibrosis, etc.)
   f. Severe arteriosclerosis
   g. Halothane anesthesia (can produce arrhythmias)
   h. In labor and delivery if an oxytocic drug has also been used (the combination can produce *severe* hypertension)
2. The pressor effect of this drug is potentiated by MAO inhibitor agents. If the patient has been receiving an MAO inhibitor, the initial dose of phenylephrine should be reduced.
3. If excessive hypertension occurs with this drug, phentolamine (Regitine) can be used. See page 273 for further information on phentolamine.
4. In hypotension secondary to hypovolemia, blood volume depletion must always be corrected before or during use of this drug.
5. When used to treat paroxysmal supraventricular tachycardia, a large dose of this drug (greater than 1 mg) can precipitate premature ventricular contractions, ventricular tachycardia, a sensation of fullness in the head and tingling of the extremities. The effects of the drug last 15–20 minutes.

Adverse Reactions
1. Excessive elevation in blood pressure

2. Ventricular irritability producing premature ventricular contractions, ventricular tachycardia and fibrillation
3. Sinus tachycardia
4. A feeling of fullness in the head
5. Tingling in the extremities

☐ Nursing Implications
1. Monitor blood pressure (direct arterial pressure is the preferred method) continuously during injection and for 15 minutes following, followed by determinations every 5 minutes for 30 minutes, and every 10–15 minutes thereafter until pressure has stabilized at a desirable level (as determined by the physician). An 0.5 mg injection will elevate systemic blood pressure for approximately 15 minutes.
   During infusions, monitor blood pressure every 2 minutes until a desirable level is reached (as determined by the physician) and every 15–30 minutes thereafter. As blood pressure is rising toward desired level, slow infusion. When level is reached, stop infusion. Continue to monitor blood pressure and heart rate for return of hypotension. See No. 5 below.
2. Administer supportive care such as replacement of fluids, maintenance of body warmth, and use of Trendelenburg position (unless contraindicated) for the patient in shock.
3. Monitor urine output hourly in the shock patient; report oliguria (output less than 30 ml in 2 consecutive hours) to the physician.
4. All patients should be observed for cardiac arrhythmias via a continuous ECG monitor. Be prepared to treat premature ventriculation contractions and ventricular tachycardia (lidocaine and defibrillator should be readily available).
5. Use an infusion pump. If unavailable, use microdrop IV tubing and do not leave the patient unattended.

phenytoin sodium ■
(Dilantin)

Actions/Indications
Anticonvulsant, antiarrhythmic
agent. Used to prevent and control
seizures of grand mal variety. Also
used to control arrhythmias such as:
• Supraventricular tachycardia
• Premature ventricular contractions
• Ventricular tachycardia
especially those arrhythmias secondary to digitalis toxicity. Exerts little
effect on atrial flutter or fibrillation
or recurrent ventricular tachycardia.
Plasma concentrations between 10
and 18 mcg/ml produce therapeutic
effects.[1]
Plasma drug concentration is the
most reliable guide for adequate
dosage.

Dosage
Adults:
Status epilepticus—150–250 mg
followed by 100–150 mg 30 min later; repeat until seizures are controlled. Do not exceed 750 mg in 1
hr.
 *Seizure prophylaxis, postsurgery or
trauma*—100–200 mg every 4 hrs.
 Arrhythmias—50–100 mg every 5
min until toxicity (nystagmus) occurs, the arrhythmia is controlled, or
1000 mg has been given. Follow
with 500 mg in 24 hrs. Place patient
on oral antiarrhythmic therapy as
soon as possible.
See Warning No. 3.
Patients with renal impairment
and uremia may require reduced
dosage according to the severity of
impairment.
Children:
Seizures and status epilepticus—3–8
mg/kg/24 hrs or 250 mg/M^2/24 hrs
in divided doses.

Preparation and Storage
Available in a premixed form, 2-ml
and 5-ml ampuls, and 2-ml prefilled
syringes, all 50 mg/ml. Discard unused portions of ampuls.
 Do not use drug solution if it is
hazy or contains a precipitate. A
faint yellow color has no effect on
potency.
 Do not add to IV fluids; see Injection under Modes of IV Administration.

Drug Incompatibilities
Do not mix with any other medication in any manner.

Modes of IV Administration

Injection
Yes
*Slowly. Do not exceed an injection rate of
50 mg/min* (25 mg/min in patients
with coronary artery disease).
 Inject either directly into the vein
or cannula, or into an injection site
in the IV tubing that is *immediately*
above the junction between the tubing and cannula. This prevents mixing of the drug with fluid.
 Flush IV line or vein with 10 ml
NS after injection. It is not necessary
to further dilute ready-mixed solution prior to injection.

Intermittent Infusion
No
This drug precipitates in *all* solutions. Effects such precipitation may
have on the patient are not known.[2]

Continuous Infusion
No
Some groups are administering this
drug as a 1-mg/ml infusion in NS.
This practice is not currently recognized by the F.D.A. or the manufacturer.

Contraindications; Warnings; Pre-
cautions; Adverse Reactions

Contraindications
1. Hypersensitivity to hydantoin
 products
2. Sinus bradycardia
3. Sinus node exit block (sinoatrial
 block)
4. Second and third degree A-V
 block
5. Stokes-Adams syndrome

Warnings
1. Intravenous injection must not

exceed 50 mg/min, or 25 mg/min in patients with coronary artery disease. See Adverse Reaction No. 1.
2. This agent is not indicated for seizures secondary to hypoglycemia.
3. There are many drug interactions associated with this agent:

Drugs That May Affect the Pharmacokinetics of Phenytoin (Diphenylhydantoin) in Man[3]

Drugs That May Increase Phenytoin Levels in the Blood

Bishydroxycoumarin	Isoniazid
Chloramphenicol	Methylphenidate
Chlordiazepoxide	Phenyramidol
Chlorpromazine	Phenobarbital
Diazepam	Prochlorperazine
Disulfiram	Propoxyphene
Estrogens	
Ethyl alcohol	

Drugs That May Decrease Phenytoin Levels in The Blood by Enzyme Induction

Carbamazepine	Phenobarbital
Ethyl alcohol	

Drugs That May Alter Plasma Protein Binding of Phenytoin

Phenylbutazone	Sulfafurazole
Salicylic acid	

Dosage requirements of phenytoin will be altered in the presence of these agents, to prevent toxicity or underdosage.
4. Use with caution in patients with coronary artery disease or hypotension. Injections may cause further lowering of pressure and possibly reduced myocardial perfusion. See injection rate in Injection section.
5. The effects of this drug in pregnancy and nursing infants are unknown. Some studies suggest the possibility of drug-related birth defects. However, anticonvulsant drugs should not be withheld in patients likely to have major seizures because of the possibility of precipitating status epilepticus.

Precautions
1. Patients with liver impairment, or the elderly may need dosage modification. Serum levels must be closely followed.
2. This drug may cause hyperglycemia in normal individuals and further elevation of serum glucose in diabetics.

Adverse Reactions
1. During injection at a rate greater than 50 mg/min: respiratory arrest, hypotension, idioventricular rhythm, asystole, ventricular fibrillation
2. This drug usually improves A-V conduction, but can also cause slowing of atrial and A-V conduction, precipitating heart block
3. Vertigo, nausea and drowsiness are side effects
4. Toxic blood levels can cause: nystagmus or lateral gaze, ataxia, lethargy
5. Can also precipitate megaloblastic anemia (responsive to folate), thrombocytopenia, leukopenia, granulocytopenia and agranulocytosis
6. Peripheral neuropathy
7. Rashes, mild and severe
8. Hyperglycemia
9. Vomiting and constipation

Management of Overdosage
Initial signs of toxicity: nystagmus, ataxia, dysarthria. Signs of advancing toxicity are coma, unresponsive pupils, hypotension. Death can occur secondary to apnea. Treatment:
1. Prevent by following serum drug levels frequently (range of therapeutic level: 10–18 mcg/ml).
2. No antidote known. Discontinue the drug with appearance of earliest signs.
3. In advanced toxicity, support respirations with airway or endotracheal tube, oxygen and respirator as needed.
4. Vasopressors to support blood pressure (dopamine).
5. Hemodialysis if necessary to clear drug from the serum.

phenytoin sodium
(continued)

☐ **Nursing Implications**
1. Follow hospital policy as to who can administer this drug intravenously, physician or nurse.
2. This medication should not be added to IV fluid for infusion.
3. Closely observe **all** patients receiving this drug intravenously, using continuous ECG monitoring during the injection. The injection should be stopped if the P-R interval becomes prolonged (normal is 0.08–.20 seconds), or if the QRS duration is prolonged beyond 0.12 seconds. Maximal effect of the drug is seen in 5 minutes after IV injection. Monitor for drug effectiveness at this time. Do not leave the patient unattended for the first 10 minutes following injection.
4. Obtain a blood pressure reading just prior to and immediately following injection of the drug. Monitor every 5 minutes for the following 30 minutes. The injection should be slowed or momentarily stopped if the patient complains of dizziness or diaphoresis. Take the blood pressure at this time. Monitor closely until return to the preinjection level and stabilization are seen.
5. Ambulate the patient with caution, after 1 hour of bed rest following an injection.
6. Observe for signs of toxicity. It is important to discontinue injections at the earliest sign: ataxia, nystagmus (constant involuntary eye movements), dysarthria (difficulty or slurring of speech), change in mental status. Notify the physician immediately on appearance of any of these signs.
7. If early signs of toxicity are present, monitor for advancing signs: hypotension, depressed mental activity, decreasing respiratory rate. Be prepared to support ventilation. Place the following equipment at the bedside and prepare it for immediate use: airways, suction, oxygen, endotracheal tubes and laryngoscope, manual breathing bag (Ambu, Hope, Puritan) with mask. Begin ventilatory support via airway and manual bag if respiratory rate falls below 8–10/minute despite verbal stimuli. Continue ventilation until patient regains an appropriate respiratory rate and arterial blood gases return to normal. Patient may require endotracheal intubation.

References
1. Winkle, Roger A., Glantz, Stanton A., and Harrison, Donald C.: Pharmacologic Therapy of Ventricular Arrhythmias. *American Journal of Cardiology*, 36:643, October 31, 1975.
2. Trissel, Lawrence Al: *Handbook on Injectable Drugs*, American Society of Hospital Pharmacists, Washington, D.C., 1980, p. 416.
3. Winkle, op. cit. p. 643.

Suggested Readings
Amsterdam, Ezra, et al.: Systemic Approach to the Management of Cardiac Arrhythmias. *Heart and Lung*, 2:747–753, September–October 1973 (references).
Levitt, Barrie, Borer, Jeffrey, and Saropa, Arleen: The Clinical Pharmacology of Antiarrhythmic Drugs. Part II: Quinidine, Propranolol, Diphenylhydantoin, and Bretylium. *Cardiovascular Nursing*, November–December, 1974, pp. 27–32.
———: Treatment of Cardiac Arrhythmias. *Medical Letter on Drugs and Therapeutics*, 16(25):101–108, December 6, 1974.

physostigmine salicylate ■
(Antilirium)

Actions/Indications
Cholinesterase inhibitor, prolongs and exaggerates the effect of acetylcholine at the myoneural junction. Produces:
• Constriction of pupil

- Increased tone of gastrointestinal muscles
- Constriction of bronchi
- Stimulation of salivary and sweat glands

Used to reverse toxic effects on the central nervous system caused by anticholinergic drugs (atropine, scopolamine, benztropine, and tricyclic antidepressants).

Toxic effects of these drugs are: hallucinations, disorientation, hyperactivity, coma, medullary paralysis. This is the only cholinesterase inhibitor that can effectively cross the blood-brain barrier.

Dosage
Adults:
0.5–2.0 mg
  Repeat 1 mg doses as needed.
  To reverse the toxic or clinical effects of anticholinergic drugs, the dose of physostigmine is twice that of the other drug in milligrams. For example, if the dose of atropine had been 2 mg, the dose of physostigmine could be 4 mg.
Children:
No data available on intravenous administration.

Preparation and Storage
Discard unused portions of vials.
  Supplied in 2 ml ampuls, 1 mg/ml.

Drug Incompatibilities
Do not mix with fluids or any other medication.

Modes of IV Administration

Injection
Yes
Inject undiluted over 1–2 minutes.

Intermittent Infusion
No

Continuous Infusion
No

Contraindications; Warnings; Precautions; Adverse Reactions

Contraindications
  1. Asthma

  2. Gangrene
  3. Diabetes mellitus
  4. Cardiovascular disease
  5. Mechanical obstruction of the intestinal or urinary tract
  6. In patients receiving choline esters or neuromuscular blocking agents (succinylcholine or decamethonium)

Precautions
  1. Patients may exhibit hyperreactivity to this agent. Keep atropine readily available as an antidote.
  2. If symptoms of excessive salivation, emesis, urination and defecation occur, injection and further use of this drug should be terminated.
  3. If excessive sweating or nausea occurs, the dosage should be reduced.
  4. Rapid administration can cause bradycardia, hypersalivation leading to respiratory difficulties and possible convulsions.
  5. An overdose of this drug will cause a full cholinergic crisis characterized by:
     a. Excessive salivation
     b. Sweating
     c. Miosis
     d. Nausea, vomiting, diarrhea
     e. Bradycardia or tachycardia
     f. Hypo- or hypertension
     g. Confusion
     h. Convulsions, coma
     i. Muscle weakness and paralysis
     In order of appearance.

☐ Nursing Implications
  1. Monitor for signs of cholinergic crises following injection of this drug; see Precautions. Be prepared to support respiration.
  2. Keep atropine at the bedside. Do not leave the patient alone for the first 15–30 minutes after injection.
  3. This drug is rapidly metabolized by the body, and additional doses may be required if the duration of the anticholinergic agent's action exceeds that of the physostigmine. Monitor for

physostigmine salicylate
(continued)
signs of the effects of the anticholinergic agent: mental confusion, stupor, nausea and diaphoresis. Notify the physician of these effects and be prepared to administer additional doses of physostigmine.

Suggested Reading
Guyton, Arthur C.: *Textbook of Medical Physiology,* Chapter 57—The Autonomic Nervous System: The Adrenal Medulla, Philadelphia: W. B. Saunders Company, 1976, pp. 768–780.

phytonadione ■
(Vitamin K₁, AquaMEPHYTON, Konakion)

Actions/Indications
Vitamin necessary for the production of active prothrombin, and clotting factors VII, IX and X, in the liver. After IV administration hemorrhage can be controlled in 3–6 hrs. Used to treat coagulation disorders caused by vitamin K deficiency or interference with vitamin K activity; as an antidote for coumarin drugs.

Dosage
IV administration should be used *only* when subcutaneous or intramuscular routes cannot be used. See Warning No. 7.
Adults:
Anticoagulant-induced prothrombin deficiency and hypoprothrombinema due to other causes—2.5–10 mg or up to 25 mg. Repeat if prothrombin time has not been shortened satisfactorily in 8 hrs.
Use smallest dose for effectiveness without lowering prothrombin time too far below an effective level. Short-acting anticoagulants will require lower dose than long-acting.
Children:
In newborn hemorrhagic disease intramuscular or subcutaneous routes must be used.

Preparation and Storage
Supplied in 2 mg/ml and 10 mg/ml solutions. Protect these vials from light
Use immediately after adding to fluids. Do not use if, when mixed with fluid, an oily layer or droplets appear.
Wrap IV bottle, bag or burette chamber with an ultraviolet light bag or aluminum foil to protect the solution from light.
Discard all unused portions of drug vials.

Drug Incompatibilities
Do not mix with any other medication in any manner.

Modes of IV Administration

Injection
Yes
In emergency, 5–25 mg over 5–10 min into the tubing of a running IV. No more than 1 mg/min.
Dilution prior to injection is not required.

Intermittent Infusion
Yes
Use only NS, D5/NS, or D5W, 50 ml. *Preferred route.* Infuse no more rapidly than 1 mg/min.
Dilute dose in enough fluid to make drip rate calculation easy.
Use an infusion pump.

Continuous Infusion
No
Short-term infusions only.

Contraindications; Warnings; Precautions; Adverse Reactions

Contraindications
Hypersensitivity

Warnings
1. An immediate coagulant effect cannot be expected even after IV push administration. Measurable effect will not be seen before 1–2 hrs. Whole blood or component therapy must be used in hypotension and hemorrhage.

2. This drug will not counteract the effects of heparin.
3. In anticoagulant-induced hypoprothrombinemia, overzealous therapy with vitamin K may restore conditions which originally permitted thromboembolic phenomena. Keep vitamin K dose as low as possible to prevent under-anticoagulation.
4. Monitor prothrombin time during therapy.
5. Repeated large doses of vitamin K are not warranted in liver disease if response to initial dose is unsatisfactory.
6. It is not known whether this drug affects fertility or fetal development.

Precautions
1. A temporary resistance to prothrombin-depressing anticoagulants (coumarin) may result, especially in larger doses. Increased doses of the anticoagulant may be required when reinitiated, or another agent such as heparin may be used.
2. Follow injection-rate limitations *absolutely.*

Adverse Reactions
1. **Deaths have occurred after IV administration.**
2. Transient flushing sensations and alterations of taste have been reported.
3. Dizziness, rapid weak pulse, profuse sweating, brief hypotension, dyspnea and cyanosis.
4. Anaphylaxis, shock and cardiac arrest.

☐ **Nursing Implications**
1. Signs and symptoms of too-rapid injection are chills and fever, chest tightness, hypotension, seizures, cyanosis.
2. Monitor blood pressure frequently during injection and infusion, every 2–5 minutes. If any of the above signs or symptoms appear, slow or stop infusion or injection. Do not leave the patient unattended.
3. Be aware of the patient's prothrombin times.

4. Monitor for bleeding until an effect is seen from the drug. Administer supportive measures as prescribed.
5. Monitor for adverse reactions and initiate appropriate care. Notify physician if tachycardia, diaphoresis, hypotension, dyspnea or cyanosis occurs.
6. Take anaphylaxis precautions; see Appendix.

polymyxin B sulfate ■
(Aerosporin)

Actions/Indications
Antibiotic; used to treat infections caused by susceptible strains of:
- *Pseudomonas aeruginosa*
- *H. influenzae*
- *E. coli*
- *Aerobacter aerogenes*
- *Klebsiella pneumoniae*

The intravenous route is indicated in infections in all locations except meningeal infections, in which case the drug should be administered intrathecally.

Dosage
Adults and Children:
15,000–25,000 units/kg/day in the presence of normal kidney function. (Do not exceed 25,000 units/kg/day.)

In all cases, one half of the daily dose is administered by infusion twice daily.
Adults and Children With Renal Failure:[1]
Mild impairment—25,000 units/kg the first day and then 10,000 units/kg every 3 *days.*
Uremia—25,000 units/kg the first day and then 10,000 units/kg every 5–7 *days.*
Infants:
Up to 40,000 units/kg/day, depending on condition of the patient, organism being treated, response to the drug.
Premature and Newborn Infants:
25,000–40,000 units/kg/day via infusion.

Preparation and Storage
Reconstitute 500,000-unit vial with 2

polymyxin B sulfate
(continued)
ml sterile water for injection, D5W or NS. Shake vial until drug is dissolved.

Store under refrigeration; discard any unused portions after 72 hrs.

Use only D5W or NS for infusion fluid, 300–500 ml.

Drug Incompatibilities
Do not mix in any manner with:
Amphotericin
Ampicillin
Cefazolin
Cephalothin
Chloramphenicol
Chlorothiazide
Chlortetracycline
Heparin
Magnesium sulfate
Penicillins
Prednisolone
Tetracycline

Modes of IV Administration

Injection
No

Intermittent Infusion
Yes
500,000 units in 300–500 ml D5W or NS with drip rate set to deliver 1/2 daily dose over 60 to 90 minutes.

Continuous Infusion
No

Contraindications; Warnings; Precautions; Adverse Reactions

Contraindications
Hypersensitivity to polymyxin or colistin.

Warnings
1. Renal function must be monitored during therapy.
2. Patients with renal impairment must have a reduced dosage.
3. Nephrotoxicity due to this drug is evidenced by albuminuria, cellular casts in the urine and increased BUN. Diminishing urine output and rising BUN are indications for discontinuation of the drug.
4. Neurotoxicity may be manifested by irritability, weakness, drowsiness, ataxia, numbness of the extremities, blurring of vision. This is usually seen in high doses or in patients with renal failure. The drug should be discontinued with the onset of these signs and symptoms.
5. Concurrent use of other neurotoxic antibiotics (kanamycin, streptomycin, polymyxin E, neomycin, gentamicin and viomycin) should be avoided.
6. Neurotoxicity can result in respiratory paralysis, especially when the drug is given soon after anesthesia and/or muscle relaxants.
7. Safety for use in pregnancy has not been established.

Precautions
1. Obtain baseline renal functions prior to use.
2. This drug can cause prolongation of the muscle-paralyzing effects of tubocurarine, succinylcholine, gallamine, and decamethonium.
3. If respiratory depression occurs, drug must be discontinued.
4. Overgrowth of nonsusceptible organism can occur; if so, this drug must be discontinued.

Adverse Reactions
1. Renal: albuminuria, cylinduria, azotemia, rising polymyxin blood levels without increase in dose.
2. Neurologic: dizziness, ataxia, drowsiness, circumoral numbness, respiratory paralysis.
3. Rash, drug fever, anaphylaxis.
4. Thrombophlebitis at injection site.

☐ Nursing Implications
1. Take anaphylaxis precautions; see Appendix.
2. Monitor for the onset of renal damage:

a. Measure urine output at least every 8 hours. A urine output less than 30 ml/hour for 2–3 consecutive hours in adults or below normal in children, according to age and size, should be reported to the physician.
b. Send urine for analysis daily or on alternate days.
c. Be aware of the patient's pretreatment BUN and any changes during therapy.
3. Monitor for the onset of signs and symptoms of neurotoxicity as listed in Warning No. 4. Notify the physician of positive findings.
4. If neurotoxicity occurs, begin monitoring for respiratory depression:
   a. Count respiratory rate and depth hourly
   b. Notify the physician if the respiratory rate falls below 8–10/minute
   c. Monitor arterial blood gases as indicated
   d. Be prepared to support ventilation
5. Monitor for signs and symptoms of nonsusceptible organisms or overgrowth infection:
   a. Fever (take rectal temperature at least every 4–6 hours)
   b. Increasing malaise
   c. Localized signs and symptoms of infection—redness, soreness, pain, swelling, drainage (change in volume or character of pre-existing drainage)
   d. Cough (change in volume or character of pre-existing sputum)
   e. Diarrhea
   f. Rash (monilial) in the perineal area or mouth (thrush) due to *Candida albicans*

Reference
1. Appel, Gerald B. and Neu, Harold C.: The Nephrotoxicity of Antimicrobial Agents. *New England Journal of Medicine*, 296(12):667, March 24, 1977.

potassium chloride and potassium lactate ■

Actions/Indications
Electrolyte solution to provide potassium ions to intra- and extracellular fluids, to maintain osmotic balance and cell membrane electrical potential.

Used to maintain serum potassium at normal levels during parenteral fluid therapy and to correct hypokalemic states.

Dosage
Dosage and rate of infusion are dependent on serum potassium (K+) levels:
Adults:
If serum K+ is *greater than* 2.5 mEq/liter, administer at a rate no greater than 10 mEq/hour in an infusion concentration less than 30 mEq/liter. The total 24-hour dose should not exceed 150 mEq.

If serum K+ is *equal to or less than* 2.0 mEq/liter with ECG changes or paralysis present, infuse at a rate of 40 mEq/hour. As much as 400 mEq can be given in 24 hours. (Use saline for infusion in this situation; dextrose solutions may lower serum K+.) **Cardiac Monitoring Is Mandatory During This Therapy.**
Do not administer in a concentration greater than 80 mEq/liter or infusion rate greater than 40 mEq/hour, **under any circumstances.**
Children:
Do not administer over 3–5 mEq/kg in 24 hours except in severe cases. Base replacement on daily need vs. deficit. Use a solution of 20–40 mEq/L.

Do not administer until patient is excreting adequate amounts of urine.

Preparation and Storage
Use any IV solution except mannitol (see reference to indications for the use of NS, in Dosage section). MIX ALL PREPARATIONS WELL AFTER ADDING POTASSIUM BY *INVERTING* BOTTLE SEVERAL TIMES TO AVOID CONCEN-

potassium chloride and potassium lactate
(continued)
TRATED ACCUMULATION OF
THE POTASSIUM AT THE BOT-
TOM OF THE CONTAINER. MIX-
ING IS ESPECIALLY IMPORTANT
IN THE USE OF PLASTIC IV
BAGS.
Use only clear solutions.
Supplied in several forms and
concentrations.

Drug Incompatibilities
Do not add to mannitol.
Do not inject diazepam (Valium)
into an IV line containing potassium.

Modes of IV Administration

Injection
No
**Potassium Should Never Be Ad-
ministered By This Mode or In an
Undiluted Form.**

Intermittent Infusion
Yes
In emergency treatment of hypokalemia—
Add 40–60 mEq to 500 ml NS.
Use cardiac monitoring during use
of this mode for emergency treat-
ment.
See Dosage section for infusion
rates.
Use infusion pump.

Continuous Infusion
Yes
Usually 20–40 mEq in 1000 ml. See
Dosage section for rate of infusion.

Contraindications; Warnings; Pre-cautions; Adverse Reactions

Contraindications
1. In conditions where high serum
   potassium levels are likely to
   develop, such as renal failure
   and shock
2. Chronic nephritis
3. In the presence of potassium retention

Warnings
1. To avoid potassium intoxica-

tion, follow infusion rate
recommendations in Dosage
section.
2. In patients with renal or adrenal
   insufficiency, serum potassium
   levels may already be elevated.
3. Monitor serum potassium and
   ECG changes frequently during
   therapy.

Precautions
1. Plasma potassium levels do not
   necessarily correlate to cell potassium levels.
2. A high serum potassium level
   may precipitate death due to
   cardiac depression or arrhythmias (such as conduction defects).
3. The patient should be well
   hydrated and should demon-
   strate adequate renal function
   prior to the parenteral administration of potassium.

Adverse Reactions
1. Gastrointestinal: nausea,
   vomiting, diarrhea, abdominal
   pains
2. Hyperkalemia:
   a. Numbness and tingling in
      the extremities
   b. Flaccid muscle paralysis
   c. Listlessness
   d. Confusion
   e. Hypotension
   f. Cardiac arrhythmias: atrio-
      ventricular block, loss of P-
      waves, widening QRS,
      peaked T-waves, bradycardia

Management of Overdosage
(serum potassium greater than 6
mEq/liter)[1]
1. Discontinue the infusion immediately; keep the vein open.
2. Reduce serum potassium:
   a. If there are ECG changes,
      administer 5–10 ml of calci-
      um gluceptate intravenously
      until ECG appears normal.
      See entry on calcium
      gluceptate, page 42. (Calci-
      um gluconate or chloride,
      10% solutions, can be used
      in place of calcium

gluceptate.) Administration of the calcium preparation should continue until definitive measures are successful in reducing serum potassium.

b. A rapid injection of 44 mEq of sodium bicarbonate over 5–10 minutes will lower the serum potassium level by increasing blood pH and subsequently moving the potassium intracellularly. This initial sodium bicarbonate should be followed by 88 –132 mEq in a continuous infusion each hour.

c. Another method for reducing serum potassium is with glucose and insulin administration. Usually 500–1000 ml of 10% dextrose and water is given over 1 hour with 10–15 units of regular insulin. As with the use of sodium bicarbonate, this technique only moves the potassium into the intracellular space.

d. To remove potassium from the body, cation exchange resins such as polystyrene sodium sulfonate (Kayexalate) should be given as a retention enema. Usually 30 gm of the polystyrene is added to 100–200 ml of water. See specific instructions accompanying the drug. Keep in mind that sodium is exchanged for the potassium. This may be a problem in patients with congestive heart failure. Sorbitol solution can also be administered to induce diarrhea and thus increase potassium loss.

e. In severe cases of hyperkalemia, hemo- or peritoneal dialysis may be indicated to rapidly reduce serum potassium.

f. In all therapy, care must be taken to closely monitor serum potassium and to prevent hypokalemia.

☐ Nursing Implications

1. Monitor the patient's ECG continuously if:
   a. The potassium infusion must be rapid in the presence of severe hypokalemia.
   b. There are ECG changes secondary to the hypokalemia.
   c. The patient has pre-existing arrhythmias.
2. Use an infusion pump for rapid infusions to prevent overdosage.
3. Be aware of the patient's serum potassium (normal is 3.5–4.5 mEq/liter) during therapy.
4. Monitor for signs and symptoms of hyperkalemia. See Adverse Reaction No. 2.
5. Avoid extravasation. See Appendix. Thrombophlebitis is common following potassium infusions, especially if the infusion rate is rapid or concentrated. To prevent this complication, use a large central vein, such as the subclavian, if possible. Discontinue if phlebitis is suspected; apply warm compresses until signs and symptoms subside.
6. The signs and symptoms of hypokalemia: weakness, muscle cramps, irritability, abdominal distention, cardiac arrhythmias.

Reference

1. Newmark, Stephen R., and Dluhy, Robert G.: Hyperkalemia and Hypokalemia. *JAMA*, 231(6):632, February 10, 1975.

pralidoxime chloride ■
(PAM, Protopam Chloride)

Actions/Indications

Anticholinesterase antagonist, reactivates cholinesterase which has been inactivated by an organophosphate (insecticides*). Used to relieve respiratory paralysis in such poisoning. Also relieves the salivation, bronchospasm, etc. Weakly antagonizes the

*Parathion, sairin, tetraum, TEPP, and Diazinon.

pralidoxime chloride
(continued)
effect of: neostigmine, pyridostigmine, and ambenonium used in the
treatment of myasthenia gravis,
where one of these agents has precipitated a cholinergic crisis.

Dosage

In poisoning: while maintaining respiratory support in the absence of
cyanosis, give *atropine* IV, 2–4 mg. If
cyanosis is present, atropine should
be given IM; administer every 5–10
minutes until signs of atropine toxicity appear (tachycardia, mental confusion). Maintain atropine effects for
at least 48 hours.

Start pralidoxime at the same time
as atropine.
Adults:
(for all indications):

Initially—1–2 gm as an infusion in
100 ml NS over 15–30 minutes. If
pulmonary edema is present, give as
an injection over not less than 5
minutes.

After 1 hour, give a second dose
of 1–2 gm if muscle weakness has
not been relieved. Additional doses
may be needed if muscle weakness
persists.

*In cholinergic crisis produced by neo-
stigmine, pyridostigmine, or ambenonium*
—1–2 gm followed by 250 mg every
5 min up to an additional 1–2 gm as
needed.
Children:
20–40 mg/kg as 5% solution; most
effective when given within a few
hours after poisoning. Little effect is
seen if given after 48 hours; but in
severe poisoning, the therapy should
be initiated regardless. Repeat
doses, titrate with recurring signs of
poisoning.

Preparation and Storage

To reconstitute, add 20 ml of sterile
water for injection to each 1-gm vial
to be used. Shake until powder cake
is dissolved. Add to NS for infusion.

Drug Incompatibilities

Do not mix with any other medication in syringe or infusion fluid.

Modes of IV Administration

Injection
Yes
Inject undiluted over not less than 5
minutes. See Dosage section for indications for this mode.

Intermittent Infusion
Yes
Preferred Mode.
Add dose to 100 ml NS. Infuse over
15–30 minutes. See Dosage section
for indications for this mode.

Continuous Infusion
No
Pharmacologically inappropriate.

Contraindications; Warnings; Precautions; Adverse Reactions

Warnings
1. Not effective in the treatment of
   poisoning due to phosphorus,
   inorganic phosphates, or organophosphates not having anticholinesterase activity. Consult
   local poison control center for
   this information.
2. No recommendation is made as
   to the use of this drug in the
   management of poisoning by
   pesticides of the carbamate class
   (Sevin). Pralidoxime can intensi-
   fy the signs of toxicity.

Precautions
1. Poisoning symptoms may mask
   side effects of this drug.
2. Rapid infusion may cause tachycardia, laryngospasm, and muscle rigidity; follow infusion
   recommendations.
3. Renal insufficiency will contribute to accumulation of the drug;
   a reduced dosage is
   recommended.
4. Use with great caution in the
   management of reversal of therapeutic drug overdose in myasthenia gravis since it may
   precipitate a myasthenic crisis.
5. Barbiturates are potentiated by
   the poisons being treated by
   this drug. Use them with cau-

tion to treat seizures produced by the poisoning.
6. Morphine, theophylline, aminophylline, succinylcholine, reserpine, and phenothiazine-type tranquilizers should be avoided in the presence of this type of poisoning.

Adverse Reactions
It is difficult to differentiate drug side effects from the effects of poison or atropine.
1. Central nervous system: excitement, manic behavior following recovery of consciousness, dizziness, blurred vision, diplopia, headache, drowsiness
2. Gastrointestinal: nausea, vomiting
3. Cardiac: tachycardias
4. Hyperventilation

☐ **Nursing Implications**
Management of Organophosphate Poisoning:
1. Signs and symptoms of organophosphate poisoning appear at varying times and in varying degrees after exposure, depending on the route of administration and degree of exposure, but always appear at least within 24 hours. In *mild* poisoning, signs and symptoms can be—fatigue, headache, dizziness, numbness of extremities, nausea and vomiting, excessive sweating, and salivation, tightness in the chest, abdominal cramps, and a serum cholinesterase activity of 20–50% above normal.
    Severe poisoning can result in unconsciousness, seizures, loss of pupillary reaction to light, muscle fasciculations, flaccid paralysis, heavy secretions from the mouth and nose, rales, cyanosis, respiratory distress, and a serum cholinesterase activity of less than 10% below normal. This degree of poisoning, if untreated, can be fatal.[1]
2. Patient must be in an ICU while receiving this drug.
3. Maintain respiratory support as indicated.
4. Monitor vital signs, including ECG, continuously during therapy in the acute states. Be prepared to treat any arrhythmia. Keep lidocaine 100 mg and atropine 1 mg at the bedside.
5. Confirm nature of poisoning and recommended treatment through the local poison control center.
6. Wear rubber gloves and use good handwashing techniques when handling patient to avoid contamination by the poison. Remove and rinse contaminated clothing and place in plastic bags for disposal. Bathe skin thoroughly with a water-baking soda solution. Rinse well. *Discard* bath linen in plastic bags; do not launder. Flush eyes well with saline. Gastric lavage will be performed if ingestion of the poison is suspected.
7. Monitor urine output hourly during the first 24 hours and every 8 hours for the next 48 hours. Notify the physician if the urine output falls below 30 ml/hours for 2–3 successive hours in adults. Monitor urine glucose and acetone every 4 hours.
8. Take precautions to prevent patient injury in the event of excitement or manic behavior on return of consciousness. Use seizure precautions.
In Myasthenia Gravis:
1. If this drug is being administered to antagonize an anticholinesterase drug in the patient with myasthenia gravis, monitor for the signs of a myasthenic crisis: drooping eyelids, slurring of speech, generalized muscle weakness, difficulty swallowing, decreasing respiratory rate.
    The patient can pass quickly from a cholinergic crisis (for which the pralidoxime is being given) to a myasthenic crisis. Keep neostigmine or pyridostigmine readily available, as well as respiratory support equipment. See neostigmine, page 239, and pyridostigmine, page 303.

pralidoxime chloride,
(continued)

Reference

1. Namba, Tatsuji, *et al.*: Poisoning Due to Organophosphate Insecticides. *The American Journal of Medicine*, 50:481, April, 1971.

Suggested Reading

Namba, Tatsuji, *et al.*: Poisoning Due to Organophosphate Insecticides. *The American Journal of Medicine*, 68(3):335–339, March, 1975.

prednisolone sodium phosphate (Hydeltrasol) and prednisolone sodium succinate ■
(Meticortelone)

Actions/Indications

Synthetic glucocorticoid (analog of hydrocortisone) that has salt-retaining anti-inflammatory properties and other profound and varied effects on metabolism. The following is a partial list of the major indications for the use of this drug:

• Endocrine disorders, such as adrenocortical insufficiency
• Rheumatic disorders
• Collagen diseases
• Dermatologic disorders
• Allergic states
• Ophthalmic diseases
• Gastrointestinal diseases
• Respiratory disorders
• Hematologic disorders
• Neoplastic diseases

Dosage

Prednisolone Sodium Phosphate:
Adults:
Initially—4–60 mg depending on condition being treated. *Usual maintenance range*—10–400 mg/day
Children:
40–250 mcg/kg or 1.5–7.5 mg/M^2 1 to 2 times daily
Prednisolone Sodium Succinate:
Adults:
Range: 4–60 mg daily in two equal doses
Children:
40–250 mcg/kg or 1.5–7.5 mg/M^2 1 to 2 times daily

Preparation and Storage

Prednisolone Sodium Succinate: To reconstitute, add 2 ml sterile water for injection or NS to the 50-mg vial, this yields as 25 mg/ml solution. Use only clear colorless solutions. Refrigerate unused portions and discard after 24 hours.

Do not autoclave or store near heat.

The sodium succinate form of prednisolone is also supplied in vials of 500 mg, this is an *investigational* form. Use accompanying literature for reconstitution, dilution and use.

Prednisolone Sodium Phosphate: Supplied in 2- and 5-ml vials, 20 mg/ml.

Drug Incompatibilities

Do not mix with any other medication in solution. Do not inject into an IV line containing:
Calcium
Metaraminol
Polymyxin B

Modes of IV Administration

Injection
Yes
At a rate of 10 mg/minute. Decrease rate if patient complains of burning or tingling at injection site.

Intermittent Infusion
Yes
Use D5W or NS for infusion; infuse over 15–30 minutes.

Continuous Infusion
Yes
Use D5W or NS for infusion. Usually in a 12-hour infusion of 1/2 the daily dose.

Contraindications; Warnings; Precautions; Adverse Reactions

Contraindications
1. Systemic fungal infections.
2. In the absence of a life-threatening condition, this glucocorticoid should be avoided in: active peptic ulcer disease, systemic or ophthalmic viral disease, infections without antibiotic treatment, active and

healed TB, myasthenia gravis, psychoses.
3. Hypersensitivity.

Warnings

1. Increase dosage before and during stress, such as surgery, which increases need for glucocorticoids.
2. There may be a decreased resistance to infection and inability to localize infection during therapy. Signs of infection may be masked by steroids.
3. In pregnancy and lactation, benefits must be weighed against the risks. Observe infants born of mothers receiving this drug for signs of hypoadrenalism.
4. Can cause elevation in blood pressure, salt and water retention and increased excretion of potassium. Dietary salt restriction and potassium supplementation may be needed, along with the use of a mild diuretic.
5. Do not vaccinate during therapy.
6. Use in active TB should be limited to fulminating, disseminated cases where antituberculosis drugs are being used.
7. Patients with positive TB reactivity, administer chemoprophylaxis and monitor for activation of disease.

Precautions

1. Gradual reduction of doses prior to discontinuation may prevent secondary adrenocortical insufficiency (may not be necessary with short-term intravenous therapy).
2. Effects of this drug are enhanced in hypothyroidism and cirrhosis; dosage should be reduced in these cases.
3. Use the lowest possible effective dose.
4. Psychic disturbances may occur ranging from euphoria to psychoses.
5. Use aspirin cautiously during use of this drug in the presence of hypothrombinemia to prevent aggravation of bleeding

problems, and to prevent gastric irritation.
6. Use with caution if there is a possibility of perforation in ulcerative colitis, or diverticulitis, fresh intestinal anastomoses, active or latent peptic ulcer disease.
7. Use with caution in renal disease and congestive heart failure because of enhanced salt and water retention.
8. Use with caution in the presence of osteoporosis; this drug increases calcium loss from bones and excretion via the kidney.
9. May precipitate a crisis in myasthenia gravis.
10. Initiate antiulcer therapy during use of this drug.
11. This drug should be used with caution in patients with glaucoma because it can increase the intraocular pressure.
12. When used in the treatment of adrenocortical insufficiency concomitant therapy with a mineralocorticoid is also required.

Adverse Reactions Seen in Short-Term Intravenous Therapy

1. Fluid and electrolyte imbalance: sodium and water retention with possible secondary hypertension, hypokalemia, hypocalcemia.
2. Gastrointestinal: peptic ulcer with possible perforation, pancreatitis, ulcerative esophagitis.
3. Dermatologic: impaired wound healing.
4. Neurologic: increased intracranial pressure, seizures (increasing frequency in patients with pre-existing seizure disorder), vertigo, headaches, mental confusion, euphoria, exacerbation of psychosis.
5. Endocrine: decreased glucose tolerance, increased hypoglycemic agent and insulin requirements in diabetics.
6. Eye: increased intraocular pressure.
7. Metabolic: negative nitrogen

**prednisolone sodium phosphate
and prednisolone sodium succinate**
(continued)
balance secondary to rapid muscle catabolism.

☐ **Nursing Implications**

1. Take precautions to prevent infections in wounds by using strict aseptic technique in dressing changes, etc. Avoid traumatic procedures such as catheterizations. The skin may become more fragile because of the steroid therapy. Patients on bed rest and those with general body weakening secondary to acute illness should be turned hourly (except during sleep, then every 2–3 hours) to prevent skin breakdown. Initiate the use of supportive measures, such as flotation pads, water mattress, etc. Administer scrupulous skin care to prevent infection.
2. Monitor blood pressure every 2–4 hours, or as the patient's condition dictates, and before, during and immediately after intravenous injection; hypotension can occur.
3. Weigh the patient daily to detect for water and sodium retention. Dietary restriction in sodium may be prescribed by the physician. Examine daily for peripheral edema.
4. There may be delayed healing of wounds; take precautions to prevent dehiscence. Sutures may be left in place longer than usual for this reason.
5. Monitor urine glucose in patients on high-dose therapy and those with diabetes. These individuals may require a larger dosage of insulin or oral agent.
6. Administer antiulcer therapy as ordered to assist in preventing peptic ulcer. Monitor for signs of the development of an ulcer and/or acute intestinal bleeding: melena, positive stool guaiac, hematemesis, epigastric pain and/or distention, anemia or falling hematocrit.

7. Monitor for signs and symptoms of hypokalemia: weakness, irritability, abdominal distention, poor feeding in infants, muscle cramps.[1] Dietary or pharmacologic potassium supplements may be ordered, guided by serum potassium levels.
8. Monitor for signs and symptoms of hypocalcemia (a serum calcium of 8.5 mg%): irritability, change in mental status, seizures, nausea, vomiting, diarrhea, muscle cramps, carpopedal spasm; late effects are cardiac arrhythmias, laryngeal spasm and apnea.[2,3] Dietary or pharmacologic supplements may be ordered, guided by serum calcium levels.
9. Patients with a history of seizure activity may have an increasing number of seizures while on steroid therapy. Apply appropriate safety precautions.
10. Monitor for behavioral changes, which may range from simple euphoria to depression and psychosis. Apply appropriate safety precautions. A change in dosage may relieve such symptoms.
11. Tuberculin testing should be carried out prior to initiation of steroid therapy, if possible. The patient's reactivity to the tuberculin is altered by the drug, giving a false result.
12. Ambulate the patient with caution if vertigo occurs, and initiate the use of side rails to prevent injury. Report the onset to the physician.
13. Be alert to the signs of increasing intraocular pressure: eye pain, rainbow vision, blurred vision, nausea and vomiting.[4] Notify the physician immediately.

References

1. Beeson, Paul, and McDermott, Walsh (editors): *Cecil-Loeb Textbook of Medicine* (14th ed.), Philadelphia: W. B. Saunders Company, 1975, p. 1587.
2. Ibid., p. 1815.
3. Guyton, Arthur C.: *Textbook of Medical Physiology* (5th ed.), Phil-

adelphia: W. B. Saunders Company, 1976, p. 1056.
4. Newell, Frank W., and Ernest J. Terry: *Ophthalmology—Principles and Concepts* (3rd ed.), St. Louis: C. V. Mosby Company, 1974, p.329.

Suggested Readings

Glasser, Ronald J.: How the Body Works Against Itself: Autoimmune Disease. *Nursing '77*, September 1977, pp. 38–39.
Melick, M. E.: Nursing Intervention for Patients Receiving Corticosteroid Therapy. In *Advanced Concepts in Clinical Nursing* (2nd ed.), K.D. Kintzel, ed., Philadelphia: J. B. Lippincott Company, 1977, pp. 606–617.
Newton, David W., Nichols, Arlene, and Newton, Marion: You can Minimize the Hazards of Corticosteroids. *Nursing '77*, June 1977, pp. 26–33.
Reichgott, Michael J., and Melmon, Kenneth L.: The Role of Corticosteroids in Shock. In *Steroid Therapy*, Daniel Azarnoff, ed., Philadelphia, W. B. Saunders Company, 1975, pp. 118–133.

procainamide hydrochloride ▆
(Pronestyl)

Actions/Indications

Antiarrhythmic. Depresses the excitability of cardiac muscle to stimulation; slows conduction in the atrium, bundle of His, and ventricles. Contractility is usually not affected.
Used to treat:
• Premature ventricular contractions
• Ventricular tachycardia
• Atrial fibrillation
• Paroxysmal atrial tachycardia
• Supraventricular tachyarrhythmias unresponsive to digitalis
Action begins almost immediately after intravenous injection. Therapeutic plasma levels have been reported to be 3–10 mcg/ml. This drug is excreted primarily in the urine.

Dosage

The intravenous mode should be used only in extreme emergencies.
Adults:
100 mg at 5-min intervals. Stop injections when desired effect is achieved, when a total dose of 1 gm is reached, or when signs of toxicity are seen (see Nursing Implications No. 1).
Begin an infusion at a rate of 2–6 mg/min simultaneously with the first injection dose. Titrate with patient response to maintain desired drug effect.
Children:
2 mg/kg/dose (maximum dose is 100 mg). Administer by slow infusion over 5 min, repeat every 10–30 min until desired effect is seen or the maximal dose is reached. Titrate with patient response.
Oral therapy should be started as soon as the cardiac rhythm stabilizes, if continuing therapy will be necessary. The first oral dose should be started 3 to 4 hours *after* the last intravenous dose.

Preparation and Storage

Available in 10-ml vials with a concentration of 100 mg/ml, and 2-ml vials with a concentration of 500 mg/ml.
Protect vials from light (keep in manufacturer's package). This drug may be stored at room temperature, but refrigeration will retard color formation. The solution is initially colorless but may turn slightly yellow over time. Discard if color is darker than pale amber.[1]

Drug Incompatibilities

Do not mix in infusion bottle with any other medication.
Do not combine in IV line with:
Diazepam (Valium)
Phenytoin (Dilantin)
Chlordiazepoxide (Librium)
Narcotics
Barbiturates

Modes of IV Administration

Injection
Yes

procainamide hydrochloride
(continued)
Dilute 500 mg/ml solution with an
equal amount of D5W or sterile water. Inject at a rate no greater than
25–50 mg/min.

Intermittent Infusion
No
See table below for dilutions and
rates for infusions.

Continuous Infusion
Yes
Use a 4 mg/ml solution (2 gm in
500 ml D5W or NS). Infuse as a secondary line and use an infusion
pump. Titrate with patient response.
See table below for dilutions and
rates for infusions.
  Infuse at a rate no greater than
25–50 mg/min. Use an infusion
pump.

**Contraindications; Warnings; Pre-
cautions; Adverse Reactions**

Contraindications
1. Myasthenia gravis (not an absolute contraindication)
2. Hypersensitivity to this drug or
   any procaine-related drugs
3. Complete atrioventricular heart
   block or second degree heart
   block in the absence of an artificial pacemaker

Precautions
1. Monitor for changes in cardiac
   function (blood pressure, cardiac output).
2. This drug produces peripheral
   vasodilatation.
3. In atrial fibrillation or flutter
   the ventricular rate may increase as the atrial rate is
   slowed, due to transient anticholinergic effect. Digitalis may
   reduce this, but not entirely.
4. Use with caution for ventricular
   tachycardia in acute myocardial
   infarction.
5. In the presence of first, second
   or third degree block, this drug
   may precipitate complete heart
   block, ventricular asystole or fibrillation.
6. ECG monitoring must be carried out during administration
   in any mode. Discontinue drug
   if A-V conduction is compromised to prevent asystole. Widening of the QRS complex or
   prolongation of the P-R interval
   suggest myocardial toxicity, and
   administration of this drug
   should be temporarily discontinued.
7. Renal or hepatic impairment
   will cause accumulation of this
   drug. Reduce dosage and monitor closely for symptoms of
   overdosage.

Dilutions and Rates for Infusions

Approximate Final Concentration	Infusion Bottle Size (ml.)	ml. of Pronestyl (100 mg./ml. solution) to be added	ml. of Pronestyl (500 mg./ml. solution) to be added	Infusion Rate (Adults)
0.2% (2 mg./ml.)	500	10	2	1–3 ml./min. (2–6 mg./min.)
	250	5	1	
0.4% (4 mg./ml.)	500	20	4	0.5–1.5 ml./min. (2–6 mg./min.)
	250	10	2	

CAUTION: The flow rate of all intravenous infusion solutions must be closely
monitored. These dilutions are calculated to deliver 2 to 6 mg. per minute at the
infusion rates listed.

8. A syndrome resembling systemic lupus erythematosus may occur with high-dose chronic therapy, producing polyarthralgias, arthritis, and pleuritic pain. There may also be fever, myalgia, rashes, pleural effusion. Rarely, thrombocytopenia, or Coombs-positive hemolytic anemia, may also be seen. Discontinue the drug if there is a rising antinuclear antibody titer, or if symptoms of the syndrome appear. This syndrome may be reversible. Steroids may relieve symptoms.
9. In the emergency treatment of ventricular arrhythmias, lidocaine is the drug of choice.
10. When initiating oral therapy, give the first oral dose 3–4 hrs after discontinuing the intravenous infusion.

Adverse Reactions
1. May produce transient but severe hypotension
2. Ventricular asystole or fibrillation
3. Lupus-like syndrome (see Precaution No. 8 above)
4. Nausea, vomiting, abdominal pain, diarrhea, bitter taste
5. Hepatomegaly, rise in SGOT
6. Weakness, mental depression, hallucinations, seizures
7. Hypersensitivity: eosinophilia, urticaria
8. Agranulocytosis with oral lesions, fever, infection

☐ **Nursing Implications**
1. Close ECG monitoring must be maintained during intravenous therapy. Monitor for onset of:
   a. Increasing A-V block (e.g., prolongation of PR interval, second degree block)
   b. Signs of toxicity (e.g., widening of QRS complex, prolongation of PR interval). If any of these signs appear, stop the infusion and notify the physician.
   c. Ineffective control of arrhythmia being treated; another agent may be needed.
2. Keep atropine, defibrillator and temporary transvenous pacemaker equipment readily available.
3. Keep patient supine during drug administration; monitor blood pressure continuously during infusion (direct arterial pressure preferred). Do not leave the patient unattended. If fall in blood pressure exceeds 15 mm Hg, discontinue infusion. Phenylephrine hydrochloride (Neo-Synephrine) or norepinephrine bitartrate (Levophed) can be used to correct hypotension.
4. Be prepared to manage vomiting to prevent aspiration.
5. Be prepared to manage hallucinations to protect patient from injury.
6. Use an infusion pump, or at least microdrop tubing to control drip rate.

Reference
1. Trissel, Lawrence A: *Handbook on Injectable Drugs* (2nd ed.) Washington DC: American Society of Hospital Pharmacists, 1980, p. 444.

Suggested Readings
Cardiac Drugs Today—Part Four: Antiarrhythmics. *Nursing '73*, August 1973, pp. 29–34.
Treatment of Cardiac Arrhythmias—Part I: The Arrhythmias. *The Medical Letter*, 16:101–108, December 6, 1974.
Amsterdam, Ezra A., et al.: Systematic Approach to the Management of Cardiac Arrhythmias. *Heart and Lung*, 2:747–753, September–October 1973 (references).
Levitt, Barrie, Borer, Jeffrey, and Saropa, Arleen: The Clinical Pharmacology of Antiarrhythmic Drugs. Part II: Quinidine, Propranolol, Diphenylhydantoin, and Bretylium. *Cardiovascular Nursing*, 10:27–32, November–December 1974 (references).
Pamintuan, Jose C., Dreifus, Leonard S., and Watanabe, Yoshio: Comparative Mechanisms of Anti-

procainamide hydrochloride
(continued)
arrhythmic Agents. *American Journal of Cardiology,* 26:512–523, November 1970 (references).
Hoffman, Brian F., Rosen, Michael R., and Wit, Andrew L.: Electrophysiology and Pharmacology of Cardiac Arrhythmias. VII. Cardiac Effects of Quinidine and Procainamide. *American Heart Journal,* 89(6):804–808, June 1975.

promethazine hydrochloride ■
(Phenergan)

Actions/Indications
Antihistamine, antiemetic, sedative (a phenothiazine derivative).
Used to manage:
- Allergic reactions to blood and plasma
- Anaphylaxis
- Preoperative, postoperative, obstetric sedation
- Nausea and vomiting
- Motion sickness

Also used to potentiate analgesics, induce sedation.

Dosage
Adults:
Allergy—25 mg every 2–4 hours.
Nausea and Vomiting—12.5–25 mg every 4–6 hours.
Sedation—25–50 mg.
Obstetrics—25–75 mg as needed. Do not exceed a dose of 100 mg in 24 hours.
Children*:
Allergy—6.25–12.5 mg every 3–4 hours.
Nausea and Vomiting—0.5–1.1 mg/kg every 4–6 hours as needed.
Sedation—12.5–25 mg (or 0.5 mg/kg).

Preparation and Storage
Supplied in 1-ml ampuls and disposable syringes of 25 mg/ml and 50 mg/ml solutions.
Refrigerate and protect from light

*Intramuscular or oral route is preferred.

(keep in individual box). Do not use if discolored darker than light yellow. Avoid contact with skin, eyes, clothing.

Drug Incompatibilities
Do not mix with any other medication in solution; and do not inject into an IV line containing the following drugs:
Aminophylline
Chloramphenicol
Chlorothiazide
Dimenhydrinate
Heparin
Hydrocortisone
Methicillin
Methohexital
Penicillin G
Phenytoin
Prednisolone sodium phosphate
Vitamin B complex with vitamin C

Modes of IV Administration

Injection
Yes
Use a 25 mg/ml concentration, further dilute with 9 ml NS. Inject at a rate no greater than 25 mg/min. If administering via a heparinized intermittent scalp vein needle (heparin-lock set), flush system with NS before and after injecting the drug.

Intermittent Infusion
Yes
Use any IV fluid at a rate no greater than 25 mg/minute.
Flush system with NS before and after infusion if heparin is present.

Continuous Infusion
Yes
Use any IV fluid; infuse at a rate to meet dosage guidelines and produce desired response.

Contraindications; Warnings; Precautions; Adverse Reactions

Contraindications
1. Hypersensitivity to this or any other phenothiazine
2. Comatose states, and when the patient has received large amounts of CNS depressants.

Warnings
1. Potentiates other central nervous system depressants. Reduce dosage of narcotics, barbiturates, hypnotics and sedatives.
2. Safety for use in pregnancy has not been established.
3. Avoid extravasation and intra-arterial injection.
4. Use with caution in children; large doses can cause hallucinations, convulsions and sudden death, especially in children who are acutely ill and dehydrated. Do not administer for uncomplicated vomiting. The extrapyramidal symptoms which can occur secondary to this drug may be confused with the CNS signs of encephalopathy or Reye's syndrome.
5. Reduce dosage in the elderly.
6. Because of this drug's anticholinergic effects, use with caution in patients with an acute asthmatic attack, narrow-angle glaucoma, prostatic hypertrophy, stenosing, peptic ulcer, or bladder-neck obstruction.
7. Use with caution in the presence of bone marrow depression; leukopenia and agranulocytosis have been reported.
8. Do not use concomitantly with epinephrine.

Precautions
1. The antiemetic actions can mask the symptoms of increased intracranial pressure, intestinal obstruction, drug toxicity.
2. Can cause dizziness and hypotension.
3. Use with caution in the presence of liver dysfunction.

Adverse Reactions Seen In Short-Term Intravenous Use
1. Neurologic:
   a. Sedation, drowsiness and deep sleep
   b. Blurred vision
   c. Extrapyramidal reactions such as motor restlessness resembling Parkinson's disease, drooling, tremors, muscle spasms, shuffling gait, dystonias (involuntary movements), difficulty swallowing
   d. Agitation and nervousness
   If these occur, dosage must be reduced or the drug discontinued. Symptoms will subside in 24–48 hours.
2. Rashes usually due to hypersensitivity
3. Hypotension (especially immediately after injection); may be postural type
4. Palpitations, especially immediately after an injection
5. Liver damage, producing jaundice (cholestatic hepatitis)
6. Anticholinergic reactions such as: dryness of the mouth, tachycardia, blurred vision, increased salivation, nasal congestion.
7. Exacerbation of seizure disorders.
8. Alterations that may be seen in laboratory tests:
   a. Pregnancy—those tests based on immunological reactions between HCG and anti-HCG may result in false negative or false positive results.
   b. Glucose tolerance—this drug can cause a false increase in glucose tolerance.

☐ **Nursing Implications**
1. Monitor for neurologic disturbances following an injection, or during an infusion; see Adverse Reaction No. 1. Report any of these reactions to the physician immediately. If the patient experiences difficulty in swallowing, discontinue infusion immediately, and remain with the patient until the severity of the reaction is determined. The patient may need parenteral hydration and nutrition until swallowing returns. Monitor children for change in mental status, hallucinations and seizures. See Warning No. 4.
2. Examine for rashes; report them to the physician.

promethazine hydrochloride
(continued)

3. Keep the patient supine during injection or infusion.
4. Monitor blood pressure before, during and after injection or infusion. If hypotension occurs during an infusion, discontinue administration and continue to take the blood pressure until stabilization occurs. Hypotension can usually be avoided with slow injection. If a patient is to be ambulated after an injection, obtain lying and standing blood pressure. If postural hypotension is significant, report the fact to the physician and keep the patient at rest. As postural effects decrease over time, begin to ambulate the patient if desirable; do so cautiously to prevent injury, especially if he is experiencing sedation or blurred vision. Warn the patient not to stand up suddenly until the effects of the drug have disappeared. Initiate safety precautions, such as side rails, to prevent injury.
5. Monitor for jaundice; notify the physician.
6. The patient may experience anticholinergic side effects; see Adverse Reaction No. 6. Inform him of the origin of the symptoms and their transient nature.
7. Initiate seizure precautions if not already in effect.
8. This drug can cause the urine to darken or turn orange for 24 hours after administration. Inform the patient of the harmlessness of this effect.
9. Intra-arterial injection and extravasation must be avoided. Gangrene and tissue sloughing can result. Inject into the tubing of an IV system known to be working. Do not inject or infuse into a scalp vein in children. If the patient complains of pain during an injection, stop administration immediately and evaluate for the possibility of intra-arterial injection or perivascular extravasation. Note that the aspiration of dark blood back into the syringe or IV tubing does not rule out intra-arterial needle placement, because blood turns dark in color upon contact with promethazine.

Notify the physician. Signs and symptoms are severe pain in the affected area, edema along the vessel tract, and possibly blanching of the extremity.

Successful management of this situation has not been described in the literature, although sympathetic nerve blockade and heparinization have been employed. See Appendix.

propranolol hydrochloride ■
(Inderal)

Actions/Indications
Beta adrenergic blocking agent. Blocks beta receptor sites, most importantly in the heart and blood vessels, similar to the effects of epinephrine and norepinephrine. The major effects produced are:

1. Decreased heart rate (decreased sinus node rate, prolongation of the A-V node refractory period, decreased ventricular automaticity)
2. Decreased cardiac contractility
3. Decreased blood pressure (secondary to decreased cardiac output, inhibition of renin release, decreased tonic sympathetic nerve outflow from the vasomotor center)

Intravenous Administration
is indicated **only** for the emergency management of life-threatening arrhythmias, or arrhythmias occuring during general anesthesia such as:

- Paroxysmal atrial tachycardias secondary to increased catecholamines, digitalis, or Wolff-Parkinson-White syndrome
- Persistent sinus tachycardia which is non-compensatory and is a hazard to the patient
- Tachycardias or other arrhythmias due to thyrotoxicosis (as an adjunct to specific thyroid therapy)

- Persistent atrial extrasystoles which are a hazard to the patient and unresponsive to other therapies
- Atrial flutter and fibrillation, to control ventricular rate, when digitalis cannot be used or is ineffective alone
- Ventricular tachycardias induced by excessive serum catecholamines and digitalis; in other situations propranolol is not the drug of first choice (lidocaine should be used)
- Persistent premature ventricular contractions which do not respond to conventional drugs
- Tachyarrhythmias during surgery for pheochromocytoma

This drug is currently *not* approved for use in hypertensive emergencies.

This is only a brief outline of the uses and effects of this drug in the intravenous mode. The clinician is encouraged to do additional reading in the current literature.

Dosage
Adults:
1–3 mg may be followed by a second dose in 2 min. Subsequent doses should *not* be given in less than 4 hrs.

There is no simple correlation between dose or plasma level and therapeutic effect. This is probably because sympathetic tone varies widely between individuals. Proper dosage, then requires titration.
Children:
Dosage has not been established.

Preparation and Storage
Available in 1-ml ampuls with a concentration of 1 mg/ml.

Do not dilute in large volumes of fluids.

Drug Incompatibilities
Do not mix with any other medication in any manner.

Modes of IV Administration

Injection
Yes

Rate of injection should not exceed 1 mg/min.

Titrate injections with antiarrhythmic response.

May be injected into Y injection site of IV tubing.

Intermittent Infusion
Yes
Add dose to 50–100 ml NS, infuse over 10–15 minutes.

Continuous Infusion
No

Contraindications; Warnings; Precautions; Adverse Reactions

Contraindications
1. Bronchial asthma (can cause bronchoconstriction)
2. Allergic rhinitis during the pollen season
3. Sinus bradycardia
4. Heart block greater than first degree
5. Cardiogenic shock
6. Right ventricular failure secondary to pulmonary hypertension
7. Congestive heart failure, unless it is secondary to propranolol-treatable arrhythmia (see Warning No. 2)
8. In the presence of adrenergic-augmenting psychotropic drugs (MAO inhibitors) and within 2 weeks of their discontinuation

Warnings
1. This drug is not currently indicated in the management of hypertensive crisis.
2. Propranolol can further depress myocardial contractility and precipitate pulmonary edema in patients with congestive heart failure. This drug may also reduce the positive inotropic effects of digitalis.
3. The effects of propranolol and digitalis are additive in depressing A-V conduction. Use propranolol with great caution in the presence of atrioventricular block secondary to digitalis.
4. At the first sign of heart failure the patient should be digita-

propranolol hydrochloride
(continued)

lized. If the progression of failure continues, propranolol must be discontinued.

5. Use in hyperthyroidism may mask continuing hyperactivity of the thyroid and its complications.

6. May cause severe bradycardia when used in Wolff-Parkinson-White syndrome.

7. Use with caution in anesthesia; hazardous myocardial depression can occur precipitating pulmonary edema or shock.

8. This drug should be discontinued 48 hours prior to surgery, except when used in pheochromocytoma. In emergency surgery, isoproterenol or norepinephrine may be used to counteract the hypotensive effects of propranolol.

9. May cause bronchoconstriction in susceptible patients (chronic lung disease, asthmatics).

10. May depress early signs and symptoms of hypoglycemia.

11. Safety for use in pregnancy has not been established.

12. This is not the first drug of choice in the management of ventricular arrhythmias.

13. Patients with angina pectoris may experience an exacerbation of the condition with abrupt withdrawal of propranolol therapy; gradually reduce dosage prior to discontinuation in these patients.

Precautions

1. Use with caution in patients receiving catecholamine-depleting drugs such as reserpine.

2. May produce hypotension, marked bradycardia, dizziness, syncopal attacks, or orthostatic hypotension due to its relaxing effect on vascular smooth muscle.

3. Use with caution in patients with hepatic or renal impairment; decreased dosage is advisable.

4. Monitor ECG continuously

during intravenous use, to observe for bradycardia and for effectiveness in abolishing arrhythmias.

Adverse Reactions

1. Cardiovascular: bradycardia, congestive heart failure, intensification of A-V block, hypotension, numbness of hands, arterial insufficiency (Raynaud type)

2. Central nervous system: lightheadedness, mental depression, insomnia, weakness, catatonia, visual disturbances, hallucinations, acute reversible syndrome of confusion, memory loss, emotional lability

3. Gastrointestinal: nausea, vomiting, diarrhea or constipation

4. Allergic: pharyngitis, agranulocytosis, rash, fever, laryngospasm, respiratory distress

5. Respiratory: bronchospasm

6. Hematologic: thrombocytopenic purpura, nonthrombocytopenic purpura

7. Reversible hair loss (rare)

8. In patients with heart disease: elevated SGOT, alkaline phosphatase, LDH, BUN

Management of Overdosage or Untoward Response

1. Bradycardia: atropine 0.25–1.0 mg; if no response, isoproterenol drip titrated cautiously; initiate temporary transvenous pacing if necessary

2. Cardiac failure: digitalization and diuretics

3. Hypotension: norepinephrine or epinephrine via transfusion; titrate with blood pressure

4. Bronchospasm: isoproterenol via infusion, aminophylline via intermittent infusion, intubation and mechanical ventilation if necessary.

☐ **Nursing Implications**

1. Monitor for signs and symptoms of cardiac failure:
   a. Elevation of CVP (or pulmonary capillary wedge pressure); measure every 15

minutes after injection for 1 hour, then hourly.

b. Shortness of breath, orthopnea, coughing; count respirations every 15 minutes after injection for 1 hour, then hourly.

c. Rales; auscultate lungs every half hour for the first 2 hours after injection.

d. Be prepared to treat as outlined above. Notify physician immediately.

2. Monitor PR interval for prolongation. The patient should be monitored continuously via cardiac monitor during and after injection. Be prepared to treat bradycardia or A-V block; see above.

3. If used to supress supraventricular tachycardia in Wolff-Parkinson-White syndrome, be prepared to treat severe bradycardia with atropine, isoproterenol and temporary pacing.

4. Monitor for respiratory distress secondary to bronchospasm. Signs and symptoms: wheezing, tightness in the chest, increased respiratory rate. Be prepared to treat with isoproterenol and aminophylline, and assisted ventilation.

5. Monitor for hypoglycemia when appropriate. This drug may mask the onset of diaphoresis and tachycardia. Observe for visual changes, dizziness, and changes in mental status. Be prepared to treat with glucose.

6. Keep patient supine during injection and monitor blood pressure continuously. Following injection monitor blood pressure every 5 minutes for 1/2 hour, then every 15 minutes for 1/2 hour, then hourly until stable. Ambulate with caution 1 hour postinjection. Check lying and standing blood pressure.

7. Hypotensive effects, cardiac failure, bradycardia, A-V block, and other adverse effects may occur in a more severe form, with greater duration in patients with hepatic or renal impairment.

8. Be prepared to manage mental confusion and hallucinations, to prevent patient injury.

Suggested Readings
Cardiac Drugs Today—Part Four: Antiarrhythmics. *Nursing '73*, August 1973, pp. 29–34.

Treatment of Cardiac Arrhythmias—Part I: The Arrhythmias. *The Medical Letter*, 16:101–108, December 6, 1974.

Amsterdam, Ezra A., et al.: Systematic Approach to the Management of Cardiac Arrhythmias. *Heart and Lung*, 2:747–753, September–October, 1973 (references).

Levitt, Barrie, Borer, Jeffrey, and Saropa, Arleen: The Clinical Pharmacology of Antiarrhythmic Drugs. Part II: Quinidine, Propranolol, Diphenylhydantoin, and Bretylium. *Cardiovascular Nursing*, 10:27–32, November–December 1974 (references).

Pamintuan, Jose C., Dreifus, Leonard S., and Watanabe, Yoshio: Comparative Mechanisms of Antiarrhythmic Agents. *American Journal of Cardiology*, 26:512–523, November 1970 (references).

Guyton, Arthur C.: *Textbook of Medical Physiology* (5th ed.) Philadelphia, W. B. Saunders Company, 1976, Chapter 57, The Autonomic Nervous System; The Adrenal Medulla, pp. 768–781.

protamine sulfate ■

Actions/Indications
Heparin neutralizer (when given in the presence of heparin). A basic protein carrying a positive charge that will neutralize the negatively charged heparin molecule. This drug has anticoagulant effects when given in the absence of heparin. Used to treat heparin overdosage or to counteract the effects of heparin on clotting time during extracorporeal circulation (hemodialysis, cardiopulmonary bypass).

protamine sulfate
(continued)

Dosage
Adults and Children:
Dosage is determined by the amount and kind of heparin that has been administered in the last 3–4 hours.

Each 1 mg of protamine neutralizes 90 units of heparin activity when the heparin has been derived from *lung tissue* and 115 units of heparin when the heparin has been derived from *intestinal mucosa.*

Do not exceed the equivalent of 50 mg of protamine in a 10-minute period.

Do not exceed a dose of 100 mg in a short period unless guided by coagulation studies.

Dosage required decreases rapidly with time elapsed following the injection of the heparin. If protamine is injected 30 minutes after heparin, one-half a dose of protamine should be given. Use anticoagulation studies to guide subsequent doses.

Preparation and Storage
Supplied in 5 ml ampuls containing 50 mg of active drug; (10 mg/ml); and 25 ml vials containing 250 mg of active drug (10 mg/ml).

Use caution; note the difference in dosage contained in the two preparations available.

Refrigerate; avoid freezing. Discard unused portions of vials.

Drug Incompatibilities
Do not mix with any other medication in any manner.

Modes of IV Administration

Injection
Yes
Dilute in an equal volume of NS prior to injection. Inject over 1–3-minute period.

Do not exceed a dosage of 50 mg over a 10 minute period.

Intermittent Infusion
Yes
Use NS as infusion fluid; add to at least an equal volume of NS. Titrate drip rate with clotting time or plasma thrombin time.

Continuous Infusion
Yes
Use NS as infusion fluid. Titrate drip rate with clotting time or plasma thrombin time.

Contraindications; Warnings; Precautions; Adverse Reactions

Contraindications
None when used as indicated.

Warnings
1. Administer additional doses titrated with anticoagulation studies (clotting time and plasma thrombin time).
2. Be prepared to treat hypotension.
3. Safety for use in pregnancy has not been established.
4. Hyperheparinemia and bleeding have occurred after cardiopulmonary bypass despite adequate doses of protamine.

Precautions
1. Do not exceed a dose of 100 mg in a short period of time unless guided by coagulation studies.
2. Patients with an allergy to fish may develop hypersensitivity to protamine.

Adverse Reactions
1. Hypotension
2. Bradycardia
3. Dyspnea
4. Transient flushing of the face
   These reactions usually occur after rapid administration.

☐ Nursing Implications
1. Assist in monitoring partial prothromboplastin time or clotting time during therapy. Observe for signs of overanticoagulation; e.g., oozing around vascular access or other surgical incisions.
2. Monitor blood pressure every 2–3 minutes during and immediately following a direct intra-

venous injection. Vasopressors may be used in the event of hypotension. Keep the patient supine during injection. Take blood pressure every 30 minutes during an infusion.

3. Monitor heart rate during and immediately after a direct intravenous injection and every 30 minutes during an infusion.

4. Heparin rebound can occur 8–9 hours after protamine neutralization. This is due to the more rapid metabolism of protamine in relation to that of heparin; i.e., heparin activity may exist after the protamine effects have diminished.[1] Monitor for sudden bleeding tendency during the first 24 hours after neutralization.

Signs of bleeding: epistaxis, gum bleeding, hemoptysis, hematemesis, melena and bright red blood in stools, vaginal bleeding, hematuria, bruising, oozing of blood at incisions, sudden appearance of blood in drainage tubes (chest, abdominal, etc.)

Reference
1. Ellison, Norig, et al.: Heparin Rebound. *Journal of Thoracic and Cardiovascular Surgery*, 67(5):724, May 1974.

pyridostigmine bromide ■
(Mestinon Injectable, Regonol)

Actions/Indications
Cholinesterase inhibitor, facilitates the transmission of impulses across the myoneural junction by inhibiting the destruction of acetylcholine by cholinesterase.

Used to treat myasthenia gravis when oral agents cannot be given, and also used as a reversal agent for curariform neuromuscular blocking agents, and gallamine triethiodide.

Dosage
Adults:
Myasthenia Gravis—1/30th of the patient's usual oral dose, this varies greatly from patient to patient.

Large parenteral doses should be given with atropine, usually 0.6 to 1.2 mg.

In labor and delivery—Give 1/30th of the patient's usual oral dose 1 hr before completion of the second stage of labor.

Reversal of Nondepolarizing Muscle Relaxants—give atropine sulfate (0.5–1.2 mg) prior to dose of pyridostigmine. Then give the pyridostigmine 10–20 mg. Full recovery is usually seen in 15 min. (See detailed information in this book on the muscle relaxant being used).

Children:
Neonates of myasthenic mothers—IM or oral route **only,** 0.05–0.15 mg/kg. See Warning No. 2.

Preparation and Storage
Supplied in 2-ml ampuls of a 5 mg/ml solution.
Discard unused portions.

Drug Incompatibilities
Do not mix with any other medications in any manner.

Modes of IV Administration

Injection
Yes
Very slowly over 2–4 min into the tubing of a running IV.

Intermittent Infusion
No

Continuous Infusion
No

Contraindications; Warnings; Precautions; Adverse Reactions

Contraindications
1. Hypersensitivity to any anticholinesterase drug
2. Mechanical intestinal or urinary obstruction

Warnings
1. Use with caution in patients with epilepsy, bronchial asthma, bradycardia, recent myocardial infarction, vagotonia, hyperthy-

pyridostigmine bromide
(continued)

roidism, cardiac arrhythmias or peptic ulcer. The secondary effects of this drug may increase the severity of these problems while the drug is being administered.

2. Overdosage may result in a cholinergic crisis—increasing muscle weakness involving muscles of respiration. This may be impossible to distinguish from worsening of myasthenia gravis itself. Crisis secondary to drugs requires immediate withdrawal of the drugs. Crisis secondary to the disease requires more drugs. An edrophonium test should be employed to distinguish them. Keep atropine available when giving this drug. (See Adverse Reaction No. 3.) This applies also to neonates of myasthenic mothers. See page 144, on edrophonium.

3. Maintain respiratory support until there is full recovery of respiratory function.

4. Safety for use in pregnancy and lactation has not been established.

5. Failure of this drug to produce reversal of neuromuscular blocking agents within 30 minutes may be seen in extreme debilitation, carcinomatosis, and with concomitant use of aminoglycoside antibiotics or anesthetic agents, such as enflurane and methoxyflurane.

Adverse Reactions

1. Side effects are most often due to overdosage.

2. Muscarinic effects: nausea, vomiting, diarrhea, abdominal cramps, increased salivation, increased bronchial secretions, constricted pupils, diaphoresis.

3. Muscarinic effects can be counteracted with atropine, but this can mask the signs of overdosage and lead to the iatrogenic induction of a cholinergic crisis.

4. Thrombophlebitis at injection site.

5. Rashes.

☐ **Nursing Implications**

1. In patients with a history of bronchial asthma, monitor for respiratory distress, wheezing, increased respiratory effort, increased rate, restlessness.

2. Monitor ECG in patients with a history of cardiac arrhythmias during and for 2 hours following injection. Be prepared to treat bradycardia with atropine.

3. In myasthenia gravis patients, notify physician immediately if signs of increasing muscle weakness occur. Be prepared to support respiration with airways, a manual breathing bag (Hope, Ambu, Puritan), suction, oxygen, endotracheal tube, and laryngoscope. Have atropine 1.0 mg and edrophonium at the bedside. Do not leave the patient alone. Begin ventilatory support if respiratory rate falls below 8–10/minute, if there is cyanosis or restlessness. Continue until physician determines that spontaneous ventilation is adequate. Monitor neonates of myasthenic mothers, for respiratory weakness.

4. In patients recovering from nondepolarizing muscle blockade (e.g., pancuronium), keep respiratory support intact until full recovery has been made from the drug, evidenced by full spontaneous respirations of adequate rate and depth and adequate arterial blood gases. A physician should discontinue respiratory support. Monitor vital signs according to recovery room policy. See detailed information in this book on the muscle relaxant being used.

5. Monitor for signs of overdosage (see Adverse Reactions above). Be prepared to manage vomiting to prevent aspiration. Keep patient in a lateral position if there is a threat of

vomiting. Suction equipment must be at the bedside. Do not leave the patient alone if there is nausea, vomiting, or abdominal cramping.

6. Patients with myasthenia gravis and their families will require self-care instruction and close nursing follow-up.

Suggested Readings

Guyton, Arthur C.: *Textbook of Medical Physiology* (5th ed.), Philadelphia: W. B. Saunders Company, 1976, Chapter 12, Neuromuscular Transmission, Function of Smooth Muscle, pp. 147–157; Chapter 15, The Autonomic Nervous System; The Adrenal Medulla, pp. 768–781.

Jones, LeAnna: Myasthenia and Me. *RN*, June 1976, pp. 50–55.

Smith, Dorothy W., and Germain, Carol P. Hanley: *Care of the Adult Patient* (4th ed.), Philadelphia: J. B. Lippincott Company, 1977, pp. 382–384.

ritodrine hydrochloride ■
(Yutopar)

Actions/Indications

Beta-receptor agonist that exerts a preferential effect on the beta-2 adrenergic receptors such as those in uterine smooth muscle. Stimulation of these beta-2 receptors inhibits contractility of the uterine smooth muscle both in intensity and frequency of contractions.

This agent is indicated in the management of preterm labor, to prolong gestation and thus decrease the incidence of neonatal mortality and respiratory distress syndrome. Therapy should be instituted as soon as the diagnosis is established in pregnancies over 20 weeks gestation. Elimination from the body is by a combination of hepatic metabolism and urinary excretion. This drug crosses the placental barrier.

Dosage

Initially: 0.1 mg/minute (0.33 ml/min, 20 microdrops/min of the suggested solution). This should be increased by 0.05 mg/min increments every 10 minutes until desired results are seen.

Maintenance: 0.15–0.35 mg/min (0.50–1.17 ml/min or 30–70 microdrops/min of the recommended solution).

Continue the infusion for 12 hours after uterine contractions cease. Oral maintenance should be continued starting with a dose of 10 mg 30 minutes before discontinuation of the infusion. For the next 24 hours the oral dose is 10 mg every 2 hours.

Thereafter, 10–20 mg every 4 to 6 hours depending on the uterine response and side effects. Do not exceed a total daily dose of 120 mg. The duration of therapy should be determined by how long the pregnancy should be prolonged.

Preparation and Storage

Supplied in 5 ml ampuls of 50 mg (10 mg/ml).

To prepare for administration, add 150 mg (3 ampuls) of drug to 500 ml of NS, D5W, 10% Dextran 40 in NS, 10% Invert Sugar, Ringer's solution or Hartmann's solution. The resulting concentration is 0.3 mg/ml. Do not use if solution is discolored or contains particulate matter. Use infusion solution immediately and never beyond 48 hours time.

Drug Incompatibilities

Do not mix with any other medication in any manner.

Modes of IV Administration

Injection
No

Intermittent Infusion
No

Continuous Infusion
Yes
Use microdrop delivery set and an infusion pump for accurate administration and titration.

ritodrine hydrochloride
(continued)

Contraindications; Warnings; Precautions; Adverse Reactions

Contraindications

1. Before the 20th week of pregnancy.
2. Antepartum hemorrhage, which demands immediate delivery.
3. Eclampsia and severe preeclampsia
4. Intrauterine fetal death
5. Chorioamnionitis
6. Maternal cardiac disease
7. Pulmonary hypertension
8. Maternal hyperthyroidism
9. Uncontrolled maternal diabetes mellitus
10. Maternal medical conditions that would be seriously affected by the properties of this drug:
    - hypovolemia
    - cardiac arrhythmias such as tachycardia or those seen with digitalis toxicity
    - uncontrolled hypertension
    - pheochromocytoma
    - asthma already treated by betamimetics and/or steroids
11. Known hypersensitivity

Warnings

1. Maternal pulmonary edema has been seen in patients concomitantly receiving corticosteroids; one death has been reported. This apparently occurs more frequently when normal saline is used for infusion. If pulmonary edema occurs, both drugs should be promptly discontinued and conventional management of the edema initiated.
2. Maternal and fetal heart rates and maternal blood pressure should be closely monitored for cardiovascular effects. Occult cardiac disease may be uncovered by the use of this drug.
3. This drug should not be used in mild to moderate preeclampsia, hypertension, or diabetes unless the benefits clearly outweigh the risks.

Precautions

1. If used in the management of the patient in preterm labor with premature rupture of the membranes, the benefits of delaying delivery should be weighed against the risk of development of chorioamnionitis.
2. Intrauterine growth retardation should be considered in the differential diagnosis of preterm labor. This is important when the gestational age is not known with certainty.
3. Monitor blood glucose and electrolytes during therapy. This drug increases blood glucose and insulin levels and decreases serum potassium. These values are especially important to monitor in patients with diabetes or in those who are on potassium depleting diuretics.
4. The effects of other sympathomimetic amines may be potentiated when concurrently administered with ritodrine. The effects may also be additive.
5. Beta-adrenergic blocking agents inhibit the action of ritodrine.
6. This drug can potentiate the hypotensive effects of anesthetics.
7. Animal studies have shown no ill effects on fertility or on the fetus. Studies have not been done on human pregnancies under 20 weeks gestation. This drug is not recommended for use before this time. Observations of children born of mothers who received this drug have not revealed harmful effects. However, the possibility cannot be ruled out.

Adverse Reactions

Undesirable effects are related to this drug's betamimetic activities and can be controlled by dosage adjustment.

1. Usual effects (80–100% of patients):
   a. Increased maternal and fetal heart rates and alterations in maternal blood pressure
   b. Increased blood glucose and insulin, which decreases to-

wards normal after 48 to 72 hours even with continued administration of the drug
c. Increased free fatty acids and cyclic AMP
d. Decreased serum potassium
2. Frequent effects (10–50% of patients):
a. Palpitation
b. Tremors
c. Nausea, vomiting
d. Headache
e. Erythema
3. Occasional effects (5–10% of patients):
a. Nervousness
b. Jitteriness
c. Restlessness
d. Anxiety
e. Malaise
4. Infrequent effects (1–3% of patients):
a. Chest pain or tightness
b. Arrhythmias
c. Anaphylaxis
d. Rash
e. Heart murmurs
f. Epigastric distress
g. Ileus, constipation, diarrhea
h. Dyspnea, hyperventilation
i. Hemolytic icterus
j. Glycosuria, lactic acidosis
k. Sweating, chills
l. Drowsiness and weakness
5. Neonatal effects:
a. Hypoglycemia
b. Ileus
c. Hypocalcemia
d. Hypotension

Overdosage
Exaggerations of the above maternal effects that do not resolve with reduced dosage may require discontinuation of the drug depending on the situation. An appropriate beta-blocking agent can be used after discontinuation as an antidote. This drug is dialyzable. The amount of drug required to produce symptoms of overdosage is variable.

☐ **Nursing Implications**
1. Monitor and chart the frequency, duration and intensity of uterine contractions as a guide for drug dosage. Increase infu-

sion rate as ordered, noting dosage when contractions cease. Accuracy of dosage delivery is essential. Monitor for vaginal bleeding, notify the physician in this event.
2. Monitor maternal heart rate and blood pressure, and fetal heart rate. Notify the physician of exaggerated increases, and decrease drug dosage as ordered. Monitor the effect of dosage reduction on vital signs and uterine contractions.
3. Maternal blood glucose should be monitored in the presence of diabetes.
4. The patient should be well hydrated before the initiation of therapy.
5. If the patient has a history of cardiac problems or arrhythmias, monitor the patient electrocardiographically. Report arrhythmias to the physician.
6. If the patient has recently received or is receiving corticosteroids, monitor for the signs and symptoms of the onset of pulmonary edema:
a. Increased respiratory rate
b. Dyspnea
c. Rales
d. Cough
e. Jugular venous distention
Notify the physician immediately.
If this occurs, ritodrine and the steroid should be discontinued. Be prepared to treat the patient with intravenous diuretics (furosemide, etc.), morphine, oxygen, rotating tourniquets, etc. Do not leave the patient unattended. Monitor fetal heart rate.
7. Be familiar with the listed adverse reactions. Reduce drug dosage as ordered for minor effects and reassure the patient of their origin and control.
8. Keep the patient on bedrest and positioned in the lateral recumbent (Simms) position preferably on the left side to prevent compression of the inferior vena cava by the gravid uterus

ritodrine hydrochloride
(continued)
(and therefore prevent maternal and fetal hypotension). Encourage frequent movement of the legs to prevent venous stasis.
9. The patient and her husband or family will be anxious about the safety of the baby because of the premature labor. Give realistic reassurance and time for the patient and husband or significant other to express their concerns, fears, and needs. See that their questions are answered.
10. The baby should be monitored for hypoglycemia and hypocalcemia after delivery. Observe for signs of paralytic ileus and systemic hypotension.

secobarbital sodium ■
(Seconal Sodium)

Actions/Indications
Central nervous system depressant, barbiturate, short-acting. Response depends on dose, and ranges from mild sedation to profound hypnosis.
Used as a sedative, anticonvulsant in:
• Status epilepticus
• Toxic reactions to strychnine or local anesthetics
• Tetanus
• Adjunct to anesthesia

Dosage
Adults:
Anesthesia—Inject at a rate not to exceed 50 mg/15 seconds; discontinue when desired effects are seen. Do not exceed 250 mg.
In dentistry for heavy sedation when nerve blocks are also used—100–150 mg.
Convulsions and tetanus—5.5 mg/kg every 3–4 hours as needed or via continuous infusion.
In general, the total IV dose should not exceed 500 mg. Doses of 1.1–1.7 mg/kg produce moderate to heavy sedation. A dose of 2.2 mg/kg will produce hypnosis. In extreme agitation, 3.3–4.4 mg/kg may be re-

quired but should be administered with caution.[1]

Preparation and Storage
Available in 1-ml and 2-ml ampuls and 50-ml multidose vials; all contain 50 mg/ml.
Also supplied in ampuls of dry powder to be reconstituted with sterile water for injection. Add 2 ml of diluent to the 100 mg vial, and 5 ml to the 250 mg vial. The resulting concentration is 50 mg/ml.
Use only clear, colorless solutions.
This is a Schedule II drug under the Controlled Substances Act of 1970. Maintain hospital or institutional regulations guiding its use.

Drug Incompatibilities
Do not mix with any other medication in any manner.

Modes of IV Administration

Injection
Yes
Rate not to exceed 50 mg/15 seconds.
Using a 5% solution (50 mg/ml) may be given undiluted or diluted 2:1 in sterile water for injection or NS.

Intermittent Infusion
Yes
Infuse in 50–100 ml NS or RL.

Continuous Infusion
No
Pharmacologically inappropriate.

Contraindications; Warnings; Precautions; Adverse Reactions

Contraindications
1. Hypersensitivity to any barbiturate
2. Porphyria (confirmed or familial history)
3. Respiratory depression
4. Severe cardiac disease
5. During labor and delivery

Warnings:
1. Do not exceed an injection rate of 50 mg/15 seconds; respirato-

ry depression, apnea, laryngospasm, or hypotension may result.
2. Use with caution in any patient with impaired hepatic function.
3. Use with caution in patients concomitantly receiving analgesics, other sedatives or hypnotics, or tranquilizers. There is a greater chance of respiratory depression.
4. The polyethylene glycol vehicle contained in this drug may be irritating to the kidneys when renal disease is present.
5. Safety for use in pregnancy has not been established. Use only if benefits outweigh risks; fetal heart rate must be monitored during administration.

Precautions:
1. When used on an outpatient basis, the patient should only be discharged after full recovery has been made, and then only in the company of a responsible adult.
2. This drug increases responsiveness to coumarin anticoagulants, i.e., there is less suppression of prothrombin time; adjust anticoagulant dose accordingly.
3. Patient must be warned against operating hazardous machinery, or participating in hazardous activities, e.g., walking near traffic or on stairs, until there is full recovery from drowsiness, etc.

Adverse Reactions:
1. Respiratory depression
2. Idiosyncrasy in the form of excitement, "hangover" or pain
3. Hypersensitivity: rashes to anaphylaxis
4. Laryngospasm with large, rapidly administered doses
5. Hypotension with rapid administration

☐ **Nursing Implications**
1. Strictly adhere to maximum injection and infusion rate suggestions and dose maximum limits. Use an infusion pump to

assist with rate control, to insure maximum benefit from the drug and to prevent overdosage. Patients with liver impairment should receive smaller doses and should be monitored more closely and for a longer period of time than usual.
2. Keep the patient supine during and after injection or infusion. Monitor blood pressure, heart rate and respiratory rate every 5 minutes for 1 hour following an injection, or every 5 minutes through the duration of an infusion. This includes fetal heart rate monitoring. (See Warning No. 5.) Do not leave the patient unattended.
3. Patients with porphyria are sensitive to barbiturates in that they may experience an acute attack of the disease secondary to the administration of a barbiturate (see Contraindications). The onset of an acute attack is indicated by severe colicky abdominal pain radiating to the back. There is usually severe vomiting, fever and leukocytosis in addition.[2]
4. Avoid extravasation; see Appendix. Extravascular or intra-arterial injection of this drug can cause tissue necrosis and gangrene of the affected extremity, respectively. Thrombophlebitis can also occur during the course of an infusion. Examine for redness and pain along the vein tract, and discontinue the infusion if signs and symptoms appear; notify the physician immediately.
5. Take anaphylaxis precautions; see Appendix.
6. Monitor for symptoms of acute overdosage (listed in order of progression):
   a. Respiratory depression, i.e., decreased respiratory rate and depth
   b. Peripheral vascular collapse, i.e., fall in blood pressure, pallor, diaphoresis, tachycardia
   c. Pulmonary edema (rare)

secobarbital sodium
(continued)
  d. Decreased or absent reflexes,
     pupillary constriction
  e. Stupor
  f. Coma
  Stop the injection or infusion
  immediately upon noting any
  one of these symptoms. Notify
  the physician. Discontinuation
  of the infusion is usually all that
  is necessary to prevent further
  problems. If not, see No. 7 below.
7. Management of acute
   overdosage:
   a. Continue to stay with the
      patient and monitor vital
      signs
   b. Maintain an open airway and
      adequate ventilation
   c. Keep the patient as alert as
      possible by verbal and physi-
      cal stimuli. Encourage the
      patient to breathe at an ade-
      quate rate (12–14 breaths/
      minute for an adult). If nec-
      essary, initiate artificial ven-
      tilation with a manual
      breathing bag (Puritan,
      Hope, Ambu, etc.) or
      mouth-to-mouth breathing
      at a rate of 12–14 breaths/
      minute
   d. Circulatory support in the
      form of fluids and drugs
      may be ordered.
8. The sedation produced by this
   drug may be preceded by transient changes in mental status,
   such as feelings of euphoria and
   confusion. If this occurs, attempt
   to calm the patient and take
   measures to prevent injury until
   the patient returns to his normal status.
9. If a patient is to be ambulatory
   following an injection, ambulate
   with assistance; there may be
   transient dizziness. Obtain lying,
   then sitting and standing blood
   pressures to detect postural hypotension. If this drug has been
   used for an outpatient procedure, a responsible adult should
   accompany the patient home.

The patient should not drive for
at least the next 8 hours.

References
1. Formulary Section 28:24. American Hospital Formulary Service, American Society of
   Hospital Pharmacists, Washington, D.C., 1979.
2. Beeson, Paul B., and
   McDermott, Walsh (editors):
   Cecil-Loeb Textbook of Medicine
   (14th ed.) Philadelphia: W. B.
   Saunders Company, 1975, p.
   1873.

sodium lactate ■
(5.0 mEq/ml)

Actions/Indications
Buffering agent to contribute material for the body to regenerate bicarbonate (HCO_3^-) from lactate. Used
for prevention and treatment of
mild to moderate metabolic acidosis
in patients with restricted oral intake
whose ability to convert lactate to
bicarbonate has not been impaired.

Dosage
Dosage must be individualized according to the patient's electrolyte
requirements.
  Usually administered in units of
50 mEq, or milliliters of a 1/6th
molar solution.
  The following formula can be
used to guide dosage:
  Dose in ml's of a 1/6th molar solution = (60–plasma CO_2) × (0.8 of
the body weight in lbs).

Preparation and Storage
Solution contains 50 mEq of sodium
and 50 mEq of lactate in 10 ml.
  Discard unused portions of vials.
  An approximately isotonic (1/6
molar) solution can be made by the
addition of 50 mEq (10 ml) sodium
lactate to 290 ml sterile water for injection.

Drug Incompatibilities
Do not mix with:
Novobiocin

Oxytetracycline
Sodium bicarbonate
Sulfadiazine

Modes of IV Administration

Injection
No

Intermittent Infusion
No

Continuous Infusion
Yes
At a rate no greater than 300 ml/hr
Add to the following solutions:
- Dextran (any form)
- D5/NS
- Any dextrose solution
- Fructose solution
- Invert sugar solutions
- Ionosol products
- Protein hydrolysate
- Ringer's solutions
- NS

Contraindications; Warnings; Precautions; Adverse Reactions

Contraindications
1. Hypernatremia
2. Fluid retention
3. Respiratory alkalosis
4. Not indicated in acidosis associated with congenital heart disease or persistent cyanosis.

Precautions
1. Must be used in diluted form.
2. Avoid rapid infusion.
3. Administer with caution to patients who may not tolerate a large amount of sodium; e.g., congestive heart failure, edematous or sodium-retaining states, and patients with oliguria or anuria.
4. This drug is not intended nor effective for correcting severe acidotic states which require immediate restoration of serum bicarbonate levels. Sodium lactate has no advantage over sodium bicarbonate and may be detrimental in the management of lactic acidosis.

☐ Nursing Implications
1. Monitor cardiac status in patients likely to decompensate (those known to have congestive heart failure; the elderly, etc.):
   a. Increasing heart rate > 110/minute in adults
   b. Elevation of central venous pressure or external jugular venous distention
   c. Increasing respiratory rate, orthopnea, rales, cough
   d. Onset of third and/or fourth heart sounds
   e. Peripheral edema (see Contraindications).
   Notify physician of the onset of any of these signs.
2. Weigh patients before and after therapy and thereafter as needed.
3. Monitor intake and output every 8 hours to detect fluid retention.
4. Be aware of the patient's serum sodium concentration, arterial blood gas values (pH, $pHCO_3$, pO_2, pCO_2). These parameters should be monitored carefully during administration of this agent to assist in preventing metabolic alkalosis. Do not administer this drug in the presence of hypernatremia or alkalosis (pH greater than 7.3).

streptokinase ■
(Streptase)

Actions/Indications
This drug is an enzyme derived from group C beta hemolytic streptococci. In the body it acts with plasminogen to produce an "activator complex" that converts plasminogen to the proteolytic enzyme plasmin. It is the plasmin that degrades fibrin clots as well as fibrinogen and other plasma proteins that make up a blood clot.

An infusion of streptokinase is followed by increased fibrinolytic activity, an effect that disappears within a few hours after discontinuation of the infusion of the drug. A pro-

streptokinase
(continued)
longed thrombin time due to a decrease in plasma levels of fibrinogen and an increase in the amount of circulating fibrinogen degradation products may last for 12 to 24 hours after discontinuation of the drug.

Streptokinase is indicated in the treatment of:

*   *ACUTE PULMONARY EMBOLISM,* involving the obstruction of blood flow to a lobe or multiple lung segments, or any embolus that is accompanied by unstable hemodynamics, i.e. inability to maintain systemic blood pressure without supportive measures. Diagnosis should be confirmed by objective means (pulmonary angiography or lung scan).
*   *ACUTE DEEP VEIN THROMBOSIS,* extensive thrombi of deep veins such as the popliteal or those more proximal. Diagnosis should be by objective means such as venography.
*   *ACUTE ARTERIAL THROMBOSIS OR EMBOLI* (see Contraindication No. 4)
*   *ARTERIOVENOUS CANNULAE OCCLUSION.*

Dosage
Adults:
In deep vein thrombosis, pulmonary embolus or arterial embolism or thrombosis:

Loading dose—250,000 IU into a peripheral vein by infusion over 30 minutes. (Human exposure to streptococci bacteria is common, antibodies to streptokinase then are found in most patients. This can be overcome in most instances with a loading dose of the drug.)
Maintenance—100,000 IU/hr via continuous infusion
Duration: Pulmonary embolus – 24 hours; pulmonary embolus with concurrent deep vein thrombosis – 72 hours; arterial thrombosis and embolism – 24 to 72 hours; deep vein thrombosis alone – 72 hours.

If thrombin time or any other parameter of clot lysis is less than 1 1/2 times the normal control value after 4 hours of therapy, discontinue therapy (this indicates excessive resistance, i.e. antibody activity, to the streptokinase).

After terminating treatment, anticoagulation is recommended, that is, a continuous infusion of heparin guided by clotting studies. This is to prevent recurrent thrombosis. Do *not* begin the heparin until the thrombin time has decreased to less than twice the normal control value (approximately 3 to 4 hours). The heparin therapy should be followed by conventional oral anticoagulant therapy.

In arteriovenous cannulae occlusion:
Before treatment, an attempt should be made to clear the cannulae manually using a syringe and heparinized saline. After the effects of this heparin have diminished, streptokinase can be initiated.

Slowly instill 250,000 IU in 2 ml normal saline into each occluded limb of the cannulae. Clamp the limbs off for 2 hours. Aspirate the contents of the cannulae and flush with saline.

Children:
Not recommended.

Preparation and Storage
This drug is supplied in vials of 250,000 IU (with the green label) and 750,000 IU (with the blue label), in powder form. Store at room temperature.

To prepare for infusion:
1. Add 5 ml of sodium chloride injection SLOWLY into the vial.
2. Roll and tilt the vial gently to reconstitute. Do NOT shake the vial to mix.
3. Further dilute the entire reconstituted contents of the vial slowly with the sodium chloride injection to a volume of approximately 45 ml. See the table below. Do not shake even if thin translucent fibers are seen in the solution, they do not interfere with safe use of the drug unless they are in large amounts. (Solutions containing large amounts of fibers should NOT

be used.) If necessary, the total volume of the solution may be increased in increments of 45 ml up to 180 ml. See the table below for infusion pump rates. The infusion time should be correspondingly increased with any increase in infusion volume.

4. This final solution can be administered through an in-line filter.

5. Use solutions within 24 hours, store in the refrigerator after reconstitution. After administration, unused portions should be discarded.

For use in A-V cannulae: Reconstitute the contents of a 250,000 IU vial with 2 ml of sodium chloride for injection.

Drug Incompatibilities

Do not mix with any other medication in any manner; use only sodium chloride for injection for dilution and normal saline for infusion.

Modes of IV Administration

Injection
No

Intermittent Infusion
No

Continuous Infusion
Yes
Use an infusion pump, see the table under Preparation and Storage for infusion rates.

Contraindications
Because this agent increases the risk of bleeding, it is contraindicated in the presence of:
1. Active internal bleeding
2. Cerebrovascular accident, intracranial or intraspinal surgery within the past 2 months
3. Intracranial neoplasm
4. Arterial emboli that have originated from the left heart (as in mitral stenosis with atrial fibrillation). This is due to the danger of new emboli phenomenon including those to the cerebral vessels.

Warnings
1. Thrombolytic therapy should only be considered in situations where the benefits to be achieved outweigh the risk of serious hemorrhage that can occur with this therapy.
2. When internal bleeding does occur, it may be more difficult to manage than that which occurs with conventional anticoagulant therapy.
3. Therapy with this agent should be initiated as soon after an embolic event as possible, preferrably no later than 7 days after onset. Delay decreases the potential for optimal outcome.
4. Fibrin deposits, which provide hemostasis at needle puncture sites, etc., are also lysed with administration of this drug and bleeding may occur. Perform

Suggested Dilutions and Infusion Rates*

Streptase (streptokinase) Dosage/Infusion Rate	Streptase (streptokinase) Vial Content Needed	Total Volume of Solution (ml)	Pump Infusion Rate (ml/hr)
A. Loading Dose 250,000 IU/30 min	a) 1 vial, 250,000 IU	45	90 for 30 min
	or		
	b) 1 vial, 750,000 IU	45	30 for 30 min
B. Maintenance Dose 100,000 IU/hr	1 vial, 750,000 IU	45	6
(depending on the type of infusion pump, dosage rate may have to be adjusted with corresponding adjustment of total volume of the solution.)			

*Courtesy of Hoechst–Roussel Pharmaceuticals, Inc. Somerville, NJ 08876

streptokinase
(continued)

venipunctures only when absolutely necessary, and apply adequate pressure at the puncture site afterward.

5. Intramuscular injections and nonessential handling of the patient must be avoided during therapy.

6. If arterial puncture is necessary use upper extremity vessels. Apply pressure to the site for at least 30 minutes, then apply a pressure dressing and monitor the site frequently for bleeding.

7. The risk of therapy is increased in the following conditions and should be weighed against the anticipated benefits:

- Major surgery, obstetrical delivery, organ biopsy, or puncture of noncompressible vessels (carotid) within the past 10 days
- Serious gastrointestinal bleeding within the past 10 days
- Recent trauma including cardiopulmonary resuscitation
- Severe uncontrolled arterial hypertension
- The likelihood of left heart thrombus
- Subacute bacterial endocarditis
- Hemostatic defects including those secondary to hepatic or renal disease
- Pregnancy
- Cerebrovascular disease
- Diabetic hemorrhagic retinopathy
- Prior severe allergic reaction to streptokinase
- Septic thrombophlebitis or occluded A-V cannulae at a seriously infected site
- Any other condition in which bleeding constitutes a significant hazard

8. Should severe spontaneous bleeding occur, streptokinase should be discontinued and the situation treated as described under Adverse Reactions.

9. Concurrent use of anticoagulants is not recommended.

Precautions
1. Safety for use in children and

during pregnancy has not been established.

2. Drugs that alter platelet function should not be used during streptokinase therapy, e.g. aspirin, indomethacin, phenylbutazone.

3. The following studies should be carried out prior to therapy: thrombin time, activated partial thromboplastin time, prothrombin time, hematocrit and platelet count. It may also be advisable to type and crossmatch the patient prior to therapy to have blood available in the event of hemorrhage. If heparin is being given, it should be discontinued and the thrombin time or activated partial thromboplastin time should be twice the normal control value before streptokinase therapy is initiated.

4. During therapy, decreases in the plasminogen and fibrinogen levels and an increase in the level of fibrin degradation products will confirm the activity of the drug (lytic state). These levels should be monitored about 4 hours after the initiation of treatment.

Adverse Reactions
1. Minor bleeding often occurs at puncture sites.

2. Severe gastrointestinal, retroperitoneal, intracerebral, genitourinary bleeding can also occur. Fatalities have been reported.

3. If uncontrollable bleeding occurs, therapy with streptokinase should be discontinued. Whole fresh blood should be given and may reverse the bleeding (packed red cells, or fresh frozen plasma can also be used).

4. The use of aminocaproic acid as an antidote has not been adequately documented, but may be considered in severe bleeding.

5. Anaphylaxis has rarely been reported. Other allergic-like reactions have ranged from minor difficulty in breathing to bronchospasm, periorbital edema or angioneurotic edema. Urticaria,

itching, flushing, nausea, headache, and musculoskeletal pain have also been seen. Mild to moderate reactions may be managed with antihistamine or corticosteroid therapy. Severe reactions should prompt the discontinuation of the streptokinase and the use of any supportive therapy required.
6. Increases in body temperature have been seen in some patients. This can be controlled with acetaminophen.

☐ **Nursing Implications**
1. Be aware of contraindications and clinical situations in which the risk of bleeding is great. Monitor even more cautiously than patients without these risks.
2. Monitor for all signs and symptoms of bleeding:
   a. Intracerebral bleeding, as indicated by change in mental status, change in neurologic signs (pupil size, hand grip, extremity motion), headache, or change in vision. Check neurologic signs every 2–4 hours.
   b. Gastrointestinal bleeding, as indicated by hematemesis, abdominal pain or tenderness, fall in blood pressure, melena or red blood in the stools.
   c. Respiratory tract bleeding by hemoptysis (may already be present secondary to pulmonary embolus) as indicated, increase in amount of hemoptysis, respiratory distress, chest pain, hypotension.
   d. Bleeding from the urinary tract as indicated by hematuria (micro- and macroscopic) or dark brown urine.
   e. Vaginal bleeding.
   f. Ecchymosis or petechiae.
   g. Retroperitoneal bleeding as indicated by severe back pain and hypotension.
3. If bleeding begins, notify the physician immediately. If it is

sudden and severe, the streptokinase infusion should be stopped without delay. Be prepared to administer supportive measures as ordered, see Adverse Reactions No. 3 and 4. Volume expanding agents and vasopressors should be available. Monitor blood pressure, usually by indirect technique, frequently. Do not leave the patient unattended, he will probably not tolerate the loss of blood volume well because of the already present stress of the embolic event.
4. Oozing from venipuncture sites is to be expected. It is advisable to avoid all such invasive procedures when possible. Pressure should be applied to all venipuncture sites until it is certain that bleeding has stopped. If arterial puncture is needed, apply pressure for *at least* 30 minutes followed by a pressure dressing. Avoid use of the femoral artery for arterial puncture. Monitor all puncture sites frequently for bleeding and/or hematoma formation.
5. Avoid other traumatic procedures such as nasogastric intubation and urinary catheterization when possible. When performing endotracheal suctioning, use low vacuum settings (below 110 mm Hg) and keep the frequency and duration of suctioning at a minimum. Watch for blood in the aspirate.
6. Handle the patient carefully to prevent bruising and hematoma formation. Use adequate numbers of personnel when turning to prevent tissue trauma. Use protective devices on the bed (flotation pad, water mattress or air mattress) when possible to lessen trauma to the skin. If a hematoma does occur, notify the physician. Pressure dressings (elastic bandage) and ice packs may be ordered.
7. Monitor blood pressure and pulse indirectly every 1–4 hours

streptokinase
(continued)
depending on the patient's overall condition. If there is an increased risk of bleeding, vital signs should be taken hourly to detect the onset of bleeding.

8. Monitor temperature every 4–6 hours. Fever can occur; acetaminophen will be ordered to control it.

9. The clinician is encouraged to read further on this drug and the conditions for which it is indicated.

Suggested Readings
Cudkowicz, Leon, and Sherry, Sol: The Venous System and the Lung. *Heart and Lung*, 7(1):91–96, January/February 1978.
——: Current Status of Thrombolytic Therapy. *Heart and Lung*, 7(1): 97–100, January/February 1978.

succinylcholine chloride ■
(Anectine, Quelicin, Sucostrin)

Actions/Indications
Neuromuscular blocking agent of the depolarizing type, ultra-short-acting. Produces flaccid paralysis of skeletal muscles.

A single paralyzing dose produces effects within one minute of injection, that last up to 8 minutes. Respirations usually return within 30 seconds to 3 minutes after discontinuation of an infusion.

Used as an adjunct to anesthesia to facilitate intubation and manipulation of abdominal wall or other skeletal muscles, usually for short surgical procedures.

Also used to reduce the intensity of muscle contractions induced pharmacologically, electrically (electro-convulsive therapy) or by disease states.

Can also be used in certain situations to control respirations when artificial ventilation is required.

Nondepolarizing neuromuscular blocking agents (pancuronium, tubocurarine) are usually preferred for controlling ventilation because they do not cause muscle fasciculations.

Dosage
Administer only after unconsciousness or a sedated state has been induced.

Adults:
A test dose of 10 mg can be given to evaluate the patient's sensitivity to the drug.

Short procedures—40 mg initially (after test dose) then titrate with response and to reaction to the test dose. (Dose range: 25–80 mg.) Alternative dosages: 0.5–1.0 mg/kg or 40 mg/M^2.

Long procedures or for prolonged control of respiration—by small intermittent doses or by infusion: 2.5 mg/minute, titrate with patient response. (Dose range: 0.5–10 mg/minute.) Use a 0.1% (1 mg/ml) or 0.2% (2 mg/ml) solution for infusion, see table under Preparation and Storage.

Infants and Children:
1.0–2.0 mg/kg, titrated with patient responses, for all indications.

NOTE: When administering this drug during electroshock therapy administer it approximately 1 minute before the shock, usually in a dose of 10–30 mg. (Atropine and a tranquilizer [barbiturate] are usually given prior to the succinylcholine.)

See Precaution No. 5 for dosage modifications.

Preparation and Storage
Available in the following solution concentrations: 20, 50, and 100 mg/ml; also supplied in dry powder form.

Most commonly used infusion concentrations are 0.1% and 0.2%. To prepare these solutions the amounts of diluent and drug shown in the table on page 317 can be used.

Store vials of liquid drug in the refrigerator, dry powder can be stored at room temperature.

Used prepared infusion solutions immediately, discard unused portions.

Preparation of Solutions for Infusion

Product	0.1% Sol. (1 mg/ml)		0.2% Sol. (2 mg/ml)	
	Volume of Drug to be Added	Volume of Diluent	Volume of Drug to be Added	Volume of Diluent
500 mg powder	—	500 ml	—	250 ml
1000 mg powder	—	1000 ml	—	500 ml
100 mg/ml injection	5 ml	500 ml	5 ml	250 ml
	10 ml	1000 ml	10 ml	500 ml
50 mg/ml injection	10 ml	500 ml	10 ml	250 ml
	20 ml	1000 ml	20 ml	500 ml

Drug Incompatibilities

Do not mix with any other medication in any manner.

Modes of IV Administration

Injection
Yes
May be given undiluted over 10–30 seconds.

Intermittent Infusion
Yes
Use a 0.1% solution (1 mg/ml) to make calculation of dose simple. (A 0.2% solution, 2 mg/ml, can be used for patients requiring fluid restriction.)
  Compatible with most IV fluids. Use D5W, NS or RL.

Continuous Infusion
Yes
Use a 0.1% solution (1 mg/ml) to make calculation of dose simple. (A 0.2% solution, 2 mg/ml, can be used for patients requiring fluid restriction.)
  Compatible with most IV fluids. Use of an infusion pump advisable.

Contraindications; Warnings; Precautions; Adverse Reactions

Contraindications
Known hypersensitivity

Warnings
1. Intubation must be performed concomitantly with the administration of this drug before anesthesia. Adequate artificial ventilation, oxygen under positive pressure and the elimination of carbon dioxide must be maintained throughout the administration of this drug and the duration of its effects. This drug's effects cannot be chemically reversed.
2. Safety for use in pregnancy has not been established. Effects on fetal development are not known. This drug does not cross the placental barrier in amounts sufficient to affect the fetus, as far as the drug's effects on skeletal muscles.

Precautions
1. Administer with caution, closely monitoring reaction to test dose, in patients with cardiovascular, hepatic, pulmonary, metabolic, or renal disorders.
2. Administer with caution to patients with severe burns, those who are digitalized or who have been severely traumatized; severe electrolyte disturbances can result, leading to cardiac arrhythmias and possibly arrest.
3. Severe hyperkalemia can occur in patients with pre-existing elevations in serum potassium, in paraplegics, spinal cord injuries, or in patients with dystrophic neuromuscular disease.
4. Myoglobinemia and myoglobinuria can occur, especially in children. Small doses of nondepolarizing neuromuscular blocking agents given before

succinylcholine chloride
(continued)

succinylcholine can decrease the incidence of myoglobinuria.
5. A low level of plasma pseudocholinesterase may be associated with prolongation of respiratory paralysis following succinylcholine. Such low plasma levels are seen in patients with severe liver impairment, anemia, malnutrition, dehydration, recent exposure to neurotoxic insecticides (organophosphates), those receiving quinine, and those with a hereditary trait.[1] Such patients should be monitored carefully during administration of the test dose. Administration of succinylcholine should be via a slow 0.1% infusion. Drugs which either inhibit plasma pseudocholinesterase (neostigmine) or compete with succinylcholine for the enzyme (intravenous procaine) should not be given concomitantly with succinylcholine, to avoid prolongation of the paralyzing effects of this drug.
6. When administered over a prolonged period of time, the block produced by this drug can assume the characteristics of a nondepolarizing block. This can result in prolonged respiratory depression or apnea. The usual nondepolarizing agent antagonists, e.g., neostigmine, plus atropine can be used to counteract the paralysis. A nerve stimulator can be used to determine if the block is a depolarizing or nondepolarizing type.
7. This drug can increase intraocular pressure during the initial stages of administration. Use with caution, if at all, during eye surgery or in patients with glaucoma or eye trauma.
8. Caution should be observed when this drug is used in patients with fractures where the muscle fasciculations produced may aggravate the trauma. Fasciculations and hyperkalemia can be reduced by the adminis-

tration of a small dose of a nondepolarizing type of neuromuscular blocking agent prior to succinylcholine.
9. MAO inhibitor drugs can increase and prolong the effects of this drug.

Adverse Reactions
1. Prolongation of effects producing respiratory depression and apnea (see Precautions and Nursing Implications for agents and conditions that can cause prolongation)
2. Hypersensitivity, rare
3. Cardiovascular: tachycardia, elevation in blood pressure, lowering of blood pressure, arrhythmias and cardiac arrest; in children, bradycardia, hypotension, arrhythmias including sinus arrest can occur during intubation following a second dose of succinylcholine; this may be due to increased vagal tone. These effects are enhanced by the presence of cyclopropane and halothane anesthetics
4. Respiratory: prolonged respiratory depression, apnea
5. Malignant hyperthermia in patients with personal or family history of the disease
6. Increased intraocular pressure
7. Postoperative muscle pain (secondary to fasciculations)
8. Excessive salivation (when atropine or scopolamine has not been given prior to surgery)

☐ **Nursing Implications**
Postanesthesia Care:
1. Equipment that should be readily available: suction, manual breathing bag, airways, endotracheal tubes and laryngoscope, oxygen.
2. Patients receiving this agent must be intubated to assist in maintaining an adequate airway and ventilation.
3. Be aware of the duration of action of this drug (See Actions/Indications section), and when

the patient received the last dose.

4. Be aware of the sequence of progression of the paralytic effects as they will occur after an injection of succinylcholine:
   a. Loss of eye movement
   b. Eyelid droop
   c. Stiffness of jaw muscles
   d. Fasciculations and then paralysis of upper trunk muscles spreading to lower trunk and then extremities
   e. Paralysis of pharyngeal muscles (tongue, muscles of swallowing, etc.)
   f. Respiratory paralysis, i.e., paralysis of intercostal muscles and finally the diaphragm.
   Recovery will occur as a complete reversal of this sequence,[2] and usually occurs rapidly.
5. Be aware of elements which may prolong the effects of this drug according to the manufacturer:
   a. Decreased circulation time, e.g., congestive heart failure or shock
   b. Decreased body temperature (especially in infants)[3]
   c. Dehydration
   d. Decreased renal function
   e. Decreased hepatic function
   f. Concomitant use of neurotoxic antibiotics such as the aminoglycosides (gentamicin, amikacin, etc.), polymyxin B or bacitracin
   g. Other drugs that effect the central nervous system, e.g., diazepam, quinine, quinidine, MAO inhibitors, magnesium salts (magnesium sulfate), procaine
   h. Extremes in age
   i. Hypokalemia and hypocalcemia
   j. Anticholinesterase agents and other depolarizing or nondepolarizing neuromuscular blocking agents
   k. Low serum pseudocholinesterase (see Precaution No. 5)
6. Discharge from the recovery room will depend on the following criteria:
   a. Grip strength
   b. Ability to lift the head
   c. Ability to open the eyes
   d. Respiratory status, e.g., vital capacity and tidal volume (it is helpful to obtain these values preoperatively for comparison)
   Patients under the effects of any one of these elements will require prolonged monitoring as described in No. 5 above, for recovery from the succinylcholine.

Maintenance Care for Controlled Ventilation:
1. Nondepolarizing agents are usually given for controlling ventilation because they do not cause fasciculations of the muscles.
2. When used, this drug is usually administered on a p.r.n. basis for control of ventilation. The criteria for when to administer succinylcholine are determined by the physician. The criteria will include such situations as:
   a. Respiratory rate limit set by the physician
   b. When the patient's respiratory effort is out of phase with the respirator
   c. When the patient is struggling against the respirator
   d. When positive-end expiratory pressure (P.E.E.P.) is in use
   Monitor for the onset of any of these situations and administer the drug or have the drug given. Who administers neuromuscular blocking agents is usually governed by hospital policy.
3. Make certain that the endotracheal tube is securely and correctly inserted. Check the connection between the endotracheal tube and the respirator; it must be tight. **Keep respirator alarm systems functioning at all times**. The patient is totally dependent on the respirator for ventilation.
4. This drug paralyzes skeletal muscles, it does not alter con-

succinylcholine chloride
(continued)

sciousness or relieve pain and anxiety. Therefore, the patient must be adequately sedated and given analgesics as indicated by his condition. These agents will also decrease discomfort caused by fasciculations. He will not be able to make his needs known; the persons caring for him must anticipate those needs. Many institutions assign one or more nurses to be in constant attendance with these patients.

5. Monitor vital signs before administration and every 5 minutes after until stabilization is seen, then every 15–30 minutes. Repeat the cycle with each dose. Succinylcholine can cause bradycardia or tachycardia, elevation of temperature and increased salivation. Monitor accordingly. Patients with cardiac disease should be observed via continuous ECG monitoring.

6. Monitor for the signs and symptoms of increased intraocular pressure, i.e., dilation of pupils, and vomiting.

7. Because this agent produces muscle paralysis, handle the patient with care to prevent trauma to joints and muscles during turning and positioning. Turn frequently to prevent skin breakdown.

8. When the patient is taken off this medication and the respirator, proceed with the nursing management as described under Postanesthesia Care.

References
1. Melmon, Kenneth L., and Morrelli, Howard F. (editors): *Clinical Pharmacology, Basic Principles in Therapeutics,* New York: Macmillan Publishing Company, 1972, p. 539.
2. Wylie, W. D., and Churchill-Davidson, H. C. (editors): *A Practice of Anesthesia* (3rd ed.), Chicago: Year Book Medical Publishers, 1972, p. 816.
3. Ibid., p. 833.

tetracycline hydrochloride ■
(Achromycin Intravenous)

Actions/Indications
Antibiotic; broad spectrum, active against a wide range of organisms:
- Rickettsiae
- *Mycoplasma pneumoniae*
- Agents of psittacosis and ornithosis
- Agents of lymphogranuloma venereum and granuloma inguinale
- Spirochetal agent of relapsing fever

The following gram-negative organisms:
- *Haemophilus ducreyi*
- *Pasteurella pestis* and *P. tularensis*
- *Bartonella bacilliformis*
- *Bacteroides* species
- *Vibrio comma* and *V. fetus*
- *Brucella* species

Indicated in the following organisms if sensitivity testing shows susceptibility:
- *E. coli*
- *Enterobacter aerogenes*
- *Shigella*
- *Mima* and *Herellea* species
- *Haemophilus influenzae* (in respiratory infections)
- *Klebsiella* species (respiratory and urinary infections)

Indicated in the following gram-positive organisms when sensitivity testing shows susceptibility:
- Streptococcus (usually not susceptible, do not use for rheumatic fever prophylaxis)
- *Diplococcus pneumoniae*
- *Staphylococcus aureus* (usually not susceptible)

When penicillin is contraindicated:
- *Neisseria gonorrhoeae*
- *Neisseria meningitidis*
- *Treponema pallidum* and *T. pertenue* (syphilis and yaws)
- *Listeria monocytogenes*
- *Clostridium* species
- *Bacillus anthracis*
- *Fusobacterium fusiforme*
- *Actinomyces* species

Dosage
Adults:
250–500 mg every 12 hours. Do not

exceed 500 mg every 6 hours.
Children (over 8 years of age):
10–20 mg/kg/day in equally divided
doses every 12 hrs (See Warning
No. 6.)
*Infants and Children (8 years and
under):*
10–15 mg/kg/day in equally divided
doses every 12 hrs (See Warning
No. 6.)
Neonates:
Not recommended.
  Therapy should be continued for
at least 24–48 hours after symptoms
and fever have subsided.

Preparation and Storage
NOTE: There are two parenteral
preparations of this drug, IV and
IM, check the label before use; IV
form supplied in vials of 250 mg
and 500 mg.
  To reconstitute from powder, add
5 ml sterile water for injection to
250-mg vial, 10 ml to the 500-mg
vial.
  Store at room temperature; discard after 12 hours.
  Use only the following fluids for
infusion:
• D5/NS
• D5W
• Protein Hydrolysate 5%, plain
  with Dextrose 5% or with Invert
  Sugar 10%
• RL
• Ringer's Injection
  Infuse immediately after preparation of solution. Darkening solution
indicates deterioration of the drug.
Discontinue and use a different infusion fluid. Discontinue if a haze or
crystals appear in solution or IV tubing.

Drug Incompatibilities
Do not mix with any other medica-
tion in the IV bottle. Do not add as
a secondary line to tubing contain-
ing:
Calcium compounds
Cephalosporins
Chloramphenicol
Chlorothiazide
Erythromycin
Heparin
Hydrocortisone

Methicillin
Novobiocin
Oxacillin
Penicillin
Phenytoin
Polymyxin B
Sodium bicarbonate
Thiopental

Modes of IV Administration

Injection
No

Intermittent Infusion
Yes
Dilute to 10 mg/ml; infuse over at
least 1–2 hours (20 mg/minute).
  See Preparation and Storage for
acceptable fluids to use for infusion.

Continuous Infusion
Yes
Preferred mode of administration.
Use a concentration of 2 mg/ml of
fluid, or add a 12-hour dose to 1000
ml of any fluid listed in Preparation
and Storage. Infuse at a rate of 1.5
ml/minute.

Contraindications; Warnings; Pre-cautions; Adverse Reactions

Contraindications
Hypersensitivity to any tetracycline

Warnings
1. Tetracycline should be avoided
   in patients with renal insufficiency. This drug may exacerbate renal dysfunction directly
   and indirectly by causing a catabolic state with acidosis and increasing azotemia.[1]
2. The use of tetracycline in
   pregnant patients with renal
   dysfunction has been associated
   with maternal death due to
   acute hepatic failure.
3. This drug is not readily removed by hemodialysis.[2]
4. May cause an elevation in BUN
   in normal individuals. This is
   not harmful and will decrease
   on discontinuation of the drug.
5. Tetracycline may cause liver
   damage in the form of fatty in-

tetracycline hydrochloride
(continued)
filtration in previously normal
individuals. Do not use other
potentially hepatotoxic agents
concomitantly. Avoid use in patients with liver disease.[3]
6. Use of this drug during the
years of tooth development can
cause permanent discoloration
of the teeth. Enamel hypoplasia
has also been reported. Do not
use tetracyclines in this age
group (last half of pregnancy,
infancy, childhood up to 8 years
of age) unless other drugs are
ineffective or contraindicated.
7. This drug can cause fetal malformations (skeletal development) in animals; safety in
pregnancy has not been
established. Also, see Nos. 6
and 8 above.
8. May cause bone growth retardation in premature infants receiving large doses. This is reversible on discontinuation.
9. This drug is secreted in breast
milk. Nursing should be discontinued when this drug is being
used.

Precautions
1. Overgrowth of nonsusceptible
organisms can occur. If a superinfection occurs, discontinue the
drug and initiate appropriate
therapy.
2. Patients on anticoagulants may
require lower doses of those
drugs while on tetracycline.
3. Monitor hepatic, renal and hematopoietic systems during
therapy.
4. Treat all group A beta hemolytic streptococcus infections for at
least 10 days.
5. Avoid concomitant use of this
drug and penicillin. Penicillin
activity may be decreased.
6. Photosensitivity may occur in
the form of an exaggerated
sunburn reaction. Warn the patient of this possibility if he is
to continue this drug as an outpatient. Treatment should be

discontinued at the first sign of
erythema.

Adverse Reactions
1. Gastrointestinal: anorexia, nausea, vomiting, diarrhea, glossitis, dysphagia, enterocolitis
2. *Candida albicans* overgrowth in
the perineal area (monilia) and
mouth (thrush)
3. Skin: rashes, exfoliative dermatitis
4. Renal toxicity: rise in BUN; see
Warnings No. 1, 2, and 4.
5. Hypersensitivity: rashes, anaphylaxis
6. In infants: bulging fontanels,
papilledema (pseudotumor cerebri); usually disappears on
discontinuation of the drug
7. Hematopoietic: hemolytic anemia, thrombocytopenia (rare)
8. Discoloration of teeth and
enamel hypoplasia if administered during tooth development.

☐ **Nursing Implications**
1. Take anaphylaxis precautions;
see Appendix.
2. If gastrointestinal disturbances
occur, notify the physician. If
disturbances such as nausea,
vomiting and diarrhea are pronounced, the drug will probably
be discontinued. Antiemetics,
antacids, and constipating agents
can be ordered to control symptoms. Monitor intake and output to assist the physician in
planning for parenteral fluid replacement. Maintain hydration
orally when possible.
3. If the patient will be taking the
oral form of this drug as an outpatient, instruct him on the possibility of photosensitivity and
the advisability of avoiding exposure to the sun (sun-block lotions may be of help if exposure
cannot be avoided).
4. Women of child-bearing age
and potential, and mothers of
children who may receive this
drug, should be informed of
Warnings No. 2, 6, and 7 by the

physician. Assist in the interpretation of these warnings to the patient.

5. Even though blood dyscrasias are infrequently caused by this agent, be aware of the patient's complete blood cell count during therapy. If the platelet count begins to fall, the drug will probably be discontinued. Bleeding secondary to a lower platelet count usually begins only after the count falls below 100,000/cu.mm.

6. Monitor for signs and symptoms of overgrowth infections:
   a. Fever (take rectal temperature at least every 4–6 hours in all patients)
   b. Increasing malaise
   c. Newly appearing localized signs and symptoms: redness, soreness, pain, swelling, drainage (increasing volume or change in character of pre-existing drainage)
   d. Monilial rash in perineal area (reddened areas with itching); red lesions on oral mucosa (thrush)
   e. Cough (change in pre-existing cough or sputum production)
   f. Diarrhea

7. Report the onset of any rash to the physician. Keep the patient's environment comfortably cool and the skin clean. Diphenhydramine (Benadryl) may be ordered to relieve itching.

8. Report the onset of jaundice to the physician.

9. Report the onset of bulging fontanels and other signs of increasing intracranial pressure to the physician.

10. Be aware of this drug's relationship with renal function. Most tetracyclines are usually not given to patients with renal impairment because:
    a. The drug accumulates in the body because of decreased excretion
    b. The presence of the drug may cause further deterioration in renal function

c. It may cause a catabolic state with metabolic acidosis, increasing BUN, and possibly death due to uremia[4] Know what the patient's pretreatment BUN and creatinine levels are. Monitor for change in these values with initiation of treatment. Monitor urine output in renal patients receiving the drug. Report increasing oliguria to the physician. Send urine for analysis at least every other day.

References
1. Barza, Michael and Schiefe, Richard: Antimicrobial Spectrum, Pharmacology and Therapeutic Use of Antibiotics. Part I: Tetracyclines. *American Journal of Hospital Pharmacists*, 34(1):51, January 1977.
2. Ibid.
3. Ibid., p. 53.
4. Ibid., p. 51.

thiamine hydrochloride ■
(Vitamin B₁, Betalin S)

Actions/Indications
Vitamin necessary for carbohydrate metabolism. Used therapeutically to treat severe vitamin B₁ depletion (associated with Wernicke's disease) or beriberi.

Direct intravenous injection is recommended *only* for the emergency treatment of wet beriberi with cardiac failure.

Thiamine is also contained in vitamin B complex preparations for intravenous administration. These agents are used to prevent vitamin B deficiencies such as beriberi during chronic illness and during prolonged periods of abstinence from food intake.

Dosage
Adults:
Beriberi—10–20 mg every 8 hours until symptoms subside.

Wernicke's—50 mg daily until a

thiamine hydrochloride
(continued)
normal diet and oral vitamins can be
taken.[1]
Children:
Beriberi—10–25 mg daily until
symptoms subside.[2]

Preparation and Storage
Supplied in 1-ml ampuls, 10-ml and
30-ml vials in a concentration of 100
mg/ml.
    Refrigerate unopened vials.
    Thiamine is compatible with most
infusion fluids.
    May be infused in plastic IV bags.

Drug Incompatibilities
Do not mix with aminophilline.
    Do not mix with alkaline solutions
of barbiturates, carbonates, sodium
bicarbonate, citrates, and acetates.
    Do not mix in any manner with:
Cephaloridine
Erythromycin
Kanamycin sulfate

Modes of IV Administration

Injection
Yes
Slowly, for acute cardiac beriberi
only

Intermittent Infusion
Yes
Use any IV fluid, 100–200 ml, infuse
over 30–60 minutes. This mode is
used in the treatment of beriberi
and Wernicke's disease.

Continuous Infusion
Yes
Use any IV fluid, in any amount.
This mode is used when thiamine is
administered as a vitamin supple-
ment, e.g. hyperalimentation.

**Contraindications; Warnings; Pre-
cautions; Adverse Reactions**

Contraindications
Hypersensitivity to thiamine.

Warnings
Serious sensitivity reactions, such as
anaphylaxis, have occurred. *Deaths
have occurred during the use of intravenous route.* An intradermal test dose
for hypersensitivity is recommended
prior to administration.

Precautions
Multiple vitamin deficiencies should
be observed for in any patient with
thiamine deficiency.

Adverse Reactions
 1. Feeling of warmth
 2. Pruritus, urticaria
 3. Weakness
 4. Diaphoresis
 5. Nausea
 6. Tightness in the throat
 7. Angioneurotic edema
 8. Cyanosis
 9. Pulmonary edema
10. Gastrointestinal hemorrhage
11. Circulatory collapse and death

☐ **Nursing Implications**
 1. Take anaphylaxis precautions;
    see Appendix.
 2. Stop infusion if any adverse re-
    action occurs; it may be the first
    sign of anaphylaxis.
 3. Signs of thiamine deficiency will
    begin to appear when the di-
    etary intake is less than 0.2 mg.
    per 1000 calories of food intake.
 4. Signs and symptoms of wet beri-
    beri (cardiac failure secondary
    to thiamine deficiency):
    a. Persistent tachycardia
    b. Severe dyspnea, rales
    c. Violent palpitations of the
       heart
    d. Intense chest pain (subster-
       nal)
    e. Heaviness, constrictive, op-
       pressive feeling in the chest
    f. Cardiomegaly, hepatomegaly
    g. Cyanosis
    h. Insomnia
    i. Vomiting
    j. Peripheral edema
    These signs should disappear
    within a few days with therapy.[3]
 5. Administer supportive care for
    cardiac failure:
    a. Monitor heart rate, respira-

tory rate, blood pressure,
C.V.P. as needed
b. Place patient in a semi-Fowler's position (patient will
probably be orthopneic)
c. Administer oxygen and supportive medications as ordered
d. Monitor weight daily
6. Patients with beriberi must
receive dietary counseling and
follow-up to prevent recurrence
of the condition.
7. Signs and symptoms of Wernicke's disease (Wernicke–Kor-
sakoff syndrome), a CNS disorder secondary to thiamine
deficiency:
a. Ocular changes, e.g. nystagmus, sixth nerve palsy, diplopia, loss of ocular movement, miotic nonreactive pupils
b. Ataxia, inability to stand
c. Global mental confusion,
apathy.[4]
Recovery can be within hours of
initiation of thiamine therapy.
Long-term effects, i.e., Korsa-
koff's psychosis (amnesia, inability to learn) may remain for up
to one year.
8. Initiate measures to prevent patient injury, e.g. side rails. Ambulate only with assistance when
the patient can stand. Promote
time and place orientation.

References

1. Kurt Isselbacher, editor. *Harrison's Principles of Internal Medicine*
(9th ed.), New York: McGraw–
Hill Book Company, 1980, p.
1987.
2. American Hospital Formulary
Service, American Society of
Hospital Pharmacists, 1981, p.
88:08.
3. Beeson, Paul B., and
McDermott, Walsh (editors):
Cecil-Loeb Textbook of Medicine
(15th ed.), Philadelphia: W. B.
Saunders Company, 1975, p.
1373.
4. Kurt Isselbacher, op. cit. p.
1985.

thiopental sodium ■
(Sodium Pentothal)

Actions/Indications
Anesthetic, ultra-short-acting barbiturate. Depresses the CNS to the
point of hypnosis and anesthesia 30–
40 seconds after IV injection.
Used in anesthesia:
• Sole agent of anesthesia
• Induction
• Adjunct to other agents
• Anticonvulsant
• Narcoanalysis
Recovery is rapid after one small
dose, with some residual somnolence and retrograde amnesia. However, repeated doses lead to prolonged anesthesia because fatty
tissues in the body act as a reservoir
to the drug, they accumulate thiopental in concentrations 6–12 times
greater than the plasma, and then
release the drug slowly to produce
prolonged anesthesia.

Dosage
Adults:
Individualized according to patient's
response, usually proportional to
body weight.
Test dose—25–75 mg injected with
60-second observation of the patient
for unusual response.
Induction—adult: average, 50–75
mg at intervals of 20–40 seconds titrated to patient's reaction. As an
initial dose, 210–280 mg (3–4 mg/
kg) is required for rapid induction in
the average 70 kg adult.
Maintenance of anesthesia—25–50
mg whenever the patient moves. Use
minimal dose to achieve desirable
level. A continuous drip of a 0.2%
or 0.4% solution can be used
throughout a procedure to maintain
anesthesia.
Convulsive states—75–125 mg, up
to 250 mg over a 10-minute period.
Also by infusion.
*To decrease intracranial pressure dur-
ing surgery*—1.5–3.5 mg/kg via intermittent injection.
Psychiatry—use a test dose (see
above), then 100 mg/min injection.
Patient should be instructed to

thiopental sodium
(continued)
count backward from 100. When confused counting occurs, injection is stopped. Infusion may also be used.
Children:
Recommendations not available.

Preparation and Storage
Supplied in vials of 500 mg and 1 g and bottles of 5 g and 10 g in 250 ml and 500 ml respectively. Some are supplied with sterile water for injection as diluent.

To reconstitute, use only sterile water for injection, NS, or D5W, or Abbott Pentothal Diluent. For volumes over 100 ml, do not use sterile water for injection, to prevent hemolysis; use D5W, NS, or Normosol-R or Abbott Pentothal diluent.

To prepare solutions for administration, follow the table below:

Concentration Desired		Amounts to Use	
%	mg/ml	Thiopental grams	Diluent ml
0.2	2	1	500
0.4	4	1	250
		2	500
2.0	20	5	250
		10	500
2.5	25	1	40
		5	200
5	50	1	20
		5	100

Never use a solution with visible precipitate.

Follow directions for dilution and transfer techniques accompanying the equipment and container.

This is a Schedule III drug under the Controlled Substances Act of 1970. Maintain hospital or institutional regulations guiding the use of this drug.

This drug contains no bacteriostatic agents. Use extreme caution to prevent contamination; use only fresh solutions; discard all stock solutions after 24 hours.

Drug Incompatibilities
Do not mix in solution with other drugs.

Ideally, other drugs should not be injected into an IV line containing thiopental, many other agents are incompatible with it.

Use only D5W, Normal Saline, Normosol-R, or Abbott Pentothal Diluent for infusions.

Modes of IV Administration

Injection
Yes
Use a 2.5% solution, slowly.

Intermittent Infusion
Yes
Use 0.2–0.4% solution.

Continuous Infusion
Yes
Use 0.2–0.4% solution; titrate with patient response.

Contraindications; Warnings; Precautions; Adverse Reactions

Contraindications
Absolute:
1. Absence of suitable veins
2. Hypersensitivity to any barbiturate
3. Status asthmaticus
4. Porphyria (confirmed or familial history)
   Relative:
1. Severe cardiovascular disease
2. Hypotension and shock
3. Conditions in which effects may be prolonged: Addison's disease, excessive premedication, hepatic or renal dysfunction, myxedema, increased BUN, severe anemia (dosage must be adjusted accordingly, if the drug is given at all)
4. Increased intracranial pressure
5. Asthma
6. Myasthenia gravis

Precautions
1. Respiratory support equipment must be readily available to maintain a patent airway and ventilation. Momentary apnea following each injection is typical, and requires assisted ventilation.

2. Repeated or continuous infusion may result in cumulative effects, e.g., prolonged somnolence, and respiratory and circulatory depression.
3. Avoid extravasation. Intra-arterial injection can cause gangrene of the extremity.
4. If used in the presence of relative contraindications, reduce dosage and administer slowly.
5. Safety for use in pregnancy has not been established. This agent is excreted in breast milk.
6. The central nervous system effects of this drug may be additive with those of other depressant agents. Dosage adjustments should be made accordingly.

Adverse Reactions
1. Respiratory depression, laryngospasm, bronchospasm
2. Myocardial depression
3. Cardiac arrhythmias
4. Prolonged somnolence and recovery
5. Sneezing, coughing, shivering
6. Hypersensitivity

Overdosage
Rapid, repeated or prolonged continuous injections or infusions may be followed by a fall in systemic blood pressure, possibly to shock levels. Apnea, laryngospasm and other respiratory difficulties may also occur. In this event, discontinue the thiopental, maintain an open airway and ventilation with oxygen until effects diminish. Administer vasopressors and fluids as needed. The lethal dose level is not known. See Nursing Implications.

☐ **Nursing Implications**
1. Strictly adhere to maximum injection and infusion rate suggestions and dosage limits. Use an infusion pump to assist with rate control, to insure maximum benefit from the drug and to prevent overdosage. Patients with liver impairment, severe cardiovascular disease, hypotension, Addison's disease, renal impairment, myxedema, or severe anemia should receive smaller doses and should be monitored more closely and for a longer period of time than usual.
2. Keep the patient supine during and after injection or infusion. Monitor blood pressure, heart rate and respiratory rate every 5 minutes for 1 hour following an injection, or every 5 minutes through the duration of an infusion. This includes fetal heart rate monitoring. Do not leave the patient unattended.
3. Patients with porphyria are sensitive to barbiturates in that they may experience an acute attack of the disease secondary to the administration of a barbiturate (see Contraindications). The onset of an acute attack is indicated by severe colicky abdominal pain radiating to the back. There is usually severe vomiting, fever and leukocytosis in addition.[1]
4. Avoid extravasation; see Appendix. Extravascular or intra-arterial injection of this drug can cause tissue necrosis and gangrene of the affected extremity, respectively. Thrombophlebitis can also occur during the course of an infusion. Examine for redness and pain along the vein tract, and discontinue the infusion if signs and symptoms appear. Notify the physician immediately.
5. Take anaphylaxis precautions; see Appendix.
6. Monitor for symptoms of acute overdosage (listed in order of progression):
   a. Respiratory depression, i.e., decreased respiratory rate and depth, apnea (intermittent apnea is expected after each injection and during induction. Respiratory depression is termed as prolonged insufficient ventilation or apnea.)
   b. Peripheral vascular collapse, i.e., fall in blood pressure,

thiopental sodium
(continued)

   pallor, diaphoresis, tachycardia
c. Pulmonary edema (rare)
d. Decreased or absent reflexes, pupillary constriction
e. Stupor
f. Coma
Stop the injection or infusion immediately upon noting any of these symptoms. Support ventilation. Notify the physician. Discontinuation of the infusion is usually all that is necessary to prevent further problems. If not, see No. 7 below.

7. Management of acute overdosage:
   a. Continue to stay with the patient, and monitor vital signs
   b. Maintain an open airway and adequate ventilation
   c. Keep the patient as alert as possible by verbal and physical stimuli. Encourage the patient to breathe at an adequate rate (12–14 breaths/minute for an adult). If necessary, initiate artificial ventilation with a manual breathing bag (Puritan, Hope, Ambu, etc.) or mouth-to-mouth breathing at a rate of 12–14 breaths/minute, use oxygen.
   d. Circulatory support in the form of fluids and drugs may be ordered
8. The sedation produced by this drug may be preceded by transient changes in mental status, such as feelings of euphoria and confusion. If this occurs, attempt to calm the patient and take measures to prevent injury until the patient returns to his normal status.
9. If a patient is to be ambulatory following an injection, ambulate with assistance. There may be transient dizziness. Obtain lying, then sitting and standing blood pressures to detect postural hypotension. If this drug has been used for an outpatient procedure, a responsible adult should accompany the patient home. The patient should not drive for at least the next 8 hours.

Reference

1. Beeson, Paul B., and McDermott, Walsh (editors): *Cecil-Loeb Textbook of Medicine* (14th ed.), Philadelphia: W. B. Saunders Company, 1975, p. 1873.

thiophosphoramide ■
(Thiotepa)

Actions/Indications
Antineoplastic agent, of the alkylating type, related to nitrogen mustard. Excreted unchanged in the urine.

   Used for palliation of many types of cancers, including:
· Adenocarcinoma
· Malignant lymphomas stages III and IV (lymphosarcoma, reticulum cell sarcoma, Hodgkin's disease and giant follicular lymphoma).
· Bronchogenic carcinoma
· Superficial papillary carcinoma of the bladder.
   Also used to control intracavitary effusions secondary to neoplastic disease, and is administered directly into tumor masses and affected body cavities (e.g., abdominal chest).

Dosage
Adults:
Initially—0.3 to 0.4 mg/kg, dosage may be reduced in patients who are markedly debilitated, who have cardiovascular or renal disease or who are in shock.
   Maintenance—adjusted on basis of blood counts, at 1- to 4-week intervals (bronchogenic carcinoma—one dose is given every 5 days).
Children:
Dosage recommendations are available from Lederle Labs, Pearl River, NY 10965.

Preparation and Storage
Supplied in vials containing 15 mg of drug. To reconstitute from powder, use 1.5 ml sterile water for injection. This produces a concentration of 10 mg/ml. Solution should be clear to slightly opaque. Grossly opaque solutions, or those with a precipitate, should not be used. Refrigerate reconstituted solution and discard after 5 days. Add to NS, D5W, D5/NS, RL, or Ringer's Injection for infusion.

Drug Incompatibilities
Do not mix with any other medication in any manner.

Modes of IV Administration
Injection
Yes
Further dilution is not necessary. Inject over 1–3 minutes.

Intermittent Infusion
Yes
Add dose to 50–100 ml D5W, NS, D5/NS, RL or Ringer's injection. Infuse over 30 minutes.

Continuous Infusion
No
Injection and intermittent infusion are the preferred modes of administration.

Contraindications; Warnings; Precautions; Adverse Reactions

Contraindications
1. Hepatic, renal or bone marrow dysfunction. If need outweighs risks, use lower dosage and monitor organ function.
2. Hypersensitivity.

Warnings
1. This drug is actively teratogenic (causes fetal abnormalities).
2. Highly toxic to hematopoietic system (blood cell production). Rapidly falling WBC should prompt discontinuation of the drug.
3. Weekly CBC and platelet counts should be performed before, during and for 3 weeks after therapy.
4. Like all alkylating agents, this drug is carcinogenic.

Precautions
1. Bone marrow depression, if not checked by discontinuation of therapy, can lead to death. Fall in white cell count may occur from 2–3 weeks after therapy has been discontinued. Therapy should be stopped when white cell count is less than 3000/cu.mm. or when the platelet count falls below 150,000/cu.mm.
2. This drug should not be administered after a course of x-ray therapy or after therapy with other radiomimetic drugs until the full effects (leukocyte count) of such treatments have been observed and the leukocyte count has returned to normal.
3. In the presence of infection, use with caution and with antimicrobial agents.
4. Prophylactic antibiotics may be used if WBC falls below 3000/cu.mm.
5. Avoid concomitant use with other bone marrow depressing drugs.
6. There is no known antidote to overdosage.

Adverse Reactions
1. Pain and thrombophlebitis at injection site
2. Nausea, vomiting, anorexia, stomatitis
3. Tightness in throat
4. Dizziness
5. Headache
6. Amenorrhea
7. Allergic reactions: rash, urticaria, anaphylaxis
8. Depression of spermatogenesis and ovarian function
9. Hyperuricemia with uric acid nephropathy
10. Fever
11. Blood dyscrasias: thrombocytopenia (may result in hemorrhage), leukopenia (may result in infection)

thiophosphoramide
(continued)

☐ **Nursing Implications**

1. The patient receiving this medication will be experiencing the emotional and physical effects of the malignancy. Knowledge of the patient's feelings about his disease and its implications will assist in helping him to tolerate the chemotherapy. The incidence of uncomfortable side effects and adverse reactions is high. It is within the nurse's role to assist the patient in coping with the discomforts of the disease and its treatment, and to help him work through depression and anger toward acceptance of the disease at his own pace. Despite the unpleasantness this drug may bring, it can be a source of hope for the patient.

2. Many patients experience fewer injection side effects (nausea, vomiting, dizziness, etc.) when they are placed in a reclining position during the administration of this drug.

3. *Management of nausea and vomiting*
   a. Usually occurs 1–3 hours after injection. Vomiting may subside after 8 hours, but nausea can persist for 24 hours.
   b. Administer this drug at night if possible to correlate with normal sleep pattern, accompanied by sedation and an antiemetic drug to combat these side effects.
   c. To be effective, antiemetics should be administered 1 hour prior to the injection of the drug.
   d. Small frequent meals, timed with periods when the patient feels his best, are advisable. Bland foods are usually better tolerated. Carbohydrate and protein content should be high.
   e. If the patient is anorexic, encourage high nutrient liquids and water to maintain hydration. Hydration will help prevent uric acid nephropathy.
   f. Keep accurate measurements of emesis volume and total intake and output to guide the physician in ordering parenteral fluids when necessary.

4. *Management of hematologic effects*
   a. Be aware of the patient's white blood cell and platelet counts prior to each injection.
   b. If the WBC falls to 2000/cu.mm., take measures to protect the patient from infection such as protective (reverse) isolation, avoidance of invasive procedures, maintenance of bodily (especially perineal) cleanliness, carrying out strict urinary catheter care when appropriate, etc. Monitor for infection by recording temperatures every 4 hours, examining for rashes, swelling, drainage and pain. Explain these measures to the patient.
   c. If the platelet count falls below 100,000/cu.mm., monitor for thrombocytopenic bleeding: petechiae, purpura, hematuria, melena, blood in stools, gum bleeding, vaginal bleeding, epistaxis, hematemesis, etc. Avoid trauma. Transfusions may be ordered.
   d. Instruct the patient and family on the importance of follow-up blood studies if the drug is being administered on an outpatient basis.

5. Thrombophlebitis can occur at the injection site. Notify the physician at onset; apply warm compresses as ordered; elevate the extremity. Protect the area from trauma. Avoid extravasation. If it occurs, apply warm compresses until symptoms subside. Monitor for tissue sloughing. See Appendix.

6. *Management of stomatitis*
   a. Administer preventive oral

care every 4 hours and/or after meals.

  b. For preventive care use a very soft toothbrush (child's) and toothpaste; avoid trauma to tissues.

  c. Examine oral membranes at least once daily (instruct patient and/or family) to detect the onset of inflammation or ulceration.

  d. If stomatitis occurs, notify the physician and begin therapeutic oral care as ordered.

  e. Order a bland mechanical soft diet for patients with mild inflammation. If stomatitis is severe, the patient may be placed on NPO status by the physician.

  f. For patients who can tolerate oral intake, administer Xylocaine Viscous or acetaminophen elixir as a mouthwash prior to meals to decrease pain (do not use aspirin rinses) as ordered by the physician.

  g. Patients with severe stomatitis may require parenteral analgesia.

7. If rashes occur, administer cool compresses as ordered. Turn the patient frequently to prevent skin breakdown.

8. Patients can experience a sensation of tightness in the throat while on this drug. Reassure them as to the origin of this reaction; notify the physician.

9. This drug is also administered directly into the tumor mass or into affected body cavities. For further information see the manufacturer's package insert.

Suggested Readings

Bolin, Rose Homan, and Auld, Margaret E.: Hodgkin's Disease. *American Journal of Nursing*, 74:1982–1986, November 1974.

Bruya, Margaret Auld, and Madeira, Nancy Powell: Stomatitis After Chemotherapy. *American Journal of Nursing*, 75(8):1349–1352, August 1975.

Foley, Genevieve, and McCarthy, Ann Marie: The Disease (Hodgkin's) and Its Treatment. *American Journal of Nursing*, 76:1109–1114, July 1976 (references).

Giadquinta, Barbara: Helping Families Face the Crisis of Cancer. *American Journal of Nursing*, 77:1583–1588, October 1977.

Gullo, Shirley: Chemotherapy— What To Do About Special Side Effects. *RN*, 40:30–32, April 1977.

Hannan, Jeanne Ferguson: Talking Is Treatment, Too. *American Journal of Nursing*, 74:1991–1992, November 1974.

Showfety, Mary Patricia: The Ordeal of Hodgkin's Disease. *American Journal of Nursing*, 74:1987–1991, November 1974.

Vietti, Teresa J., and Valeriote, Frederick: Conceptual Basis for The Use of Chemotherapeutic Agents and Their Pharmacology. *Pediatric Clinics of North America*, 23:67–92, February 1976.

ticarcillin disodium ■
(Ticar)

Actions/Indications

Antibiotic, synthetic penicillin.

  Indicated for the treatment of the following infections due to susceptible strains of the designated organisms:

- Bacterial septicemia and skin and soft-tissue infections: *Pseudomonas aeruginosa*, *Proteus* species (indole positive and negative) and *E. coli*.

- Acute and chronic respiratory infections: *Pseudomonas aeruginosa*, Proteus (indole positive and negative) and *E. coli* (bacteriological cures cannot be expected in patients with chronic infections or cystic fibrosis).

- Genitourinary tract infections: *Pseudomonas aeruginosa*, Proteus species (indole positive and negative), *E. coli*, *Enterobacter* and *Streptococcus faecalis* (enterococcus).

  This drug is also indicated in the treatment of the following infections due to susceptible anaerobic organisms:

ticarcillin disodium
(continued)
- Bacterial septicemia
- Lower respiratory tract infections
- Intra-abdominal infections
- Infections of the female pelvis and genital tract
- Soft-tissue and skin infections

Dosage
Adults:
*Bacterial septicemia, pulmonary infections, skin and soft tissue infections—*200–300 mg/kg/day by intermittent infusions, every 3, 4 or 6 hrs divided doses.

*Urinary tract infections—*Uncomplicated cases: 1 gm every 6 hours by direct intravenous injection. Complicated cases: 150–200 mg/kg/day by injections or intermittent infusions every 3, 4, or 6 hrs in divided doses.
Children:
Under 40 kg or 88 lbs of body weight, do no exceed adult dose.

*Bacterial septicemia, pulmonary infections, skin and soft-tissue infections, intra-abdominal infections, infections of the female pelvis and genital tract—*200–300 mg/kg/24 hr in divided doses every 4 or 6 hours by infusion.

*Urinary tract infections—*Complicated: 150–200 mg/kg/24 hr in divided doses every 4 or 6 hours, by intermittent infusion. Uncomplicated: 50–100 mg/kg/24 hr in divided doses every 6 or 8 hours by direct IV injection.

*In renal insufficiency—*Children over 40 kg or 88 lbs should receive dosages based on adult table below. For those under 40 kg or 88 lbs no recommendations are available.

Adults With Renal Impairment*

Neonates:
For severe infections (sepsis) due to susceptible strains of Pseudomonas, Proteus, and E. coli—(less than 1 week of age): *Infants under 2000 gm—*100 mg/kg initial dose, followed by 75 mg/kg every 8 hours, by intermittent infusion.

*Infants over 2000 gm—*100 mg/kg initial dose, followed by 75 mg/kg every 4–6 hours, by intermittent infusion.
Infants Over 1 Week of Age:
100 mg/kg every 4 hours, by intermittent infusion.

Reduce dosage in renal insufficiency. No data available for exact dosage.

For adults and children gentamicin and tobramycin may be administered concurrently with ticarcillin, both initially and if susceptibility tests are positive.

Higher doses of ticarcillin may be necessary in any age patient who also has an impaired immunologic system.

Preparation and Storage
Supplied in 1, 3 and 6 gram vials.
Reconstitute vials with 4 ml. of sterile water for injection for each *gram* of drug, or for the 3 gm and 6 gm piggyback bottles, reconstitute with sterile water for injection to make the following solutions:
3-Gram Bottles

Amount of Diluent	Concentration of Solution
100 ml	1 gm/34 ml
60 ml	1 gm/20 ml
30 ml	1 gm/10 ml

Creatinine clearance ml/min	Initial loading dose of 3 gm, followed by: Dosage and frequency
>60	3 gm every 4 hours
30–60	2 gm every 4 hours
10–30	2 gm every 8 hours
<10	2 gm every 12 hours
<10 with hepatic dysfunction	2 gm every 24 hours
With peritoneal dialysis	3 gm every 12 hours
With hemodialysis	2 gm every 12 hours *and* 3 gm after each dialysis

*Manufacturer's dosage suggestion. (The drug half-life is 13 hours in patients with renal failure.)

6-Gram Bottles

Amount of Diluent	Concentration of Solution
100 ml	1 gm/17 ml
60 ml	1 gm/10 ml

These solutions can then be used for intermittent infusion. This drug can be combined with most common IV fluids.

Refrigerate reconstituted solutions; discard after 72 hours.

Drug Incompatibilities

Do not mix in solution with any other medication, and do not add to an IV line containing gentamicin or other aminoglycosides.

Modes of IV Administration

Injection
Yes
Slowly, over at least 3–5 minutes.

Intermittent Infusion
Yes
Use D5W, NS, Invert Sugar 10% in Water, Ringer's Injection or similar fluid; or use manufacturer's piggyback preparations.
Infuse over 30 min to 2 hrs time.

Continuous Infusion
Yes
Intermittent infusion is the preferred mode in most instances.
Use D5W, NS, Invert Sugar 10% in Water, Ringer's Injection, RL, or similar fluids.

Contraindications; Warnings; Precautions; Adverse Reactions

Contraindications
Hypersensitivity to any penicillin.

Warnings
1. In the presence of impaired renal function and/or high doses of this drug, patients may develop hemorrhagic conditions associated with abnormal clotting and prothrombin times. This disappears on withdrawal of the drug.

2. There can be cross-allergenicity in patients who are allergic to any cephalosporin antibiotic.

Precautions
1. Because of this drug's high sodium content, 6.5 mEq/gm, monitor cardiac status carefully for the onset of decompensation in susceptible patients.
2. Hypokalemia may occur.
3. Monitor renal, hepatic and hematopoietic function with appropriate blood studies during therapy, as with any antibiotic.
4. Overgrowth of nonsusceptible organisms can occur.
5. This drug has not been shown to produce fetal abnormalities in laboratory animals, but should be used in pregnant women only when clearly indicated.
6. Gentamicin or tobramycin are usually administered with this drug until specific organism sensitivity tests are available.

Adverse Reactions
1. Hypersensitivity: skin rashes, pruritus, urticaria, anaphylaxis, drug fever
2. Gastrointestinal: nausea, vomiting
3. Blood dyscrasias: anemia, thrombocytopenia, leukopenia; inhibition of platelet aggregation
4. Hepatic: elevated SGOT, SGPT
5. Central nervous system: convulsions, neuromuscular irritability (especially in patients with impaired renal function)
6. Phlebitis at injection site
7. Hypokalemia

☐ Nursing Implications

1. Take anaphylaxis precautions; see Appendix.
2. Patients with impaired renal function require a reduction in dosage based on creatinine clearance; see Dosage section. Be aware of the patient's BUN and creatinine clearance during therapy. Monitor for signs of bleeding that can be produced by alteration in clotting and

ticarcillin disodium
(continued)

prothrombin times in these patients:

a. Melena, or red blood in stools (guaiac tests can be done periodically to detect occult blood)
b. Hematuria
c. Ecchymosis, especially on trunk, inner thighs and inner arms
d. Nose bleeding
e. Gum bleeding
f. Vaginal bleeding
g. Petechiae
h. Fall in blood pressure
i. Hematemesis

Bleeding could also occur secondary to a reduction in platelet count. Such bleeding usually begins only after the count falls below 100,000/cu.mm. If this occurs, monitor for the signs of bleeding listed above and avoid traumatic procedures.

3. In patients with pre-existing congestive heart failure, infants and children with cardiac lesions, the elderly, or critically ill, monitor for signs of cardiac decompensation secondary to the high sodium content of the drug, if dosage is high. Signs and symptoms:
   a. Increasing weight (weigh daily, compare to baseline weight)
   b. Increasing heart rate (take every 4–6 hours or as patient's condition dictates)
   c. Increasing respiratory rate (take with heart rate), dyspnea, orthopnea, rales
   d. Peripheral and sacral edema
   e. Increasing jugular venous distention
   f. Onset of third or fourth heart sounds.

4. Monitor for signs of hypokalemia: weakness, lethargy, irritability, abdominal distention, poor feeding in infants, muscle cramps.

5. Monitor for signs and symptoms of nonsusceptible organism overgrowth infection:
   a. Fever (take rectal temperature at least every 4–6 hours)
   b. Increasing malaise
   c. Localized signs and symptoms of a new infection: redness, soreness, pain, swelling, drainage (change in volume or character of pre-existing drainage)
   d. Cough (change in sputum volume or character)
   e. Diarrhea
   f. Perineal or oral rash (*Candida albicans* colonization)

6. In patients with impaired renal function, monitor for signs of neuromuscular irritability, e.g., tremors, spasticity, difficulty moving, convulsions. Report any suspicious sign to the physician.

7. Monitor for signs and symptoms of thrombophlebitis at the injection site, e.g., redness, swelling and pain along the vein tract. If this occurs, discontinue the infusion and use another vein. Apply warm compresses to the affected area and keep the limb elevated until symptoms subside. Avoid other venipunctures in this extremity until the inflammation resolves.

8. If nausea and vomiting occur and are pronounced, the drug will probably be discontinued. Antiemetic agents can be ordered to control these symptoms. Monitor intake and output to assist the physician in planning for parenteral replacement if it is needed to maintain hydration.

9. Adhere to direct intravenous injection rates suggested under "Injection" above to prevent vein irritation.

tobramycin sulfate ■
(Nebcin and Nebcin Pediatric)

Actions/Indications
Aminoglycoside antibiotic, active against:
• *Pseudomonas aeruginosa*

- *Proteus* species
- *E. coli*
- *Klebsiella-Enterobacter-Serratia* group
- *Citrobacter* species
- *Providencia* species
- Staphylococci
- Group D streptococci

This drug is indicated in the treatment of septicemia; central nervous system infections such as meningitis; neonatal sepsis; lower respiratory tract infections; gastrointestinal infections; skin, soft-tissue and bone infections; serious and complicated infections of the urinary tract.

Sensitivity tests should be performed. This drug is used in combination therapy with penicillins in serious gram-negative infections.

Dosage

Obtain body weight in kilograms before dosage calculations.

Normal Renal Function:
Adults, Children and Older Infants:
Serious infections—1 mg/kg every 8 hours. (3 mg/kg/24 hrs)

Life-threatening infections—1.66/kg every 8 hours (5 mg/kg/24 hr). Reduce to 1 mg/kg every 8 hrs as soon as possible.

Do not exceed 5 mg/kg/24 hr unless serum levels are monitored, see Warning No. 6.

Neonates (One Week of Age or Less):
Up to 4 mg/kg/day divided into 2 doses every 12 hrs.

The usual duration of therapy is 7 to 10 days. A longer course of treatment may be necessary in severe infections.

Impaired Renal Function: Follow serum concentration if possible. *Loading dose*—1 mg/kg. Subsequent doses based on serum levels. Reduce amount of doses or the frequency of administration:

Reduced dosage technique (manufacturer's suggestion): When the creatinine clearance is 70 ml or less/minute or when the serum creatinine level is known, multiply the normal dose (as listed above) by the "percent of normal dose" from the following nomogram:

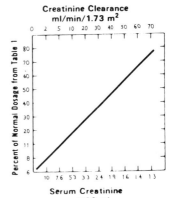

REDUCED DOSAGE NOMOGRAM

Creatinine Clearance
ml/min/1.73 m²

Serum Creatinine
mg/100 ml

*Scales have been adjusted to facilitate dosage calculations.

Courtesy of Eli Lilly and Co.
307 E. McCarty Street
Indianapolis IN 46285

An alternative when patient's serum creatinine is known is to divide the normal dose by the serum creatinine value.

Normal dosage at prolonged intervals: The dosage frequency in hours can be obtained by multiplying the patient's serum creatinine by 6. The normal dosage is then given at that frequency.

Preparation and Storage

This drug is supplied in 2 ml (40 mg/ml) vials, as well as 1.5 ml (60 mg) and 2 ml (80 mg) disposable syringes. The pediatric injection is in 2 ml vials, 10 mg/ml.

Store vials at room temperature. Use intravenous solutions within 24 hours. Store them in the refrigerator until use.

Drug Incompatibilities

Do not mix with any other medication in solution.

Do not add to IV tubing containing:
Calcium
Carbenicillin
Cephalosporins
Heparin
Magnesium

tobramycin sulfate
(continued)
Penicillin
Ticarcillin

Modes of IV Administration

Injection
No

Intermittent Infusion
Yes
Use D5W, N5, D5/NS, D10W,
Normosol-R, RL, Ringer's Injection,
Sodium Lactate 1/6 M. for infusion.
Add dose to 50–100 ml of one of
the above diluents, infuse over 30–
60 minutes.
Children—add dose to 25–50 ml of
diluent and infuse over 20–60 min.
Do not infuse in less than 20 min.

Continuous Infusion
No

Contraindications; Warnings; Precautions; Adverse Reactions

Contraindications
Hypersensitivity

Warnings
1. This drug can cause hearing
   and equilibrium disturbances
   due to eighth cranial nerve
   damage. This is more likely to
   occur in patients with pre-
   existing impaired renal function
   or when the drug is given for
   long periods of time (over 2
   weeks) or at higher than
   recommended doses. The ototoxic effects of this drug are increased by concomitant use of
   ethacrynic acid, furosemide, and
   mannitol.[1]
2. Renal damage can also result
   from administration of
   tobramycin, and is indicated by
   casts in the urine, proteinuria,
   oliguria, rising BUN and creatinine. Renal function should be
   monitored closely during therapy and the drug discontinued
   when the above signs of renal
   damage appear. The possibility
   of renal damage may be increased by the presence of dehydration, the use of potent
   diuretics, and certain other antibiotics such as polymyxins, amphotericin B, and vancomycin.[2]
3. Patients with impairment in renal function require a modified
   dosage schedule because of
   compromised excretion of the
   drug (see Dosage section).
4. This drug should be used with
   caution in premature and full-
   term neonates (up to 1 week of
   age) because of the immaturity
   of their renal function. Follow
   recommended dosage schedules.
5. Peritoneal and hemodialysis can
   remove this drug from the serum in the event of overdosage.
6. Avoid serum concentrations
   greater than 12 mcg/ml.
7. Concurrent or sequential use of
   other nephrotoxic or ototoxic
   drugs should be avoided; e.g.,
   streptomycin, neomycin, kanamycin, gentamicin, cephaloridine, paromomycin, viomycin,
   polymyxin B, colistin, and vancomycin.
8. Safety for use in pregnancy has
   not been established.
9. Some groups advocate strict adherence to suggested infusion
   rate to prevent renal and eighth
   cranial nerve toxic effects.[3]

Precautions
1. Neuromuscular blockade and
   respiratory paralysis may occur,
   especially in patients with myasthenia gravis, in the presence of
   severe hypocalcemia, or when
   neuromuscular blocking agents
   have been given. This may be
   reversed by the administration
   of calcium salts.
2. Cross-allergenicity may occur
   with other aminoglycoside antibiotics including streptomycin,
   neomycin, paromomycin, kanamycin, gentamicin, amikacin.
3. Overgrowth of nonsusceptible
   organisms can occur.

Adverse Reactions
1. Renal damage (see Warning No.
   2 above)

2. Neurotoxicity causing eighth cranial nerve damage (see Warning No. 1); symptoms include dizziness, vertigo, tinnitus, roaring in the ears, and hearing loss
3. Increased serum SGOT, SGPT, bilirubin
4. Granulocytopenia, thrombocytopenia
5. Fever
6. Allergic reactions; rash, urticaria, anaphylaxis (1–3%)
7. Gastrointestinal disturbances: nausea, vomiting; these may be secondary to vestibular damage (inner ear)
8. Headache
9. Lethargy

☐ Nursing Implications

1. Monitor for the onset of eighth cranial nerve damage, especially in patients with renal impairment. Signs and symptoms: dizziness, disequilibrium, nystagmus (involuntary movement of the eyes), nausea, and vomiting, tinnitus (ringing in the ears), roaring sound in the ears, hearing loss. Notify the physician at the onset of any one of these signs and symptoms. Give reassurance to the patient and take precautions to prevent patient injury.
2. Keep the patient appropriately hydrated to assist in preventing renal toxicity.
3. Monitor for the onset of renal damage, especially in patients who are critically ill and on high doses:
   a. Intake and output recordings at least every 4–8 hours, depending on the patient's condition. Fall in urine output may or may not occur with the onset of renal damage. Notify physician if the average urine output falls below 30 ml/hour for more than 2 consecutive hours.
   b. Urinalysis should be done daily to detect the presence of protein and casts in the urine.
   c. Be aware of the patient's serum BUN (normal values: 10–20 mg/100 ml) and serum creatinine (0.7–1.5 mg/100 ml). Renal damage is usually reversible if the drug is discontinued at the first sign of impairment.
4. Monitor for the onset of neuromuscular blockade, especially in patients with myasthenia gravis, hypercalcemia, or in patients who have received a neuromuscular blocking agent (tubocurarine, pancuronium, etc.). Signs and symptoms:
   a. Generalized muscle weakness
   b. Difficulty controlling movements
   c. Respiratory depression as evidenced by a decreased respiratory rate (adults: less than 8–10/minute) and shallow respirations (muscular weakness inhibits movements of chest muscles and diaphragm).
   Notify the physician at the onset of any one of these signs or symptoms, place the patient on bed rest, observe closely and administer respiratory support as indicated (do not leave the patient alone if respirations are less then 8/minute).
5. Monitor for nonsusceptible organism overgrowth infection:
   a. Fever (take rectal temperature at least every 4–6 hours)
   b. Increasing malaise
   c. Newly appearing localized signs and symptoms of infection: redness, soreness, pain, swelling, drainage (increasing volume, or change in character of pre-existing drainage)
   d. Monilial rash (redness and itching) in the perineal area and/or candidal lesions in the mouth (reddened areas with overlying white patches especially on inner cheeks)
   e. Cough (change in pre-

tobramycin sulfate
(continued)
existing cough and sputum
production)
f. Diarrhea
6. Take anaphylaxis precautions,
see Appendix.

References

1. Barza, Michael, and Scheife,
Richard: Drug Therapy Re-
views: Antimicrobial Spectrum,
Pharmacology and Therapeutic
Use of Antibiotics. Part 4:
Aminoglycosides. *American Jour-
nal of Hospital Pharmacy*, 34:730,
July 1977.
2. Ibid., p. 729.
3. Vanderveen, Timothy W.:
Aminoglycoside Antibiotics.
*American Journal of Intravenous
Therapy*, July 1977, p. 6.

trimethaphan camsylate ■
(Arfonad)

Actions/Indications

Antihypertensive, ganglionic blocking agent, may also have a direct peripheral vasodilator effect to lower
blood pressure. Used to treat hypertensive crisis. May also be used to
control hypertension during surgery
and in cases of dissecting aneurysm.

Onset of action is within 1–2 minutes after injection. Maximum effect
is seen after 2–5 minutes, and the
duration is 10 minutes.

Dosage

Titrate with blood pressure response. Initial infusion rate can be
3–4 mg/min. The range is as low as
0.3 mg/min to 6.0 mg/min.

Use an 0.1% solution for infusion.
Dosage recommendations for children are not available.

Delivery of an 0.1% (1 mg/ml) Solution of Trimethaphan Camsylate

Calibration of Administration Set (Drops/ml)	Drops/min. to provide 3–4 mg/min of drug
10	30–40
15	45–60
60	180–240

Preparation and Storage

Supplied in ampuls of 50 mg/ml,
10-ml ampuls. Store in refrigerator.
Use IV solutions promptly; discard
unused portions.

Each infusion should be used for
a maximum of 6 hours. Mix a fresh
solution after that.

Drug Incompatibilities

Do not mix with other medications
in IV bottle; drug should be titrated
alone. Do not add to IV tubing con-
taining:
Aminophylline
Sodium iodide
Sodium bicarbonate
Tubocurarine

Modes of IV Administration

Injection
No

Intermittent Infusion
No

Continuous Infusion
Yes
Use a solution of 1 mg/ml (1 gm in
1000 ml D5W or NS). Titrate with
blood pressure response. Use an infusion pump and microdrop tubing.

Contraindications; Warnings; Pre-
cautions; Adverse Reactions

Contraindications
1. When hypotension may produce
a risk, e.g., in severe anemia,
hypovolemic shock, asphyxia,
uncorrected respiratory insufficiency.
2. When fluids and blood are not
available to replace blood volume as needed.

Warnings
1. Use only as infusion.
2. Adequate direct (preferable) or
indirect blood-pressure monitoring must be available.
3. Maintain arterial oxygenation.
4. Use with extreme caution in patients with arteriosclerosis,
cardiac disease, hepatic, or central nervous system disease, Ad-

dison's disease, diabetes mellitus, steroid therapy.
5. Induced hypotension may have adverse effects on the fetus.

Precautions
1. Use with caution in patients who have been receiving other antihypertensive agents; in combination with anesthetic agents; during spinal anesthesia; in the elderly or debilitated.
2. This drug liberates histamine; use with caution in patients with any form of allergy, can produce bronchospasm.
3. Diuretics can potentiate this drug.
4. Causes pupillary dilatation.
5. This drug can decrease renal blood flow and glomerular filtration rate.[1] Use with caution in the presence of renal impairment of any degree.
6. May produce bowel and/or bladder atony, and a meconium ileus in the newborn of a mother who has received this drug during labor.[2]

☐ **Nursing Implications**
1. Be prepared to accurately monitor arterial blood pressure, preferably by direct arterial cannulation. If this type of monitoring is unavailable, indirect readings using a sphygmomanometer can be used.
2. Patients with a history of cardiac disease including arrhythmias must be monitored electrocardiographically during an infusion of this drug.
3. Keep the patient on bed rest in a supine position during therapy.
4. Be prepared to manage vomiting to prevent aspiration.
5. Keeping in mind the patient's pretreatment blood pressure (indirect and direct), start the infusion at 3–4 mg/minute (using a solution of 1 mg/ml, the drip rate or pump rate would be 3–4 ml/minute). Smaller initial doses may be ordered by the physician for patients with

renal failure. Observe arterial pressure recordings continuously (indirect readings every 2 minutes). Do not allow the blood pressure to fall too rapidly. The physician should set the blood pressure goal to be reached, and a time limit for when the goal should be reached. If the pressure does not begin to decrease with the initial infusion rate (3–4 mg/minute) within 10 minutes, begin increasing the rate by 0.5 mg (0.5 ml) every 10 minutes until a response is seen.
6. Monitor for the consequences of severe elevation of blood pressure:
   a. Encephalopathy: confusion, stupor, nausea, vomiting, visual changes, reflex asymmetries
   b. Cerebrovascular accident: muscle weakness, change in mental status
   c. Myocardial ischemia and/or infarction: chest pain, ECG changes, arrhythmias
   d. Left ventricular failure: shortness of breath, orthopnea, elevated central venous pressure or pulmonary capillary pressure, tachycardia, rales, third and/or fourth heart sound
   e. Renal failure: oliguria, rising BUN and creatinine[3]
   Note that a sudden fall in blood pressure below normal levels for the patient can also produce these complications. Be prepared to manage hypotension due to an exaggerated response to the drug. Phenylephrine or mephentermine can be used. Dopamine should be used if these milder vasopressor agents are ineffective.
7. Monitor for respiratory difficulties produced by bronchospasm, such as tachypnea and wheezing. Notify the physician of this reaction. Keep aminophylline and epinephrine readily available.
8. Monitor for paralytic ileus and

trimethaphan camsylate
(continued)

urinary retention. Examine for meconium ileus in newborns of mothers who have received this drug during labor.

9. If the patient will be receiving oral antihypertensive agents on a chronic basis, instruct him on hypertensive self-care.

References
1. American Medical Association Committee on Hypertension: The Treatment of Malignant Hypertension and Hypertensive Emergencies. *JAMA*, 228 (13):1675, June 24, 1974.
2. Ibid., p. 1675.
3. Romankiewicz, J. A.: Pharmacology and Clinical Use of Drugs in Hypertensive Emergencies. *American Journal of Hospital Pharmacy*, 34(2):185, February 1977.

Suggested Readings
American Medical Association Committee on Hypertension: The Treatment of Malignant Hypertension and Hypertensive Emergencies. *JAMA*, 228:1673–1679, June 24, 1974.
Dhar, Sisir K. and Freedman, Philip: Clinical Management of Hypertensive Emergencies. *Heart and Lung*, 5:571–575, January–April, 1976.
Keith, Thomas: Hypertensive Crisis. Recognition and Management, *JAMA*, 237(15):1570–1577, April 11, 1977.
Koch-Weser, Jan: Hypertensive Emergencies. *New England Journal of Medicine*, 290:211–214, January 24, 1974.
Long, M. L., et al.: Hypertension: What Patients Need to Know. *American Journal of Nursing*, 76:765–770, May 1976.
Romankiewicz, J. A.: Pharmacology and Clinical Use of Drugs in Hypertensive Emergencies. *American Journal of Hospital Pharmacy*, 34(2):185–193, February 1977 (references).

trimethoprim and sulfamethoxazole ■
(Bactrim Intravenous Infusion)

Actions/Indications
Synthetic, antibacterial combination agent (trimethoprim with sulfamethoxazole), used to treat the following situations: Pneumonitis due to *pneumocystis carinii*; shigellosis enteritis caused by susceptible strains of *Shigella flexneri* and *Shigella sonnei*; severe urinary tract infections due to susceptible strains of *E. coli, Klebsiella–Enterobacter* and *Proteus* species. Appropriate culture and susceptibility studies should be performed. This drug is metabolized in the liver and excreted chiefly by the kidneys.

Dosage
Adults and Children Over 2 Months of Age (based on trimethoprim component):
Pneumocystis carinii Pneumonitis—15 to 20 mg/kg per 24 hours given in equal doses every 6 to 8 hours up to 14 days.
Urinary Tract Infections and Shigellosis—8 to 10 mg/kg per 24 hours given in equal doses every 6, 8, or 12 hours for up to 14 days for severe urinary tract infections and 5 days for shigellosis.
Children under 2 months:
Not recommended.
In Impaired Renal Function:
(Manufacturer's suggested dosage modification)

Creatinine Clearance (ml/min)	Dosage
Above 30	usual dose
15–30	1/2 usual dose
Below 15	use not recommended

Preparation and Storage
Supplied in 5 ml ampuls containing 80 mg of trimethoprim (16 mg/ml) and 400 mg of sulfamethoxazole (80 mg/ml). Store at room temperature, DO NOT REFRIGERATE.
Each 5 ml should be added to 125 ml of D5W (only) for administration,

use within 6 hours. If fluid restriction is necessary, each 5 ml of drug can be added to 75 ml of D5W. In this case the solution should be mixed just prior to use. Do not use solution if there is cloudiness or a precipitate.

Do not use this preparation for intramuscular administration.

Drug Incompatibilities

Do not mix with any other medications in any manner. Use D5W *only* for dilution.

Modes of IV Administration

Injection
No

Intermittent Infusion
Yes
Infuse over no less than 60 to 90 min.

Continuous Infusion
No

Contraindications; Warnings; Precautions; Adverse Reactions

Contraindications
1. Hypersensitivity to either component.
2. Documented megaloblastic anemia due to folate deficiency.
3. Pregnancy at term and during the nursing period. (These drugs pass through the placenta, are excreted in the milk and may cause displacement of bilirubin from binding sites and thus cause kernicterus in the infant.
4. Infants less than two months of age.

Warnings
1. *This drug should not be used in the treatment of streptococcal pharyngitis.*
2. Severe hypersensitivity reactions can occur, deaths have been reported due to drug induced agranulocytosis, aplastic anemia, and other blood dyscrasias. Trimethoprim may interfer with

hematopoiesis in some patients. Elderly patients who are concurrently receiving thiazide diuretics have an increased incidence of thrombocytopenia with purpura.

Precautions
1. Administer with caution to patients with impaired renal or hepatic function, those with possible folate deficiency and those with severe allergies or asthma.
2. Hemolysis may occur in patients with glucose-6-phosphate dehydrogenase deficiency.
3. Adequate fluid intake must be maintained in order to prevent crystalluria and urinary stone formation.
4. Local tissue irritation and inflammation can occur with extravasation.
5. Culture and organism susceptibility studies should be performed before and throughout therapy.
6. Significant reduction in any formed blood element should prompt discontinuation of therapy. If this occurs, it is recommended that the patient also receive leucovorin 3 to 6 mg IM daily for 3 days to assist in restoring normal hematopoiesis.
7. Frequent urinalysis should be performed to detect casts and crystal formation.
8. This drug may prolong the prothrombin time in patients on warfarin.
9. Chromosomal damage has not been seen in human leukocyte cultures or samples taken from patients treated with this drug. Studies on the effects of this agent on fertility have not been carried out.
10. This drug should only be used in pregnancy when potential benefits to the mother outweigh the potential risk to the fetus. See Contraindication No. 3.

**trimethoprim and
sulfamethoxazole**
(continued)

11. In an overdose, hemodialysis is
only moderately effective in removing this compound from the
body.

Adverse Reactions

1. Most frequently seen: nausea,
vomiting, thrombocytopenia
and rash.
2. Thrombophlebitis at infusion
site.

Major reactions to sulfonamides
and trimethoprim are listed below;
not all have been reported with
sulfamethoxazole infusion:

1. Allergic reactions include:
rashes, pruritus, urticaria, erythema multiforme, Stevens–
Johnson syndrome, epidermal
necrolysis, serum sickness, exfoliative dermatitis, anaphylaxis,
periorbital edema, conjunctival
and scleral redness, photosensitivity, arthralgia and allergic
myocarditis. Cross-sensitivity
may exist with some goitrogens,
acetazolamide and thiazide diuretics, and oral hypoglycemic
agents or any drug with a sul-
fonamide base.
2. Blood dyscrasias: megaloblastic
anemia, hemolytic anemia, purpura, thrombocytopenia, leukopenia, agranulocytosis, aplastic
anemia, hypoprothrombinemia
and methemoglobinemia.
3. Gastrointestinal: Glossitis, stomatitis, nausea, vomiting, abdominal pains, hepatitis,
diarrhea, pseudomembranous
colitis and pancreatitis.
4. Central nervous system: headache, peripheral neuritis, mental
depression, ataxia, convulsions,
hallucinations, tinnitus, vertigo,
insomnia, apathy, fatigue, muscle weakness and nervousness.
5. Miscellaneous: drug fever,
chills, and toxic nephrosis with
oliguria and anuria, periarteritis
nodosa and lupus erythematosis
phenomenon, diuresis and hypoglycemia.

☐ **Nursing Implications**

1. Take anaphylaxis precautions
(see Appendix). Monitor for the
onset of rashes. Take an accurate allergy history with empha-
sis on past reactions to thiazide
diuretics, acetazolamide, goitrogens or any agent with a sulfon-
amide base.
2. Frequent complete blood
counts should be performed
during therapy. Be aware of the
results. Monitor for the onset of
sore throat, fever, pallor, purpura or jaundice. Except for purpura, these may be *early*
indications of a blood dyscrasia.
3. Monitor renal function; e.g., urinary output (every 8 hours), urinalysis (every other day or so),
serum creatinine and BUN levels. Notify the physician of a
urine output less than 240 ml in
8 hours in adults. Maintain a
high fluid (preferably water) intake to prevent crystalluria or
stone formation. Modifications
in intake will have to be made
in patients with congestive heart
failure or renal failure; follow
physician directives.
4. Prevent extravasation, monitor
for signs of vein irritation or
thrombophlebitis at infusion
site. Move site as necessary and
begin local care to the area of
inflammation. See Appendix.
5. Be aware of the patient's prothrombin time if he is receiving
a warfarin drug. The dosage of
warfarin may have to be reduced.
6. Be prepared to manage nausea
and vomiting. Monitor emesis
and diarrhea volumes if problems are severe, to assist in fluid and electrolyte replacement.
Antiemetics and antiperistaltics
can be used to control these
problems. Diarrhea may become
more severe when this drug is
used to treat shigellosis enteritis. Patients may experience
changes in their sense of taste
during therapy. Reassure them
of the temporary nature of this
effect.

tubocurarine chloride ■
(Curare, d-Tubocurarine)

Actions/Indications
Neuromuscular blocking agent, nondepolarizing type. Produces flaccid paralysis of skeletal muscles within 2–3 minutes after injection. Effects last 25–90 minutes. There may be prolongation of effects after large or repeated doses.

Used to induce muscle relaxation for tracheal intubation, surgery, electroconvulsive therapy, and mechanical ventilation. Also used to diagnose myasthenia gravis when other tests have been inconclusive.

Dosage
Dosage must be individualized in each patient after evaluation of all factors that might alter the action of the drug.

The following doses are for the average patient without altered sensitivity to the drug. (7 units = 1 mg)
Adults and Children:
In Surgery—0.1–0.3 mg/kg; do not exceed 27 mg. Subsequent doses should be based on patient response; may be 1/4–1/2 of the initial dose every 45–60 minutes. (A test dose 2–3 mg less than the calculated dose may be given to detect hyperactivity.)

Electroconvulsive therapy—0.1–0.3 mg/kg with an initial dose 2–3 mg less, then titrate as needed.

Diagnosis of myasthenia gravis—very small doses of this drug cause an exaggerated response in myasthenia patients. Give 1/15–1/5 of above calculated doses, or 4.1–16.5 mcg/kg.

Lower dosage will be required by patients on aminoglycoside antibiotics, or who have renal impairment; titrate with patient response.

When methoxyflurane or fluroxene anesthetics are used, reduce the initial dose by 33%. If halothane or cyclopropane is used, reduce by 20%.[1]

For controlled respiration—16.5 mcg/kg (average dose: 1 mg) initially; titrate with patient response thereafter.

Preparation and Storage
Supplied in 3 mg/ml, 5 mg/ml, and 15 mg/ml concentrations.

Do not use if more than faintly discolored.

Drug Incompatibilities
Do not mix with any other drug in syringe; do not inject into IV tubing containing sodium bicarbonate, methohexital, trimethaphan camsylate.

Modes of IV Administration

Injection
Yes
Inject over a 1- to 1 1/2-minute period.

3 mg/ml and 5 mg/ml preparations can be injected undiluted. If 15 mg/ml solution is used, dilute to a concentration of 3 or 5 mg/ml with NS.

Intermittent Infusion
Yes
But, direct IV injection preferred method because of drug's long duration of action.

Continuous Infusion
No
Pharmacologically inappropriate.

Contraindications; Warnings; Precautions; Adverse Reactions

Contraindications
1. Hypersensitivity
2. When histamine release is a hazard

Warnings
1. Respiratory support must be immediately available, e.g., positive pressure ventilation, intubation, oxygen.
2. Use with extreme caution in patients with documented myasthenia gravis.
3. Administration of quinidine during postoperative recovery after tubocurarine has been used may result in recurarizing and respiratory paralysis.

tubocurarine chloride
(continued)

Precautions
1. The skeletal muscle paralyzing effects (secondary to *normal* dosage) can be reversed with cholinesterase inhibitors (neostigmine, pyridostigmine).
2. Use with caution in patients with respiratory depression, renal or hepatic insufficiency. Respiratory and pulmonary patients will require lower and less frequent doses. Patients with hepatic insufficiency sometimes require a larger dosage to produce adequate paralysis.[2]
3. Hypotension can result following large doses.
4. Repeated doses may have a cumulative effect.
5. The paralyzing effects of this drug are potentiated and depressed by a variety of factors. See Nursing Implication No. 7.
6. Rapid injection or a large dosage can precipitate the release of histamine which can cause bronchospasm and/or hypotension.
7. Safety for use in pregnancy has not been established. This drug has no direct effect on the uterus or other smooth muscles, and is not thought to cross the placental barrier.[3]

Adverse Reactions
1. Extension of the drug's pharmacologic actions. Profound and prolonged muscle relaxation may occur, with respiratory depression and possible apnea
2. Hypersensitivity (rare)
3. Histamine release producing bronchospasm
4. Hypotension

☐ **Nursing Implications**
Postanesthesia Care:
1. Equipment that should be readily available: suction, manual breathing bag, endotracheal tubes and laryngoscope, oxygen.
2. Patients receiving this agent

must be intubated to assist in maintaining an adequate airway and ventilation.
3. Be aware of the duration of action of this drug (see Actions/Indications section), and when the patient received the last dose.
4. Be aware of the sequence of progression of the paralytic effects as they will occur after an injection:
   a. Loss of eye movement
   b. Eyelid droop
   c. Stiffness of jaw muscles followed by relaxation
   d. Paralysis of upper trunk muscles spreading to the lower trunk muscles and then to the extremities
   e. Paralysis of pharyngeal muscles (tongue, swallowing, etc.)
   f. Total respiratory paralysis
   Recovery will be a complete reverse of this sequence.[4]
5. Management of the patient postoperatively is centered around the use of the reversal agent (neostigmine or pyridostigmine) and respiratory support until adequate ventilation has returned. See Nursing Implication No. 10.
6. During recovery, observe for return of the paralytic effects and for incomplete reversal of the effects by the antagonist agent. Keep reversal (antagonist) agents and atropine readily available. See Precaution No. 1.
7. Be aware of elements which may PROLONG the paralytic effects of this drug:
   a. Decreased circulation time as seen in congestive heart failure or shock
   b. Low arterial blood pH (less than 7.35)[5]
   c. Decreased hepatic function (the drug is excreted in the bile) and severe renal impairment
   d. Concomitant use of aminoglycoside antibiotics (gentamicin, amikacin, etc.), polymyxin B, or bacitracin.

e. The presence of other drugs such as diazepam (Valium), halothane anesthetics, quinidine, MAO inhibitors.
The intensity of the drug's effects are *increased* with diethyl ether, methoxyflurane, enflurane. No increase in intensity is seen with thiobarbiturates, narcotics, nitrous oxide, or droperidol.

f. Extremes of age

g. The presence of myasthenia gravis

Patients under the influence of any one of these conditions will require prolonged monitoring for recovery from the effects of tubocurarine.

8. The hypotension that can be precipitated by tubocurarine can be treated by withholding additional doses of the drug, fluids, and if necessary, vasopressors. Reversal agents (neostigmine and pyridostigmine) will not reverse the effects that cause hypotension. Monitor blood pressure every 3–5 minutes or as operating room policy or patient condition dictates.

9. Bronchospasm may be serious enough to require treatment with aminophylline or other bronchodilating agents. Monitor for wheezing and decreased lung compliance, cyanosis, etc.

10. Discharge from the recovery room will depend on the following criteria:
a. Grip strength
b. Ability to lift the head
c. Ability to open the eyes
d. Respiratory status, e.g. vital capacity and tidal volume (it is helpful to have preoperative values for comparison).

Maintenance Care for Controlled Ventilation:

1. This drug is usually administered on a p.r.n. basis for control of ventilation. The criteria for when to administer it will be determined by the physician, and will include such situations as:
a. Respiratory rate

b. When the patient's respiratory effort is out of phase with the respirator
c. When the patient is struggling against the respirator
d. When positive end-expiratory pressure (P.E.E.P.) is in use

Monitor for the onset of any of the criteria and administer the drug in the amount ordered. (Be aware of hospital regulations governing the administration of a neuromuscular blocking agent, i.e. storage of the drug, and who may administer it.)

2. Make certain that the endotracheal tube is securely and correctly inserted. Check the connection between the tube and the respirator; it must be tight. KEEP RESPIRATOR ALARM SYSTEMS FUNCTIONING AT ALL TIMES. The patient is totally dependent on the respirator for ventilation.

3. This drug paralyzes skeletal muscles, *it does not alter consciousness or relieve pain and anxiety.* Therefore, the patient must be adequately sedated and given analgesics appropriate for his condition. He will not be able to make his needs known; the persons caring for him must anticipate those needs. Many institutions assign one or more nurses to stay in constant attendance with these patients.

4. Monitor vital signs before administration and every 5 minutes thereafter until stabilization is seen, then every 15–30 minutes. Repeat the cycle with each dose. Tubocurarine can lower blood pressure initially. Monitor for signs of bronchospasm, such as wheezing (by auscultation). Bronchodilator drugs such as aminophylline should be readily available. Notify the physician if bronchospasm is suspected. This agent can cause an increase in tracheobronchial secretions. More frequent suctioning may be re-

tubocurarine chloride
(continued)

quired, guided by auscultation of the chest.

5. Patients with a history of cardiac arrhythmias should be observed for exacerbation of those arrhythmias via a continuous ECG monitor. Be prepared to treat tachy- and bradyarrhythmias.

6. Because this agent produces muscle paralysis, handle the patient with care to prevent trauma to joints and muscles during turning. Turn and/or position frequently to prevent skin breakdown. Use water mattresses, flotation pads etc., as indicated.

7. When this drug is discontinued, a reversal agent (neostigmine) may be used. Proceed with the nursing management as described under Postanesthesia Care.

8. See page 239 on neostigmine, and page 303 on pyridostigmine.

References
1. Formulary 12:20. American Hospital Formulary Service, American Society of Hospital Pharmacists, Washington, D.C., 1977.
2. Ibid.
3. Wylie, W. D., and Churchill-Davidson, H. C. (editors): *A Practice of Anesthesia* (3rd ed.), Chicago: Year Book Medical Publishers, 1972, p. 877.
4. Ibid., p. 816.
5. Ibid., p. 834.

urokinase for injection ■
(Abbokinase, Breokinase)

Actions/Indications
An enzyme, potent direct activator of the endogenous fibrinolytic system. Converts plasminogen to the proteolytic enzyme plasmin. Plasmin degrades fibrin clots as well as fibrinogen and other plasma proteins associated with clotting.

Administration is followed by increased fibrinolytic activity. This effect disappears within a few hours after discontinuation, but a decrease in plasma levels of fibrinogen and plasminogen and an increase in the amount of circulating fibrinogen degradation products may persist for 12 to 24 hours. There is no correlation between embolus resolution and levels of coagulation and fibrinolytic assay.

This drug is indicated in adults in the treatment of:
- Acute massive pulmonary emboli (obstruction or significant filling defects involving a lobe or multiple segments)
- Acute massive pulmonary emboli accompanied by unstable hemodynamics; i.e., failure to maintain blood pressure without supportive measures

In these two clinical situations, urokinase is used for the lysis of these clots. Diagnosis must be confirmed by objective means; e.g., pulmonary angiogram or scan.

Treatment should be initiated as soon as possible after onset of symptoms and no later than 7 days after onset. Delay decreases the potential for optimal efficacy.

Dosage
Check the thrombin time prior to administration. The value should be *less* than two times the normal control value. See Warning No. 3.

Obtain the patient's weight in kilograms.

This drug is measured in International Units (IU) which is a standardized measure of its ability to cause lysis of a fibrin clot in vitro. **This drug is available from Abbott Laboratories and Breon Laboratories. The method of preparation and administration is different for each. For correct dosing and administration, consult the package literature.**
Adults:
Loading dose—4,400 IU/kg infused over 10 minutes.
Remaining dose—4,400 IU/kg/*hour* as a continuous infusion over a 12-hour period.

At the end of urokinase therapy a continuous intravenous infusion of heparin is recommended. This should be initiated when the thrombin time has decreased to *less* than twice the normal control value (usually 3 to 4 hours after completion of the urokinase). Heparin therapy should be followed by oral anticoagulation.
Children:
Not recommended.

Preparation and Storage
Supplied in vials containing 250,000 IU in dry powder form. To prepare, follow guidelines in the package literature. Preparation varies for the two manufacturers' preparations. Use syringe filter to aspirate drug from vial if there is particulate matter present.
Prepare immediately prior to use; discard unused portions.
For infusion add reconstituted solution only to normal saline in amounts shown in the table under Dosage.
Refrigerate unopened vials (2–8 C).

Drug Incompatibilities
Do not mix with any other medication in any manner.

Modes of IV Administration

Injection
No

Intermittent Infusion
Yes
Use only NS as infusion fluid. Use an infusion pump with rate as prescribed under Dosage.

Continuous Infusion
No

Contraindications; Warnings; Precautions; Adverse Reactions

Contraindications
This drug, through its effects on the blood coagulation system, increases the risk of bleeding and is contraindicated in:
1. Active internal bleeding

2. Recent (within 2 months) cerebrovascular accident, intracranial or intraspinal surgery
3. Intracranial neoplasm.

Warnings
1. Bleeding
   a. This agent causes a more profound alteration of the hemostatic status than does heparin or coumarin drugs. In its action of stimulating the production of plasmin for lysis of intravascular fibrin deposits, such deposits that provide control of bleeding at needle puncture sites and other trauma will also be subject to lysis, and bleeding may occur. There is a great possibility of bruising or hematoma formation, especially with intramuscular injections. Intramuscular injections must be avoided during urokinase therapy, as should arterial punctures and venipunctures. If an arterial puncture is absolutely necessary, the femoral artery must be avoided in preference to the radial or brachial. Following the procedure, pressure must be applied to the site for at least 30 minutes, a pressure dressing applied, and the site checked frequently for bleeding.
   b. In the following clinical situations, the risk of therapy may be increased. This risk should be weighed against potential benefits:
      (1) Surgery within the past 10 days, including liver or kidney biopsy, lumbar puncture, thoracentesis or paracentesis, extensive or multiple cutdowns.
      (2) An intra-arterial diagnostic procedure within 10 days.
      (3) Ulcerative wounds.
      (4) Recent trauma with the possibility of internal injuries.

urokinase for injection
(continued)

(5) Visceral malignancy.

(6) Pregnancy and the first 10 days of the postpartum period.

(7) Ulcerative colitis, diverticulitis, or an actively bleeding lesion (or one with the potential for bleeding) of the gastrointestinal or genitourinary tract.

(8) Severe hypertension.

(9) Acute or chronic hepatic or renal insufficiency.

(10) Uncontrolled hypocoagulable state, including one that may be caused by a coagulation factor deficiency, thrombocytopenia, spontaneous fibrinolysis, or other purpuric or hemorrhagic disorder.

(11) Chronic lung disease with cavitation; e.g., tuberculosis.

(12) Subacute bacterial endocarditis or rheumatic valvular disease.

(13) Any other condition in which bleeding might constitute a significant hazard or be particularly difficult to manage because of its location. These are not absolute contraindications, but situations in which the risk of hemorrhage must be weighed carefully against the anticipated benefits of using the drug. The risks and benefits of using urokinase must be weighed against those associated with other forms of therapy.

c. Spontaneous bleeding from internal sites can occur. The risk is greater in patients with pre-existing hemostatic defects such as abnormalities in platelet count, prothrombin time, partial thromboplastin time, or bleeding time.

d. Besides its fibrinolytic action, plasmin also degrades fibrinogen Factor V, VII and other proteins. Products of plasmin degradation of fibrinogen and fibrin possess an anticoagulant effect, making any bleeding difficult to control. If serious spontaneous bleeding occurs, the urokinase infusion should be terminated immediately and treatment instituted as described under Adverse Reactions.

2. In patients with a predisposition to cerebral embolism such as in cases of atrial fibrillation, the use of urokinase may be hazardous because of the possibility of bleeding into an infarcted area.

3. Concurrent use of anticoagulants is not recommended and may be hazardous. If the patient has been on heparin, its effects must be allowed to diminish until the thrombin time is less than twice the normal control value before starting urokinase. Also, heparin should not be restarted following urokinase therapy until the thrombin time has returned to less than twice the normal control value. Rethrombosis has occurred after termination of urokinase treatment. To lessen this risk, heparin followed by oral anticoagulants (warfarin) should be part of therapy.

4. Safety and effectiveness of this therapy in children and during pregnancy has not been established, and therapy with urokinase is not recommended.

Precautions

1. Concurrent use of drugs that may alter platelet functions such as aspirin, indomethacin and phenylbutazone should be avoided.

2. Dosage of this drug should *not* be based on, or altered by, knowledge of the patient's level of fibrinogen, plasminogen, Factor V and Factor VII, fibrinogen

degradation products and thrombin time. Changes in these factors *only* serve as a confirmation of the existence of the lytic state, not to guide dosage adjustment.

Adverse Reactions

1. Bleeding: Occurs in two general forms:
   - Surface bleeding from invaded or disturbed sites (punctures, incisions, etc.)
   - Internal bleeding of the gastrointestinal tract, genitourinary tract, vagina, intramuscular, retroperitoneal, or intracerebral sites

   Fatalities due to cerebral or retro-peritoneal hemorrhage have occurred.

   Management of severe bleeding: Discontinue urokinase therapy. If blood loss is large, packed red cell transfusion is indicated. Plasma volume expanders such as fresh plasma and fluids (other than dextran) should be used along with whole blood. If hemorrhage is unresponsive to blood replacement, aminocaproic acid (see page 7) can be used and may act as an antidote to urokinase effects.

2. Allergic reactions are rare and usually in the form of rash, bronchospasm, anaphylaxis.

3. Fever can occur and should be symptomatically controlled with acetaminophen rather than aspirin.

☐ Nursing Implications

1. Be aware of contraindications and of clinical situations in which the risk of bleeding is great. Monitor even more cautiously than patients without these risks.

2. Monitor for all signs of bleeding:
   a. Intracerebral bleeding, as indicated by change in mental status, change in neurologic signs (pupil size, hand grip, extremity motion), headache, or change in vision. Check neurologic signs every 2–4 hours.
   b. Gastrointestinal bleeding, as indicated by hematemesis, abdominal pain or tenderness, fall in blood pressure, melena or red blood in the stools.
   c. Respiratory tract bleeding (hemoptysis may already be present secondary to pulmonary embolus) as indicated by hemoptysis, respiratory distress, chest pain.
   d. Bleeding from the urinary tract as indicated by hematuria (micro- and macroscopic) or dark brown urine.
   e. Vaginal bleeding.
   f. Ecchymosis or petechiae. Oozing from venipuncture, arterial puncture and intramuscular injections is to be expected. It is advisable to avoid these procedures during urokinase therapy when possible. Pressure should be applied to all venipuncture sites for 15 minutes. Arterial puncture should be performed in the upper extremities only; avoid the femoral artery. Apply pressure to the site for 30 minutes and apply a pressure dressing. These sites should be inspected hourly for continued bleeding for the duration of therapy.

3. Avoid other traumatic procedures such as nasogastric intubation and urinary catheterization when possible. When performing endotracheal suctioning, use low vacuum settings (below 110 mm Hg) and keep the frequency and duration of suctioning at a minimum. Watch for increasing blood in the aspirate.

4. Handle the patient carefully to prevent bruising and hematoma formation. Use adequate numbers of personnel when turning to prevent tissue trauma. Use protective devices on the bed (flotation pad, water mattress,

urokinase for injection
(continued)

or air mattress) when possible
to lessen trauma to the skin. If a
hematoma does occur, notify
the physician. Pressure dressings (elastic bandage) and ice
packs may be ordered.

5. Monitor blood pressure and
pulse indirectly every 1–4 hours
depending on the patient's
overall condition. If there is an
increased risk of bleeding, vital
signs should be taken hourly to
detect the onset of bleeding.
Avoid taking blood pressure
readings on the lower extremities to avoid dislodging intravenous thrombi.

6. Monitor temperature every 4–6
hours. Fever can occur; acetaminophen will be ordered to
control it.

7. The clinician is encouraged to
read additional materials on this
drug and the conditions for
which it is indicated.

Suggested Readings

Cudkowicz, Leon, and Sherry, Sol:
The Venous System and the
Lung. *Heart and Lung* 7(1):91–96,
January/February 1978.

————: Current Status of Thrombolytic Therapy, *Heart and Lung*,
7(1):97–100, January/February
1978.

vancomycin hydro-
chloride ■
(Vancocin)

Actions/Indications

Antibiotic. Useful against gram-positive bacteria such as streptococci
and staphylococci. To be used in
life-threatening infections that cannot be treated with less toxic drugs
or where there has been insufficient
response with other drugs.

Used in the treatment of staphylo-
coccal (including methicillin-resis-
tant) and streptococcal endocarditis,
osteomyelitis, pneumonia, septicemia, and soft-tissue infections.

Therapeutic response is usually
seen within 48–72 hours.

Dosage

Adults:
2 gm/day in 4 equally divided doses
or via continuous infusion.
*In the Presence of Renal Impair-
ment:[1]*
Mild impairment—1 gm/day in divided doses.
Uremia—1 gm every 7 days, (with
hemodialysis and peritoneal dialysis,
dosage is the same as in uremia), in
divided doses.
Children:
20 mg/lb (44 mg/kg) in 2–4 divided
doses or via continuous infusion.
Neonates (Premature and Full-Term):
10 mg/kg/day in 2 divided doses every 12 hrs.

Length of therapy is determined
by severity of infection and patient
response.

Preparation and Storage

Available in 500-mg vials. To reconstitute, add 10 ml sterile water for
injection. Refrigerate and discard after 96 hours.

Drug Incompatibilities

Do not mix in solution with any oth-
er drug; do not infuse into an IV
tubing containing:
Aminophylline
Amobarbital
Chloramphenicol
Chlorothiazide
Heparin
Methicillin
Novobiocin
Penicillin G
Pentobarbital
Phenobarbital
Phenytoin
Secobarbital
Sodium bicarbonate
Sulfisoxazole diolamine
Vitamin B complex with vitamin C
Warfarin

Modes of IV Administration

Injection
No

Intermittent Infusion
Yes
Dilute dose to *at least* a 5 mg/ml solution (500 mg/100 ml of fluid) using D5W or NS.
  Infuse over 20–30 min.
Preferred Mode of Administration.

Continuous Infusion
Yes
Use D5W or NS. Add 12- or 24-hr dose to 1000 ml. D5W or NS and infuse over 12 or 24 hours. (Smaller or larger volumes of fluid may be used depending on patient's fluid needs.)

Contraindications; Warnings; Precautions; Adverse Reactions

Contraindications
Hypersensitivity

Warnings
1. Avoid use in patients with renal insufficiency. This drug may be ototoxic and nephrotoxic in these patients. The risk of toxicity is increased by high serum concentrations for prolonged periods. If this drug must be used, doses of less than 2 gm/day are recommended.
2. Avoid use in patients with pre-existing hearing loss. If it must be used, monitor serum levels. Deafness may be preceded by tinnitus.
3. The elderly are more susceptible to auditory damage.
4. Cessation of therapy may not halt hearing loss.
5. Concurrent or sequential use with other ototoxic-nephrotoxic agents should be avoided (e.g., kanamycin, streptomycin, neomycin, gentamicin, cephaloridine, paromomycin, viomycin, polymyxin B, colistin, tobramycin).
6. This drug is not removed by hemodialysis or peritoneal dialysis.[2]

Precautions
1. Perform serial auditory function tests and serum drug levels

(when possible) in the elderly, in patients with impaired renal function, and in patients on large doses of this drug.
2. Monitor renal, hepatic, and bone marrow function in all patients and discontinue administration if abnormal values develop. Nephrotoxicity in patients with previously normal renal function is rare. If it does occur, it will produce proteinuria, hematuria, and/or rise in BUN.[3]
3. Prevent extravasation; tissue necrosis and sloughing can result.
4. May cause phlebitis at injection site; this can be prevented with correct dilution of the drug.
5. Overgrowth infections may occur, if so, discontinue vancomycin and initiate appropriate therapy.

Adverse Reactions
1. Nausea
2. Chills and fever
3. Urticaria and macular rashes
4. Anaphylaxis
5. Rarely, renal impairment
6. Hearing loss secondary to eighth cranial nerve damage

☐ **Nursing Implications**
1. Monitor for ototoxicity: dizziness, vertigo, tinnitus (most frequent symptom), roaring in the ears, hearing loss. Report onset to the physician.
2. Monitor for nephrotoxicity:
   a. Be aware of the patient's pretreatment BUN.
   b. Measure urine output every 4 hours; report oliguria of 120 ml or less per 4-hour period.
3. Prevent extravasation; see Appendix. If it occurs, apply warm compresses continuously for 2 hours and then for 20 minutes every 4 hours. Protect the area from trauma. Observe for tissue breakdown.
4. Change IV site promptly if phlebitis occurs.
5. Monitor for signs and symptoms

vancomycin hydrochloride
(continued)
of nonsusceptible organism
overgrowth infection:
a. Fever (take rectal temperature every four hours)
b. Increasing malaise
c. Signs and symptoms of newly developing localized
infection—redness, sore-
ness, pain, swelling, drainage (change in volume or
character of pre-existing
drainage).
d. Cough (change in volume or
character of pre-existing
drainage)
e. Diarrhea
f. Oral lesions (thrush) or perineal rash and itching (monilia) secondary to *Candida
albicans* infection.
6. Take anaphylaxis precautions;
see Appendix.

References
1. Appel, Gerald B., and Neu,
Harold C.: The Nephrotoxicity
of Antimicrobial Agents. *New
England Journal of Medicine*,
296(12):667, March 24, 1977.
2. ———: The Nephrotoxicity of
Antimicrobial Agents. *New England Journal of Medicine*,
296(13):722, March 31, 1977.
3. Ibid.

verapamil hydrochloride ■
(Isoptin IV)

Actions/Indications
Antiarrhythmic. Acts by inhibiting
the inflow of calcium into conductile
and contractile cells of the heart
muscle; this in turn slows AV conduction, prolongs the effective refractory period in the AV node and
reduces the rapid ventricular rate in
supraventricular tachycardias.
Peak therapeutic effects occur 3 to
5 minutes after injection.
Indicated for: rapid conversion to
sinus rhythm of paroxysmal
supraventricular tachycardias including Wolff–Parkinson–White (WPW)
and Lown–Ganong–Levine (LGL)
syndromes; temporary control of
rapid ventricular rate in atrial flutter
or atrial fibrillation.

Dosage
Adults:
Initial Dose—5–10 mg (.075–0.15
mg/kg). If initial response is inade-
quate, give 10 mg (0.15 mg/kg) 30
minutes after first dose.
Infants and Children:
Initial Dose—
• Newborn–1 Yr.—0.1–0.2 mg/kg
(usual dose range 0.75–2 mg).
Provide CONTINUOUS ECG
MONITORING DURING AD-
MINISTRATION.
• 1–15 Yrs.—0.1–0.3 mg/kg (usual
dose range 2–5 mg). DO NOT
EXCEED 5 mg.
Repeat Dose—
• Newborn–1 Yr.—0.1–0.2 mg/kg
(usual dose range 0.75–2 mg) under CONTINUOUS ECG MONI-
TORING. Give 30 minutes after
first dose if initial response inadequate.
• 1–15 Yrs.—0.1–0.3 mg/kg (usual
dose range 2–5 mg) 30 minutes
after first dose if initial response
is inadequate. DO NOT EXCEED
10 mg AS A SINGLE DOSE.

Preparation and Storage
Available in 2 ml ampuls containing
5 mg of drug.

Drug Incompatibilities
Do not mix with any other medication in any manner.

Modes of IV Administration

Injection
Yes
*Administer Undiluted, Slowly Over at
Least 2 Minutes.*
For older patients, administer over
at least 3 minutes to minimize unto-
ward effects.

Intermittent Infusion
No

Continuous Infusion
No

Contraindications; Warnings; Precautions; Adverse Reactions

Contraindications
1. Severe hypotension or cardiogenic shock.
2. Second or third degree (complete) AV block.
3. Sick sinus syndrome (SA nodal disease)
4. Severe congestive heart failure (unless secondary to supraventricular tachycardia).
5. Patients receiving intravenous beta adrenergic blocking drugs (e.g., propranolol).

Warnings
1. Transient hypotension (systolic < 90 mm Hg; diastolic < 60 mm Hg) can occur. This is generally asymptomatic but if dizziness or other symptoms occur vasopressors may be required.
2. A very rapid ventricular rate can occur in patients with atrial flutter or fibrillation *and* an accessory AV pathway (WPW or LGL syndromes). Electrical cardioversion may be needed.
3. This drug may produce second or third degree AV block, bradycardia and asystole; this is more likely in patients with sick sinus syndrome.
4. Mild CHF should be controlled before verapamil is given; more severe CHF may be exacerbated with this drug.
5. When given concurrently with digitalis drugs, monitor for AV block or marked bradycardia.
6. Use with caution in patients receiving any cardioactive drug, particularly oral beta adrenergic blockers, since both depress AV conduction and contractility. Avoid use of disopyramide within 48 hours of verapamil administration.
7. Development of AV block or bundle branch block requires that verapamil be reduced or discontinued.
8. Avoid repeated doses in patients with hepatic or renal failure since accumulation of the drug can occur. If required, reduce dosage and monitor blood pressure and PR interval.

Precautions
1. Safety for use in pregnancy, labor, and delivery has not been established; use only when clearly needed.
2. It is not known whether this drug is secreted in human milk, but breast-feeding should be discontinued if this drug is required.

Adverse Reactions
1. Cardiovascular: symptomatic hypotension, AV block, bradycardia, severe tachycardia, asystole.
2. Central Nervous System: dizziness, headache.
3. Gastrointestinal: nausea, abdominal discomfort.
4. Other (rare): depression, nystagmus, sleepiness, vertigo, muscle fatigue, diaphoresis.

☐ Nursing Implications
1. Maintain close ECG monitoring on all patients during and following administration. Observe for:
   a. Control of arrhythmia being treated and conversion of ventricular tachycardia to normal sinus rhythm or reduction of ventricular rate in atrial fibrillation or flutter.
   b. Increasing ventricular rate.
   c. Development of any degree of AV block (increasing PR interval or dropped beats), bundle branch block, bradycardia or asystole.
2. Notify physician of changes in cardiac rate or rhythm. Be prepared to treat AV block with atrophine or isoproterenol. Keep temporary transvenous pacing equipment and defibrillator readily available.
3. Monitor blood pressure every 15 minutes for the first hour, and then every 30 minutes for the next 2 hours after each injection. Be prepared to treat

verapamil hydrochloride
(continued)

symptomatic or marked hypotension with vasopressors or atropine.
4. Monitor for increased severity of CHF: increasing dyspnea, increasing heart rate, fatigue, rales, etc.

vidarabine monohydrate ■
(Vira-A)

Actions/Indications
Antiviral agent (a purine nucleoside), is active against *Herpesvirus* simplex, types 1 and 2. The antiviral mechanism is unknown. Indicated in the treatment only of Herpes simplex virus encephalitis. This agent may reduce mortality but does not appear to alter morbidity and the neurologic sequelae in the comatose patient.

Dosage
15 mg/kg/day for 10 days.

Preparation and Storage
Supplied in vials of 200 mg/ml. Solubility in fluids is limited. Each mg of drug requires 2.22 ml of intravenous fluid for solubilization (1000 ml of fluid will carry a maximum of 450 mg of drug). For example:

70 kg patient: dosage = 1050 mg of drug; 2400 ml of intravenous fluid will be required to dilute this dose and deliver it over 24 hours in the following manner:

1st bottle: 1000 ml + 450 mg drug, run 100 ml/hr
2nd bottle: 1000 ml + 450 mg drug, run 100 ml/hour
3rd bottle: 400 ml (use 500-ml bottle) + 150 mg drug, run 100 ml/hour

Any intravenous solution may be used (type can be tailored to patient's fluid, electrolyte, and caloric needs) except colloidal fluids or blood components.

To prepare, warm intravenous fluid to 95°–100° F (35–40 C). Shake drug vial, add to fluid. Agitate new mixture until solution is clear (do not use any solution that is not clear). An in-line membrane filter (0.45 micron pore size or smaller) *must* be used for infusion. Use the solution within 48 hours.

Drug Incompatibilities
Do not mix with any other medication in any manner.

Modes of IV Administration

Injection
No

Intermittent Infusion
No

Continuous Infusion
Yes
Infuse prepared solution slowly at a constant rate over a 12 to 24 hour period. Use an infusion pump and in-line filter (0.45 micron or smaller).

Contraindications; Warnings; Precautions; Adverse Reactions

Contraindications
Hypersensitivity to vidarabine.

Warnings
This agent should not be administered via the subcutaneous or intramuscular routes.

Precautions
1. Treatment should be discontinued if a brain biopsy is negative for herpes simplex.
2. Administer with caution to patients who may be susceptible to fluid overloading or cerebral edema; e.g., in central nervous system infections or impaired renal function.
3. In renal insufficiency there may be an accumulation of this drug in the body. Dosage may need to be adjusted accordingly.

4. Patients with impaired liver function should be monitored for adverse reactions such as a rise in SGOT.
5. Laboratory studies suggest that allopurinol may interfere with vidarabine metabolism.
6. Hemoglobin, hematocrit, white cells, and platelets may be depressed during therapy. Monitor these elements carefully.
7. Some degree of immuno-competence must be present to achieve a clinical response with this agent.
8. Use in pregnancy should be limited to life-threatening situations. This agent has caused fetal abnormalities in animals.
9. It is not known whether or not vidarabine is excreted in human milk. Nursing should be discontinued.

Adverse Reactions
1. Gastrointestinal: anorexia, nausea, vomiting, and diarrhea; seldom severe.
2. Central nervous system: tremor, dizziness, hallucinations, confusion, pyschosis, ataxia.
3. Hematologic: decreased hemoglobin, hematocrit, white cell count, platelet count, elevation in SGOT and total bilirubin.
4. Miscellaneous: weight loss, malaise, pruritus, rash, hematemesis, pain at infusion site.

Overdosage
In case of overdosage, hematologic, hepatic of renal functions must be carefully monitored for signs of organ damage.

☐ **Nursing Implications**
1. This drug will not alter the central nervous system changes seen in acute encephalitis; e.g., altered mental status, seizures, etc. Do not expect improvement in these problems as an indication of drug effectiveness. If central nervous system status deteriorates, notify the physician.

2. Take anaphylaxis precautions; see Appendix.
3. Monitor fluid balances in patients who are susceptible to fluid overload or intolerance (patients with renal failure, cerebral edema, or congestive heart failure):
   a. Measure urine output at least every 8 hours; the amount should average over 30 ml/hr.
   b. Weigh every 24 hours; note any gain.
   c. Signs of overload:
      (1) Peripheral edema (periorbital, sacral, lower extremities).
      (2) Increased intracranial pressure (increasing somnolence, changes in reflexes, increasing blood pressure, decreasing pulse).
      (3) Rales in the lungs, jugular venous distention, increased respiratory rate and effort.
      (4) Ascites (increased abdominal girth).
      Notify the physician at the onset of any of these findings.
4. Be prepared to manage vomiting to prevent aspiration. Record volume of output.
5. Warn the patient that there may be pain at the infusion site.

vinblastine sulfate ■
(Velban, VLB)

Actions/Indications
Antineoplastic, mitotic inhibitor (cell-cycle specific).
Used for palliative treatment of a variety of malignant conditions:
Frequently responsive—
- Generalized Hodgkin's disease, Stages III and IV
- Lymphocytic lymphomas
- Histocytic lymphomas
- Mycosis fungoides (advanced)
- Carcinoma of testis (advanced)
- Kaposi's sarcoma

vinblastine sulfate
(continued)

- Letterer–Siwe disease (histocytosis X)
  Less frequently responsive—
- Choriocarcinoma resistant to other agents
- Carcinoma of the breast unresponsive to other therapy

Usually administered concurrently with other antineoplastic agents.

Dosage

Doses are administered 7 days apart. The first dose should be administered followed by close monitoring of the white-blood-cell count to determine the patient's sensitivity. Then the second dose is administered and so on as follows:

Adults	Children
First Dose	
3.7 mg/M²	2.5 mg/M²
Second Dose	
5.5 mg/M²	3.75 mg/M²
Third Dose	
7.4 mg/M²	5.0 mg/M²
Fourth Dose	
9.25 mg/M²	6.25 mg/M²

Administer until a maximum dose (not exceeding 18.5 mg/M² for adults, and 12.5 mg/M² for children) is reached. The dose should not be increased after that dose which reduces the white-cell count to 3000/cu. mm.

In some adults, 3.7 mg/M² may produce this leukopenia, others will require more. The average weekly dose is usually 5.5–7.4 mg/M² .
Maintenance:
When the dose which will produce the above degree of leukopenia has been established, a dose one increment *smaller* should be administered at approximately 1-week intervals for maintenance, so that the patient receives the maximum dose that does *not* cause leukopenia. However, subsequent doses should *not* be administered unless the WBC is greater than or equal to 4000 cells/cu mm.

Duration of therapy depends on other agents used and the clinical condition of the patient.

Preparation and Storage

Supplied in 10-ml vials of 10 mg, in dry powder form. Refrigerate.

To reconstitute add 10 ml NS (*with preservative*). This will yield a solution of 1 mg/ml.

Refrigerate and discard after 30 days. Protect powder and reconstituted forms from light.

Drug Incompatibilities

Do not mix with any other medication in any manner.

Modes of IV Administration

Injection
Yes
Into the tubing of a running IV over 1 minute.

Prior to withdrawal of the needle from the vein, rinse the syringe with venous blood. Leaving needle in place, remove the syringe and flush vein well after injection with 10 ml NS from a separate syringe. Then remove the needle.

Intermittent Infusion
No
This mode increases the risk of extravasation and vein irritation.

Continuous Infusion
No

Contraindications; Warnings; Precautions; Adverse Reactions

Contraindications
1. Leukopenia
2. Bacterial infection

Warnings
1. This drug may cause fetal abnormalities.
2. May cause a depression of spermatogenesis.

Precautions
1. Monitor for infection if WBC falls below 2000/cu. mm.
2. There may be a more pro-

nounced leukopenic response in cachectic patients, and in the presence of skin ulcers. The drug should be avoided in both conditions.

3. White cell and platelet counts may fall in the presence of malignant infiltration of the marrow. If this occurs, further use of the drug is inadvisable.
4. Do not administer on a daily basis.
5. Do not exceed recommended dosage.
6. Avoid contact with skin and eyes. Rinse well with running water to prevent irritation.
7. Avoid extravasation, see Nursing Implication No. 2.

Adverse Reactions

1. Blood: bone marrow suppression, of short duration; leukopenia is usually more severe than thrombocytopenia
2. Skin: hair loss, rashes
3. Gastrointestinal: nausea, vomiting, diarrhea, ulceration of the mouth, pharyngitis, ileus, hemorrhagic colitis, abdominal pain, constipation can also occur in some patients.
4. Neurologic: numbness, paresthesias, peripheral neuritis, mental depression, headache, convulsions (all of these effects are usually seen only with high dose therapy)
5. Miscellaneous: malaise, weakness, dizziness, pain at tumor site

☐ Nursing Implications

1. The patient receiving this medication will be experiencing the emotional and physical effects of the malignancy. Knowledge of the patient's feelings about his disease and its implications will assist in helping him tolerate the chemotherapy. The incidence of uncomfortable side effects and adverse reactions is high. It is within the nurse's role to assist the patient in coping with the discomforts of the disease and its treatment, and to help him work through depression and anger toward acceptance of the disease at his own pace. Despite the unpleasantness this drug may bring, it can be a source of hope for the patient.
2. Prevent extravasation; see Appendix. Follow injection procedure described under Injection section. If it occurs, local injection of hyaluronidase and application of moderate heat will be prescribed by the physician to disperse the drug, help prevent cell damage, and reduce discomfort. Protect the area to prevent further trauma.
3. Management of gastrointestinal disturbances:
   a. Nausea and vomiting are usually mild and of short duration.
   b. Administer an antiemetic, if needed, to correspond to the time when the most uncomfortable symptoms occur.
   c. Small frequent meals, timed with periods when the patient feels his best, are advisable. Bland foods are usually tolerated most easily. Carbohydrate and protein content should be high.
   d. If the patient is anorexic, encourage high nutrient liquids and water. Maintain hydration.
   e. Keep an accurate measurement of emesis and stool volumes and total intake and output to guide the physician in ordering parenteral fluids when necessary.
   f. Administer constipating agents as needed for diarrhea. Monitor for signs of hypokalemia (weakness, muscle cramps). Maintain hydration.
   g. Monitor for the onset of obstructive ileus (abdominal pain, distention, obstipation).
   h. Monitor stools for visible and occult blood.

vinblastine sulfate
(continued)

i. Administer laxatives and stool softeners if constipation occurs.

4. Management of hematologic effects:

  a. Be aware of the patient's white blood cell and platelet count prior to each injection.

  b. If WBC falls to 2000/cu. mm. (rare), take measures to protect the patient from infection such as: protective (reverse) isolation, avoidance of invasive procedures; maintenance of bodily (especially perineal) cleanliness; carrying out strict urinary catheter care when appropriate, etc. Monitor for infection: temperature every 4 hours, examination for rashes, swellings, drainage and pain. Explain measures to the patient.

  c. If platelet count falls below 100,000/cu. mm., monitor for thrombocytopenic bleeding: petechiae, purpura, hematuria, melena, blood in stools, gum bleeding, vaginal bleeding, epistaxis, hematemesis, etc. Avoid trauma. Transfusions may be ordered.

  d. Instruct the patient and/or family on the importance of follow-up blood work and the reporting of the signs and symptoms listed in "b" and "c" above, to the physician if the drug is being administered on an outpatient basis.

5. Management of neurologic side effects:

  a. Instruct patient and/or family to report numbness, paresthesias, pain, headaches. Inform the physician at the onset.

  b. If the patient is on high-dose therapy, monitor for seizures.

  c. Monitor for signs and symptoms of mental depression that are related to drug administered. Inform the physician and administer supportive care. Knowing the etiology can relieve the patient of some anxiety.

6. Management of stomatitis:

  a. Onset of stomatitis may indicate the presence of more serious intestinal ulceration.

  b. Administer preventive oral care every 4 hours and/or after meals.

  c. For preventive care use a very soft toothbrush (child's) and toothpaste; avoid trauma to tissues.

  d. Examine oral membranes at least daily (instruct patient and/or family) to detect the onset of inflammation and erythema.

  e. If stomatitis occurs, notify the physician and begin therapeutic oral care as ordered.

  f. Order a soft, bland diet for patients with inflammation. If stomatitis is severe, the patient may be placed on NPO status by the physician.

  g. For patients who can tolerate oral intake, administer Xylocaine Viscous or acetaminophen elixir as a mouthwash prior to meals to decrease pain (do not use aspirin rinses), as ordered by the physician.

  h. Patients with severe stomatitis may require parenteral analgesia.

7. If rashes occur, administer cool compresses and topical agents as ordered. Keep the patient's environment cool. Turn frequently to prevent skin breakdown.

8. Management of hair loss:

  a. Use scalp tourniquet, if ordered, to help prevent hair loss.

  b. Counsel the patient on the possibility of hair loss to enable him to prepare for this disfigurement.

c. Reassure him of regrowth of hair following discontinuation of the drug.
d. Provide privacy and time for the patient to discuss his feelings.

Suggested Readings

Bruya, Margaret Auld, and Madeira, Nancy Powell: Stomatitis After Chemotherapy. *American Journal of Nursing*, 75(8):1349–1352, August 1975.

Giadquinta, Barbara: Helping Families Face the Crisis of Cancer. *American Journal of Nursing*, 77:1583–1588, October 1977.

Gullo, Shirley: Chemotherapy — What to Do About Special Side Effects. *RN*. 40:30–32, April 1977.

vincristine sulfate ■
(Oncovin)

Actions/Indications
Antineoplastic agent (cell cycle specific). Used alone to treat acute leukemias, and in combination with other agents in the treatment of Hodgkin's disease, lymphosarcoma, reticulum-cell sarcoma, rhabdomyosarcoma, neuroblastoma, and Wilms' tumor.

Dosage
Adults:
1.4 mg/M^2 weekly. Other dosage schedules have been used.
Children:
1.5 mg–2.0 mg/M^2 at weekly intervals.

Preparation and Storage
Supplied in multidose vials of 1 mg and 5 mg of drug. Reconstitute with solution provided (bacteriostatic sodium chloride solution). Add 10 ml to each. This results in solution concentrations of 0.1 mg/ml and 0.5 mg/ml respectively.

Store in refrigerator, discard after 14 days. Protect stock solutions from light.

Drug Incompatibilities
Do not mix with any other medication in any manner.

Modes of IV Administration

Injection
Yes
Into the tubing of a running IV, over 1 minute. Flush vein well after injection.

Intermittent Infusion
Yes
In enough NS to make a concentration of at least 1 mg/ml (at least 50 ml). Infuse within 15 minutes.

Continuous Infusion
No

Contraindications; Warnings; Precautions; Adverse Reactions

Contraindications
None currently known.

Warnings
1. This drug may have adverse effects on the developing fetus.
2. There is insufficient information as to whether this drug may affect fertility in men and women.

Precautions
1. Acute hyperuricemia and uric acid nephropathy may occur.
2. Use with caution in the presence of leukopenia or infection.
3. If CNS leukemia is diagnosed, additional agents and routes of administration may be required, since this drug does not cross the blood-brain barrier.
4. Use caution in monitoring neurologic side effects, if this drug is used in patients with pre-existing neuromuscular disease or who are on other agents that have neurotoxic effects.
5. **Overdosage may cause death.** Use extreme caution in determining dose and in administering this drug.

Adverse Reactions
1. Blood: bone marrow suppression, producing mild leukopenia beginning on the fourth day of therapy and resolving by the fifth.

vincristine sulfate
(continued)

2. Neurologic: changes are frequently seen and can be dose-related, begin with loss of Achilles tendon reflex; parasthesias are common, as are neuritic pain, difficulty walking secondary to muscle weakness; these effects may last through the duration of therapy; seizures have been reported, cranial nerve deficits in the form of ptosis, abducens nerve palsy, seventh cranial nerve dysfunction and vocal cord paralysis.
3. Gastrointestinal: constipation secondary to adynamic ileus (occurs more frequently in elderly patients); impaction formation is common; stool softeners should be given prophylactically; nausea and vomiting are rare
4. Hair loss: mild but common, reversible
5. Antidiuretic syndrome: high loss of sodium in the urine followed by hyponatremia
6. Stomatitis: rare

☐ **Nursing Implications**
1. Management of hematologic effects (see Adverse Reaction No. 1):
   a. Bone marrow depression will be minimal and usually does not require special intervention.
   b. Be aware of the patient's white cell and platelet counts.
2. Management of constipation:
   a. Be aware of the patient's previous bowel habits and attempt to maintain them.
   b. Administer stool softeners and laxatives as ordered; keep the patient hydrated.
   c. Monitor stool frequency.
   d. Observe for abdominal distention and pain.
3. Monitor for signs and symptoms of hyponatremia (see Adverse Reaction No. 5) such as:
   a. Weakness

   b. Changes in mental status such as confusion and drowsiness
4. Stomatitis rarely is a problem with this drug. If the patient develops inflammation of oral mucosa with ulceration, notify the physician and begin therapeutic care as ordered. Order a soft, bland diet, and administer Xylocaine Viscous as a mouth rinse prior to meals.
5. Management of hair loss:
   a. Use a scalp tourniquet during injection of this drug, if ordered by the physician, to help prevent hair loss.
   b. Counsel the patient on the possibility of hair loss to enable him to prepare for this disfigurement.
   c. Reassure him of probable regrowth of hair following discontinuation of the drug.
   d. Provide privacy and time for the patient to discuss his feelings.
6. Monitor for neurologic changes (see Adverse Reaction No. 2). Notify physician of onset. Take safety precautions to prevent injury. Reassure him of the reversible nature of these reactions.
7. Prevent extravasation; see Appendix. If it occurs, discontinue injection or infusion promptly. Administer the remainder of the dose in another vein. A local injection of hyaluronidase and the application of moderate heat to the affected area may help to disperse the drug in the tissues to decrease pain and tissue reaction.

Suggested Readings

Bolin, Rose Homan, and Auld, Margaret E.: Hodgkin's Disease. *American Journal of Nursing*, November 1974, pp. 1982–1986.

Bruya, Margaret Auld, and Madeira, Nancy Powell: Stomatitis After Chemotherapy. *American Journal of Nursing*, August 1975, pp. 1349–1352.

Foley, Genevieve, and McCarthy, Ann Marie: The Disease (Hodgkin's) and Its Treatment, *American Journal of Nursing*, July 1976, pp. 1109–1114 (references).

————: The Child With Leukemia In a Special Hematology Clinic. *American Journal of Nursing*, July 1976, pp. 1115–1119.

Giadquinta, Barbara: Helping Families Face the Crisis of Cancer. *American Journal of Nursing*, October 1977, pp. 1583–1588.

Gullo, Shirley: Chemotherapy— What to Do About Special Side Effects. *RN*, April 1977, pp. 30–32.

Hannan, Jeanne Ferguson: Talking Is Treatment, Too. *American Journal of Nursing*. November 1974, pp. 1991–1992.

Martinson, Ida: The Child With Leukemia: Parents Help Each Other. *American Journal of Nursing*, July 1976, pp. 1120–1122.

Showfety, Mary Patricia: The Ordeal of Hodgkin's Disease. *American Journal of Nursing*, November 1974, pp. 1987–1991.

Vietti, Teresa J., and Valeriote, Frederick: Conceptual Basis for the Use of Chemotherapeutic Agents and Their Pharmacology. *Pediatric Clinics of North America*, 23:67–92, February 1976, pp. 67–92 (references).

Appendix

Table 1. Table of Metric and Apothecaries' Systems

(Approved *approximate* dose equivalents are enclosed in parentheses. Use *exact* equivalents in calculations.)

Conversion Factors

Metric	Apothecaries	Metric	Apothecaries
1 milligram (mg.)	1/64 grain	3.888 cubic centimeters or grams	1 dram (4 cc. or grams)
64.79 milligrams	1 grain (65 mg.)	31.103 cubic centimeters or grams	1 ounce (30 cc. or grams)
1 gram	15.43 grains (15 grains)	473.167 cubic centimeters	1 pint (500 cc.)
1 cubic centimeter (cc.)	16 minims		

WEIGHTS

Metric			Apothecaries	Metric			Apothecaries
0.0001	gram—0.1	mg.—	1/640 grain (1/600 grain)	0.057	gram —57	mg.—7/8	grain
0.0002	gram—0.2	mg.—	1/320 grain (1/300 grain)	0.06	gram —60	mg.—9/10	grain (1 grain)
0.0003	gram—0.3	mg.—	1/210 grain (1/200 grain)	0.065	gram —65	mg.—1	grain (60 mg.)
0.0004	gram—0.4	mg.—	1/150 grain	0.07	gram —70	mg.—11/20	grains
0.0005	gram—0.5	mg.—	1/120 grain	0.08	gram —80	mg.—11/5	grains
0.0006	gram—0.6	mg.—	1/100 grain	0.09	gram —90	mg.—11/3	grains
0.0007	gram—0.7	mg.—	1/90 grain	0.097	gram —97	mg.—11/2	grains (0.1 gram)
0.0008	gram—0.8	mg.—	1/80 grain	0.12	gram —120	mg.—2	grains
0.0009	gram—0.9	mg.—	1/75 grain	0.2	gram —200	mg.—3	grains
0.001	gram—1	mg.—	1/64 grain (1/60 grain)	0.24	gram —240	mg.—4	grains (0.25 gram)
0.0011	gram—1.1	mg.—	1/60 grain	0.3	gram —300	mg.—41/2	grains
0.0013	gram—1.3	mg.—	1/50 grain (1.2 mg.)	0.33	gram —330	mg.—5	grains (0.3 gram)
0.0014	gram—1.4	mg.—	1/48 grain	0.4	gram —400	mg.—6	grains
0.0016	gram—1.6	mg.—	1/40 grain (1.5 mg.)	0.45	gram —450	mg.—7	grains
0.0018	gram—1.8	mg.—	1/36 grain	0.5	gram —500	mg.—71/2	grains
0.0020	gram—2	mg.—	1/32 grain (1/30 grain)	0.53	gram —530	mg.—8	grains
0.0022	gram—2.2	mg.—	1/30 grain	0.6	gram —600	mg.—9	grains
0.0026	gram—2.6	mg.—	1/24 grain	0.65	gram —650	mg.—10	grains (0.6 gram)
0.003	gram—3	mg.—	1/20 grain	0.73	gram —730	mg.—11	grains
0.004	gram—4	mg.—	1/16 grain (1/15 grain)	0.80	gram —800	mg.—12	grains (0.75 gram)
0.005	gram—5	mg.—	1/12 grain	0.86	gram —860	mg.—13	grains
0.006	gram—6	mg.—	1/10 grain	0.93	gram —930	mg.—14	grains
0.007	gram—7	mg.—	1/9 grain	1	gram —1000	mg.—15	grains
0.008	gram—8	mg.—	1/8 grain	1.06	grams—1060	mg.—16	grains
0.009	gram—9	mg.—	1/7 grain	1.13	grams—1130	mg.—17	grains
0.01	gram—10	mg.—	1/6 grain	1.18	grams—1180	mg.—18	grains
0.013	gram—13	mg.—	1/5 grain (12 mg.)	1.26	grams—1260	mg.—19	grains
0.016	gram—16	mg.—	1/4 grain (15 mg.)	1.30	grams—1300	mg.—20	grains
0.02	gram—20	mg.—	1/3 grain	1.50	grams—1500	mg.—22	grains
0.025	gram—25	mg.—	3/8 grain	2	grams—2000	mg.—30	grains (1/2 dram)
0.03	gram—30	mg.—	1/2 grain (1/2 grain)	4	grams	—1	dram (60 grains)
0.032	gram—32	mg.—	1/2 grain (30 mg.)	5	grams	—75	grains
0.04	gram—40	mg.—	3/5 grain (2/3 grain)	8	grams	—2	drams (7.5 grams)
0.043	gram—43	mg.—	2/3 grain (40 mg.)	10	grams	—21/2	drams
0.05	gram—50	mg.—	3/4 grain	15	grams	—4	drams
				30	grams	—1	ounce

LIQUID MEASURES*

Metric		Apothecaries	Metric		Apothecaries
0.03	cubic centimeter —1/2	minim	8	cubic centimeters—2	fluid drams
0.05	cubic centimeter —3/4	minim	10	cubic centimeters—21/2	fluid drams
0.06	cubic centimeter —1	minim	15	cubic centimeters—4	fluid drams
0.1	cubic centimeter —11/2	minims	20	cubic centimeters—51/2	fluid drams
0.2	cubic centimeter —3	minims	25	cubic centimeters—5/6	fluid ounce
0.25	cubic centimeter —4	minims	30	cubic centimeters—1	fluid ounce
0.3	cubic centimeter —5	minims	50	cubic centimeters—13/4	fluid ounces
0.5	cubic centimeter —8	minims	60	cubic centimeters—2	fluid ounces
0.6	cubic centimeter —10	minims	100	cubic centimeters—31/2	fluid ounces
0.75	cubic centimeter —12	minims	120	cubic centimeters—4	fluid ounces
1	cubic centimeter —15	minims	200	cubic centimeters—7	fluid ounces
2	cubic centimeters—30	minims	250	cubic centimeters—8	fluid ounces
3	cubic centimeters—45	minims	360	cubic centimeters—12	fluid ounces
4	cubic centimeters—1	fluid dram	500	cubic centimeters—1	pint
5	cubic centimeters—11/4	fluid drams	1000	cubic centimeters—1	quart

(From Culver, V. M.: Modern Bedside Nursing. Philadelphia, W. B. Saunders, 1969)

* Note: A cubic centimeter (cc.) is the approximate equivalent of a milliliter (ml.). The terms are used interchangeably in general medicine.

TABLE 2. Comparative Scales of Measures, Weights and Temperatures*

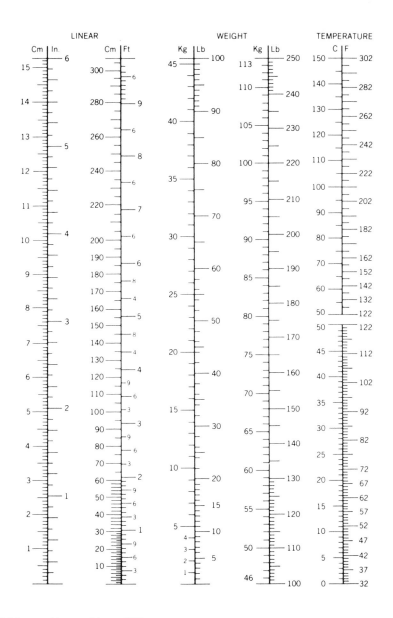

* 2.5 cm = 1 in.   1 kg. = 2.2 lb.

(From Brunner, L. S., and Suddarth, D. S.: The Lippincott Manual of Nursing Practice (2nd ed.). Philadelphia, J. B. Lippincott, 1978, p. 1833.)

TABLE 3. Nomogram for Estimating Surface Area of Infants and Young Children

HEIGHT		SURFACE AREA	WEIGHT	
feet	centimeters	in square meters	pounds	kilograms

To determine the surface area of the patient draw a straight line from the point representing his height on the left vertical scale to the point representing his weight on the right vertical scale. The point at which this line intersects the middle vertical scale represents the patient's surface area in square meters. (Courtesy, Abbott Laboratories.)

TABLE 4. Nomogram for Estimating Surface Area of Older Children and Adults

HEIGHT		SURFACE AREA	WEIGHT	
feet	centimeters	in square meters	pounds	kilograms

(Courtesy, Abbott Laboratories.)

Table 5. Normal Vital Sign Values and Ranges In Children

Temperature
Oral 36.4–37.4°C. (97.6–99.3°F.)
Rectal 36.2–37.8°C. (97–100°F.)
Axillary 35.9–36.7°C. (96.6–98°F.)

Pulse and Respiratory Rates

Age	Pulse	Respirations
Newborn	70–170	30–50
11 months	80–160	26–40
2 years	80–130	20–30
4 years	80–120	20–30
6 years	75–115	20–26
8 years	70–110	18–24
10 years	70–110	18–24
Adolescence	60–110	12–20

Blood Pressure

Age	Mean Systolic	Range in 95% of Normal Children	Mean Diastolic	Range in 95% of Normal Children
6 months–1 year	90	±25	61	±19
2–3 years	95	±24	61	±24
4–5 years	99	±21	65	±15
6 years	100	±15	56	± 8
8 years	105	±16	57	± 9
10 years	109	±16	58	±10
12 years	113	±18	59	±10
15 years	121	±19	61	±10

(Source: The Harriet Lane Handbook, 7th edition, Dennis L. Headings, ed., Copyright © 1975 by Year Book Medical Publishers, Inc., Chicago, 1975, p. 265. Used by permission.)

Hypersensitivity (Drug Allergy): Prevention, Recognition and Management

I. Identifying susceptible patients
A. Obtain history of previous allergies, especially to drugs, on admission and prior to giving any intravenous drug.
    1. Determine type of allergy (drug, food, hay fever, etc.).
    2. Note type and severity of previous symptoms.
    3. Questionable allergies should be evaluated by a physician.
B. With seriously ill or unresponsive patients, seek information from medical record, family members, medical identification tag or wallet ID card.

II. Instituting preventive measures
A. List specific drugs (and other substances) to which the patient is allergic on the front of the chart and in other pertinent parts of the medical record (nursing history, problem list, medication record, kardex, etc.)
B. Instruct patient regarding advisability of wearing a medical identification tag and assist in obtaining one as needed.
C. Be aware of related drugs that can produce cross-reactions: patients with penicillin allergies may also be allergic to ampicillin or semisynthetic penicillin (such as carbenicillin), or to the cephalosporins. Patients with known allergies to one aminoglycoside (gentamicin, kanamycin, amikacin, etc.) may be allergic to others.
D. Be aware that individuals with multiple drug allergies are also prone to developing allergies to chemically unrelated drugs.
E. When an intravenous drug, especially penicillin, is ordered, determine whether the patient

has received it previously. Prior exposure may have sensitized the person; subsequent doses can elicit an allergic response.

F. Avoid administering a drug to which the patient is known to be allergic, even if previous reactions were mild. In rare instances when such a drug must be given, follow the procedure below.

III. Monitoring for signs of allergic reactions

A. For patients with *no* history of allergy:
1. Remain with the patient for 5–10 minutes during infusion of the initial dose.
2. Observe for and report: urticaria (hives), dyspnea, edema (especially on the face) or local reactions at the IV site.
3. Without unduly alarming them, instruct appropriate patients to report any such symptoms. Patients who are unable to report symptoms should be checked periodically until dose has infused.
B. For patients with a positive history of allergies *or* when administering a drug that is likely to be allergenic (as indicated for specific drugs in this text):
1. Have emergency medications and supplies readily available (see treatment section).
2. Stay with patient throughout infusion of the first dose (or for 10–20 minutes if drug is in large volume infusion). Both for efficiency and to lessen patient apprehension, try to plan patient care that can be given while observing for allergic signs and symptoms.
3. After infusion of medication, check the patient every 30 minutes or so for the next few hours. Reactions occurring later are less likely to be severe. Check the temperature every four hours for 24 hours to detect occurrence of drug fever.
4. Instruct the patient to report any of the symptoms mentioned above, particularly breathing difficulties, swelling of the face or other parts of the body, or skin reactions.
5. At the first appearance of any allergic symptom, discontinue the drug and notify the physician immediately. Keep the intravenous line open in case any emergency medications are required. If allergic symptoms appear, consider any other drugs the patient is receiving concurrently, particularly parenteral ones that may be the source of the reaction.
6. If no allergic manifestations occur, observe the patient for 5–10 minutes during the administration of subsequent doses. Observe for late signs: fever, arthralgia, lymph-node enlargement, skin eruptions (maculopapular type), and neuritis.

IV. Administering a drug to which a patient is known to be allergic

A. In rare instances, the benefits of giving a drug outweigh the risks of a potentially serious allergic reaction. For example, penicillins, including some penicillinase-resistant semisynthetic penicillins such as nafcillin, are the treatment of choice in specific kinds of bacterial endocarditis and septicemia. In rare instances, the patient may also be allergic to an unrelated second-line drug. In such a case, the first-line drug is given and steps are taken to minimize reactions.
B. The *physician* performs appropriate skin tests (first, a scratch test; if negative, then an intradermal test).
1. If results of both tests are negative, administer the

drug, taking precautions outlined in III B above.

2. If either test is positive, one of the following measures must be performed before the drug can be given:

   (a) *Rapid hyposensitization*— ALWAYS DONE BY THE PHYSICIAN, involves giving small, increasing doses of the drug every 2–6 hours.

   (b) *Drug suppression*—using either antihistamines or glucocorticoids. This requires a day of pretreatment followed by a test dose before the drug is started.

C. When the course of therapy is started, the first dose, and ideally the first several doses, should be administered by the physician. Emergency medications and equipment that must be kept close at hand throughout both the testing and drug therapy include:

- Epinephrine, 1:1,000 and 1:10,000 solutions
- Antihistamines, such as diphenhydramine (Benadryl) for intravenous use
- Glucocorticoids, hydrocortisone (Solu-Cortef) and methylprednisolone (Solu-Medrol)
- Calcium preparations in case cardiac arrest should occur
- Vasopressors (dopamine [Intropin], levarterenol [Levophed], isoproterenol [Isuprel])
- Lidocaine
- Airway and manual resuscitation bag (Puritan, Hope, Ambu, etc.)
- Endotracheal tube and laryngoscope
- Tracheostomy tray, in case laryngeal edema or spasm prevents oral intubation
- Intravenous fluids

V. Treatment of allergic reactions

A. *Anaphylactic Shock.* Should anaphylaxis occur in spite of all possible precautions, it is essential that treatment be instituted immediately, because death can ensue in a matter of minutes. While specific regimens may vary slightly according to physician preference, essential elements of treatment generally include:

1. Aqueous epinephrine, 1:10,000, given intravenously by *slow* injection. The initial dose is 2 to 5 milliliters. For milder symptoms such as urticaria, 0.2 to 0.5 milliliters of 1:1,000 strength can be initially given subcutaneously, repeated at three-minute intervals if required. A continuous infusion of epinephrine diluted with normal saline or 5 percent dextrose in water may be given.

2. Establish and/or maintain a patent airway. Endotracheal intubation or emergency tracheostomy may be required if airway obstruction, due to either laryngeal edema or bronchospasm, is present. In these instances, either antihistamines such as diphenhydramine (Benadryl) 50 to 80 milligrams IV or IM, or chlorpheniramine (Chlor-Trimeton), 10 milligrams IV; or aminophylline, 0.25 to 0.50 grams IV (6 milligrams per kilogram over a 20-minute period), may be given as adjunctive measures.

3. Establish a secure, preferably central, intravenous line if the one already present is at risk of dislodgement or infiltration.

4. Provide intravenous volume expansion with agents, such as dextran, saline, or albumin, and treat acidosis as needed.

5. If bronchospasm or hypotension persists, corticosteroids may be used.

6. Maintain close nursing observation of the patient for at least 24 hours after

the reaction or until stable. Monitoring of vital signs, particularly blood pressure, respiration, and pulse rate, is essential for the assessment of the patient's progress.

7. Following anaphylactic shock or any significant allergic reaction, it is vital that the patient, or the parent or responsible person when indicated, be informed of the allergy and its significance. With a school-aged child, the parents should be advised to inform the child's teacher or school nurse of the allergy so that the information can be entered into the health record. Another important aspect of the nurse's teaching responsibility includes explaining the value of wearing a medical identification tag and assisting the patient in obtaining one if indicated.

B. *Treatment of Less Severe Allergic Manifestations.* The primary measure is to discontinue the drug. In cases of mild reactions, this is often the only measure required; symptoms subside spontaneously. For more severe reactions, epinephrine may be given. Antihistamines may also be used, both to relieve symptoms and as a prophylaxis against serum sickness. If signs of exfoliative dermatitis appear, steroids are used. Drug fever and other isolated symptoms are often treated symptomatically. Nursing intervention in drug allergy includes:

1. Providing psychological support to help allay the patient's anxiety. Asthmatic or other symptoms which interfere with breathing, as well as extensive skin reactions, are particularly anxiety provoking.

2. Continuing close observation following discontinuation of the drug to be sure that the symptoms are not worsening.

3. Providing symptomatic relief for skin reactions, such as urticaria and rashes, with such measures as tepid baths, use of a bed cradle to prevent pressure and irritation from the bed linen and, unless the skin is broken, application of lotion to relieve itching.

Drug Extravasation

Prevention

1. When possible, select the largest vein available and use an appropriately sized needle or cannula for that vein.

2. If the drug is to be administered by infusion, avoid needle appliances such as scalp vein needles.

3. Ideally, the appliance should be inserted for infusion into the vein at a point away from elbow, wrist, and hand joints. Motion at these areas contributes to cannula displacement.

4. Avoid using scalp veins in babies.

5. Be certain that the cannula or needle is within the lumen of the vein before initiating an infusion or injecting the drug. There should be free return of venous blood, and a test injection of normal saline or another isotonic solution should not produce pain or swelling.

6. If an infusion is to be administered, the cannula must be secured with tape to prevent movement. If a vein that is near a joint must be used, use an armboard. Anchor tubing to prevent pull on the cannula. The taping technique should be designed to allow visibility of the skin surrounding the vein and insertion site.

7. When possible, instruct the patient on the importance of the drug, as well as on the hazards of extravasation and how he can participate in its prevention.

Recognition

1. Instruct the patient to report *undue* pain at the injection site. Some drugs normally cause burning along the vein tract; help him differentiate this from unusual pain.
2. Examine the tissues proximal to the injection or infusion site for blanching, swelling, or coolness. Do this every 30 minutes, or more frequently if an infusion pump is in use.

Management

1. If extravasation is suspected, stop the infusion or injection immediately. With infusion, if the drug is non-life-supporting, remove the cannula or needle. If the drug is life-supporting, quickly restart the infusion at another site.
2. Elevate the extremity.
3. Notify the physician immediately. Treatment must begin as soon as possible after detection of the problem.
4. Be prepared for the specific treatment for the drug in use. If a treatment is known for a drug, it will appear in the text of this book; otherwise, consult the pharmacist or drug-information department of your institution.
5. After treatment, continue to monitor the affected area for signs and symptoms of tissue damage:
   a. Continuing pain or numbness
   b. Redness
   c. Swelling
   d. Cyanosis or continuing blanching
   e. Loss of pulses distal to the area
   f. Bleb formation or tissue sloughing
6. Protect the area from further trauma and from infection.

Index

Drugs are indexed by generic (initial letter, lower case) or trade (initial letter, capital) name with the corresponding trade (generic) name in parentheses: acetazolamide (Diamox); Diamox (acetazolamide).

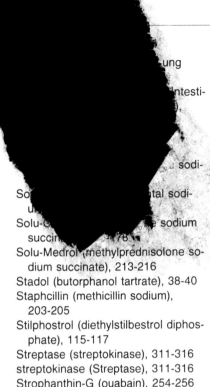

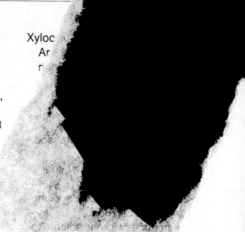